Clinical Gynaecological Oncology

To Alison and Maggie, Emily,
Katy, David, Hannah and Ruth
for continuing to recognize their fathers,
despite the late nights and
missed weekends
God bless you all

Clinical Gynaecological Oncology

EDITED BY

JOHN H. SHEPHERD

FRCS, MRCOG
*Consultant Gynaecological Surgeon, St Bartholomew's and
the Royal Marsden Hospitals, London*

AND

JOHN M. MONAGHAN

MB, FRCS(Ed), FRCOG
*Consultant Surgeon,
Queen Elizabeth II Hospital, Gateshead*

FOREWORD BY

Sir GEORGE PINKER

FRCS(Ed), PRCOG, MBPS
*President Royal College of
Obstetricians and Gynaecologists*

SECOND EDITION

OXFORD

BLACKWELL SCIENTIFIC PUBLICATIONS

LONDON EDINBURGH MELBOURNE
PARIS BERLIN VIENNA

© 1985, 1990 by
Blackwell Scientific Publications
Editorial Offices:
Osney Mead, Oxford OX2 0EL
25 John Street, London WC1N 2BL
23 Ainslie Place, Edinburgh EH3 6AJ
3 Cambridge Center, Suite 208
  Cambridge, Massachusetts 02142, USA
107 Barry Street, Carlton
  Victoria 3053, Australia

First published 1985
Second edition 1990

Set by Setrite Typesetters, Hong Kong
Printed in Great Britain by
The Alden Press, Oxford
Bound by Hartnolls Ltd, Bodmin, Cornwall

DISTRIBUTORS
  Marston Book Services Ltd
  PO Box 87
  Oxford OX2 0DT
  (*Orders*: Tel: 0865 791155
        Fax: 0865 791927
        Telex: 837515)

USA
  Year Book Medical Publishers
  200 North LaSalle Street
  Chicago, Illinois 60601
  (*Orders*: Tel: (312) 726−9733)

Canada
  The C.V. Mosby Company
  5240 Finch Avenue East
  Scarborough, Ontario
  (*Orders*: Tel: (416) 298−1588)

Australia
  Blackwell Scientific Publications
  (Australia) Pty Ltd
  107 Barry Street
  Carlton, Victoria 3053
  (*Orders*: Tel: (03) 347−0300)

British Library
Cataloguing in Publication Data

Clinical gynaecological oncology. − 2nd. ed.
  1. Woman. Reproductive system. Cancer
  I. Shepherd, John H. (John Henry) II.
  Monaghan, John M. (John Michael)
  616.99465

ISBN 0-632-02733-9

Contents

Contributors

MALCOLM C. ANDERSON MB, FRCPath, *Senior Lecturer in Gynaecologic Histopathology, Department of Histopathology, University Hospital, Queens Medical Centre, Nottingham WG7 2UH*

RICHARD H.J. BEGENT MD, FRCP, *Reader in Medical Oncology, Charing Cross and Westminster Medical School, Honorary Consultant Physician, Charing Cross Hospital, Fulham Palace Road, London W6 8RF*

VALERIE BERAL MRCP, *Senior Lecturer in Epidemiology, Imperial Cancer Research Fund's Cancer Epidemiology and Clinical Trials Unit, Radcliffe Infirmary, Oxford OX2 6HE*

GEORGE BLACKLEDGE MD, PhD, MRCP, *Director, West Midlands Cancer Research Campaign Clinical Trials Unit, Queen Elizabeth Hospital, Queen Elizabeth Medical Centre, Edgbaston, Birmingham B15 2TH*

JOHN BUXTON MRCOG, *Research Fellow, West Midlands Cancer Research Campaign Clinical Trials Unit, Queen Elizabeth Hospital, Queen Elizabeth Medical Centre, Edgbaston, Birmingham*

SIR JOHN DEWHURST FRCOG, FRCS(Ed), HonFACOG, *Professor, Institute of Obstetrics and Gynaecology, Queen Charlotte's Maternity Hospital, Goldhawk Road, London W6 0XG*

HAROLD FOX MD, MB, ChB, FRCPath, *Professor of Reproductive Pathology, Department of Pathology, University of Manchester, Stepford Building, Oxford Road, Manchester M13 9PT*

MICHAEL J.G. FARTHING MB, FRCP, *Reader in Gastroenterology, Honorary Consultant Physician, Department of Gastroenterology, The Royal Hospital of St Bartholomew's, West Smithfield, London EC1A 7BE*

BRYAN J. FEHILLY MB, MRCP, *Research Fellow, Department of Gastroenterology, The Royal Hospital of St Bartholomew's, West Smithfield, London EC1A 7BE*

JOE A. JORDAN MD, FRCOG, *Birmingham and Midland Hospital for Women, Showell Green Lane, Sparkhill, Birmingham B11 4HL*

CHARLES A.F. JOSLIN MBBS, FRCR, FFR, DMRT, *Professor, University Department of Radiotherapy, Tunbridge Building, Regional Radiotherapy Centre, Cookridge Hospital, Leeds LS16 6QB*

MICHAEL KEARNEY MB, MRCPI, *Consultant in Palliative Medicine, St Christopher's Hospice, 51–59 Lawrie Park Road, Sydenham, London SE26 6D2*

JOHN M. MONAGHAN MB, FRCS(Ed), FRCOG, *Consultant Surgeon, Regional Department of Gynaecological Oncology, Queen Elizabeth II Hospital, Sheriff Hill, Gateshead, Tyne and Wear NE9 6SX*

DAVID ORAM MB, MRCOG, *Consultant Obstetrician and Gynaecologist, The London Hospital, Whitechapel Road, London E1 1BB*

JOHN H. SHEPHERD MB, FRCS, MRCOG, FACOG, *Consultant Gynaecological Surgeon, Department of Gynaecological Oncology, The Royal Hospital of St Bartholomew's, West Smithfield, London EC1A 7BE, UK and The Royal Marsden Hospital, Fulham Road, London SW3 6JJ*

EVE WILTSHAW MD, FRCP, *Consultant Medical Oncologist, The Royal Marsden Hospital, Fulham Road, London SW3 6JJ*

Foreword

This second edition of Shepherd and Monaghan's *Clinical Gynaecological Oncology* is timely: some 5 years after the very successful first edition. Mr Shepherd indicates in his preface that gynaecological oncology as a subspecialty is becoming established in the United Kingdom and it is opportune that this excellent guide to early diagnosis and to all forms of management should become available now when development is occurring so rapidly. The joint authors, two of the leading gynaecological oncologists in the United Kingdom are the most able exponents, in their breadth of experience, their dedication to teaching and training, and as will be seen by the reader, their clarity of presentation. Each has stressed the importance of a multidisciplinary approach drawing from the experience and expertise of colleagues in allied disciplines and supportive therapies. They have, as editors, gathered together a group of internationally renowned specialists in individual areas to enhance the overall variety and authority of the text.

It is to be hoped in the changes occurring in the developing health service, that national and regional support will be available to enable the vital work of such units to develop and flourish. It is only by these means that can we expect the benefits of modern techniques to make an impact on the well being of patients with gynaecological cancer. The second edition is a must for anyone working in the field of gynaecological oncology and is a most valuable reference book for all those working in the field of gynaecological surgery.

Sir George Pinker

Preface to Second Edition

This second edition of Clinical Gynaecological Oncology serves as a timely reminder that sub-specialization in our specialty of obstetrics and gynaecology is slowly coming of age. There are now five recognized units in the United Kingdom with training programmes approved by the Council of the Royal College, having been assessed by the sub-specialization committee, for training Fellows in Gynaecological Oncology. The two editors are both directors of their respective recognized units. With one notable exception, regional referral centres are still not accepted mainly due to the lack of funds. However, tertiary and quaternary referrals are to be encouraged for the centralization of treatment as only in this way will a comprehensive management plan be developed for the overall care of women with gynaecological malignancy.

The theme throughout this book once more emphasizes the need for a multi-disciplinary approach to the subject. Although it is vital for a gynaecological oncologist to be a committed 'sub' or 'super' specialist with a thorough training in all aspects of pelvic surgery, it is most important for him to also have more than a working knowledge of all cancer treatment modalities, including radiotherapy and medical oncology. Only thus, will he be able to contribute to the overall care of his patients and co-ordinate views from other members of the team. Continuing clinical and scientific research is an integral part of such a unit, with a combined approach. Patient conferences and histopathological review sessions form an extension of the basic clinical workload, allowing thorough and thoughtful discussion. Outside referrals may be reviewed and opinions sought and discussed to the benefit of patients and general gynaecologists alike, who know an experienced yet logical opinion may be obtained from a team of cancer specialists. This is a very different situation to the days when isolated individuals were left to soldier on and try to obtain extra advice from other specialists who themselves were in fact generalists in another field.

Pelvic cancer kills more than half the women it afflicts. Earlier diagnosis and screening are to be encouraged but for the established case, surely the time has come for earlier referral to a specialist unit to give the individual patient the best overall chance of a cure. This would also allow the disease to be studied in every way, not only clinically but also for scientific research purposes. The complete management of cancer must depend on absolute referral. For cervical and vulval cancer, this is gradually becoming accepted in both early and advanced disease. Now the time has come to deal with ovarian cancer in the same way and end once and for all the nihilistic attitude that still prevails in many parts of the world. Coupled with this, must be a realistic management plan adapted for the individual patient that can only be developed by such large referral centres.

We two, and our units depend on our colleagues and friends from within and without gynaecology for our enormous referral practices. Only thus are we able to function and have such comprehensive policies for our patients with the help of all members of our team. We are both eternally grateful to all those who seek our advice and for the privilege bestowed upon us.

This edition has become British, and we believe that this confirms the maturing process and coming of age talked of earlier, of gynaecological oncology in Great Britain. The British Gynaecological Cancer Society has reproduced and multiplied. Links are being forged with Europe, both with multi-centre clinical trials as well as a free exchange of fellows in training and other personnel. The International Gynaecological Cancer Society has a large British and Commonwealth membership with active participation. We hope this edition will keep interested gynaecologists abreast of current developments as well as inform them of clinical practice in answer to their management dilemmas.

We both continue to learn ourselves from each other, from our mentors who we still need for advice and encouragement, and also from our fellows. We may train them but now we learn from them also. To our long suffering nursing, medical, para-medical and lay colleagues whose quietly efficient yet immeasurable contribution is invaluable to our units, we are utterly grateful.

We thank Blackwell Scientific Publications for their support enabling production of this text 5 years after the first edition. We are especially grateful to our long suffering secretaries, Carol and Lee, and Eileen Smith for without their perseverance, patience and continual harassment, we could not have produced this whilst still continuing our heavy clinical commitment.

J.H.S. and J.M.M.
June 1990

Preface to First Edition

Gynaecological oncology is already an accepted subspecialty in the United States and is now rapidly developing in Britain and Europe. The two editors are established as gynaecological oncologists serving large populations in their own respective areas. They have drawn on their own experience and that of leading authorities in oncology to provide a comprehensive and balanced view of the whole of this rapidly expanding subject. Each contributor has taken advantage of their own expertise and has thoroughly reviewed the world literature, providing an up to date authoritative text which will stimulate the reader to further study, critically analyse and possibly reassess his management of individual patients.

The book stresses the importance of an accurate clinical and histopathological assessment before any treatment is considered. It is a distillate of all that is best in British and American medicine, with a little leavening of Irish and South African. It is intended for the post-graduate physician who is developing an interest in the subject, as well as the more experienced doctor who may wish for an up to date comment on current practice. It is designed to cross specialty barriers so that there is something here for the gynaecologist, pathologist, radiotherapist, medical oncologist and surgeon. Although edited and mainly written by two practising surgeons the book clearly indicates the necessity for a multidisciplinary approach, reflecting their attitudes towards the care of the unfortunate women who develop gynaecological cancer.

The text conveys the dynamism of the subject as shown by the emphasis on the changing role of various disciplines; for example the marked decline in the use of inpatient surgery for the management of cervical precancer, the important role of surgery in the care of the woman with carcinoma of the vulva and body of the uterus and the increased importance of surgery in the care of primary ovarian and recurrent carcinoma of the cervix. The altering application of radiotherapy with improved techniques is realized in conjunction with the expanding possibilities for chemotherapy.

The interdisciplinary team of writers also confirms the importance of an extensive basic training and knowledge required for the gynaecological oncologist. At the present time in Britain although there are many individuals extremely skilled in certain aspects of gynaecological oncology, we have not yet begun to bring them all together to form the teams which are so important for the complete care of the patient with cancer. There is only one such health service funded unit in Britain at present (J.M.M.). With grit and determination however, others have been formed (J.H.S.) all be they at first unofficial within the confines and limitations of general obstetric and gynaecology departments. This has occurred to a certain extent throughout the country with the co-operation of medical and radiation oncologists. We hope that this book will stimulate and encourage the development of more units that are officially recognized and supported in order to bring a higher quality of co-ordinated care to all our patients.

We would like to thank all of our colleagues who have sought our advice to discuss their unusual and complicated cases, and for entrusting us with the care of their patients. All our past and present junior staff, without whom we could not function, deserve our deepest gratitude and especially our gynaecological oncology Fellows who have suffered us with fortitude. They, in the guise of learning, have taught us so much whilst becoming, we hope, the new generation of gynaecologists. We are greatly appreciative of the quiet assistance of all our laboratory staff and particularly grateful to all those wonderful nurses for the skill, compassion, support and love they extend to all our patients, and the understanding they have given to those terrible people, we two.

We recognize and are eternally grateful to all our mentors, especially Jack Dewhurst in London, Denis Cavanagh in Tampa, Tony Anderson (now sadly deceased) in Edinburgh and Ronnie Hamilton in Inverness, for guiding and encouraging us so often. They have all bestowed upon us an enthusiasm for enquiry as well as the stimulus to develop and improve this challenging subject.

For the help and advice during the preparation of the text we thank Blackwell Scientific Publications, especially Peter Saugman and Jane Grisdale.

J.H.S. and J.M.M.
August 1985

1

Epidemiology and Aetiology of Cancers of the Female Genital Tract

VALERIE BERAL

At present in England and Wales approximately one woman in 20 will develop cancer of the genital tract during her lifetime and one in 40 will die of the disease.

It has long been suspected that hormonal influences, reproductive factors and sexual behaviour are important for all these malignancies, but it is only in recent years that the way in which they affect cancer risk has been studied in detail. This chapter reviews briefly the epidemiological distribution of cancers of the female genital tract in the population and the findings from a number of studies designed to elucidate their causes. A recently published monography by Kelsey & Hildreth (1982) provides an extensive literature review of the subject.

Occurrence of malignant neoplasms of the female genital organs

Of the 99 000 malignant neoplasms registered among women in England and Wales in 1984, the primary site was the female genital tract for 13 000 — or 1 in 7 of all cancers (Office of Population Censuses and Surveys 1988). A similar proportion of deaths from cancer in 1984 were ascribed to lesions of the female genital tract (Office of Population Censuses and Surveys 1985).

The table below (Table 1.1) shows the numbers of new cases and deaths from cancers of specified reproductive sites among women in England and Wales in 1984.

It can be seen from Table 1.1 that cancer of the ovary is the most common cancer registered and also the most common cause of death — accounting for more deaths than from carcinoma of the uterine cervix and body combined.

About one woman in 20 is likely to develop cancer of the genital tract in her lifetime. Table 1.2 indicates the cumulative risk of developing or dying from these cancers before age 80.

Each malignancy has its characteristic age distribution, as is shown in Fig. 1.1. There are some similarities for cancers of the ovary, uterine corpus and uterine cervix, the age-specific incidence rates for all three increasing rapidly during the reproductive years and then reaching a plateau after the menopause.

Table 1.1. Number of new cases and deaths from cancers of the female genital tract in England and Wales in 1984

International classification of disease code (9th revision)	Site of malignancy	Number of new cases	Number of deaths
183.0	Ovary	4473	3932
180	Cervix uteri	4043	1917
182	Body of uterus	3329	952
184.1−184.4	Vulva	790	419
179	Uterus, part unspecified	430	529
184.0	Vagina	217	97
183.1−183.9	Fallopian tube and other uterine adnexa	66	28
184.9	Other and unspecified female genital organs	25	0
181	Choriocarcinoma	11	1
179−184	All female genital tract	13018	7807

Sources: Office of Population Censuses and Surveys, 1985 and 1988

Table 1.2. Cumulative risk of developing or dying from various cancers of the female genital tract before the age of 80 years

International classification of disease code	Site	Percent developing the cancer	Percent dying from the cancer
183	Ovary	1.5	1.3
180	Uterine cervix	1.3	0.7
182	Body of uterus	1.1	0.4
184.1−184.4	Vulva	0.2	0.1
184.0	Vagina	0.07	0.04
179−184	All female genital tract	4.5	2.7

Sources: Office of Population Censuses and Surveys, 1985 and 1988

The incidence of vulval and vaginal cancer increases with age and does not level off after the menopause. Choriocarcinoma shows the age pattern which might be expected for a malignancy of prègnancy.

Unfortunately, only limited information about disease trends is available. Mortality data for ovarian cancer and uterine cancer (cervix and corpus combined) date from 1911, data for cervix and corpus cancer having only been separated since 1951. Incidence data and information about other genital tract cancers were not published routinely until around 1960. Nevertheless, it does appear that the incidence of malignancies of the genital tract has not been stable over time. As is

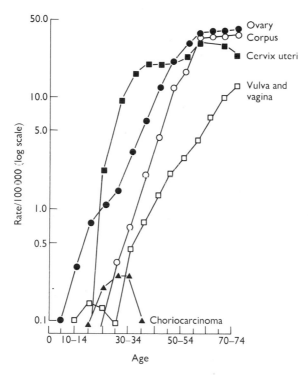

Fig. 1.1. Age-specific incidence of cancers of the female genital tract. England and Wales 1980 (Office of Population Censuses & Surveys).

shown in Fig. 1.2 mortality from ovarian cancer has increased considerably during this century and mortality from cancer of the uterus (cervix and corpus combined) has fallen. After 1951 when cervix and corpus cancer were recorded separately, it can be seen that mortality from both conditions has been falling — except perhaps until recently for corpus cancer.

Figure 1.3 shows the geographical distribution in England and Wales of cancer of the ovary, cervix uteri and other cancers of the uterus. Mortality rates from all these cancers are higher in the west and north than in the south-east.

Cervix cancer is a condition of the unskilled and semi-skilled, whereas ovarian cancer is a condition of the upper social classes (Fig. 1.4).

In the remainder of this chapter cancers of each site and the factors which are important in their aetiology are discussed separately.

Ovarian cancer

Cancer of the ovary is a malignancy of industrialized societies, and of the affluent within any country (Figs 1.4 and 1.5). It carries the worst prognosis of all the malignancies of the female genital tract — national figures indicating that only 25% survive for 5 years or longer (Toms et al. 1981).

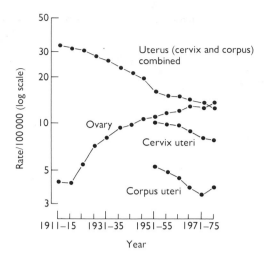

Fig. 1.2. Trends in mortality from cancers of the ovary and uterus. England and Wales 1911–78 (Toms *et al*. 1981, reproduced with permission).

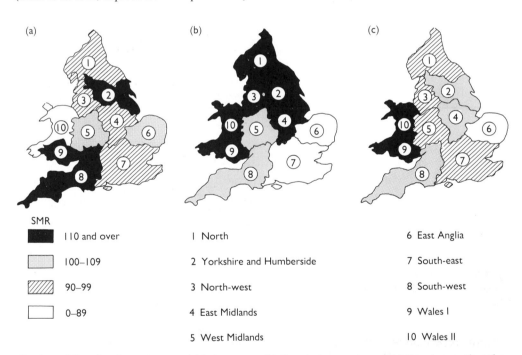

Fig. 1.3. Mortality from cancers of (a) the ovary; (b) the uterine cervix and (c) the uterus other than cervix by standard region in England and Wales 1970–72 (Toms *et al*. 1981, reproduced with permission).

As is described in Chapter 10, malignant disease of the ovary includes a multitude of histological types, which are grouped together in most epidemiological analyses. Where they have been separated it would seem that the major

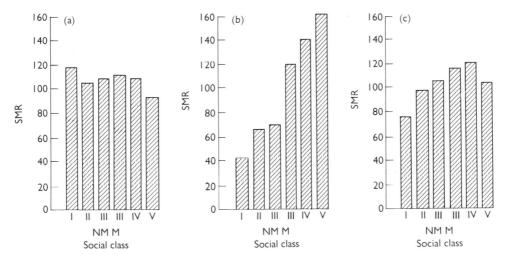

Fig. 1.4. Mortality from cancers of (a) the ovary; (b) the uterine cervix and (c) the uterus other than cervix (Toms *et al.* 1981, reproduced with permission).

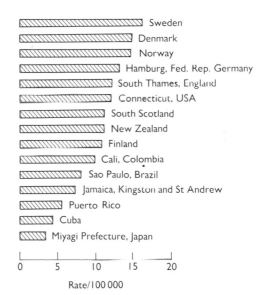

Fig. 1.5. Age-standardized incidence of ovarian cancer in selected countries (IARC 1982).

tumour types have a similar distribution and aetiology. Diagnostic differences make comparisons difficult, but Berg and Baylor (1973) showed, for instance, that the geographical distribution of epithelial carcinomas, granulosa cell tumours and malignant teratomas were similar. Only dysgerminomas had a different pattern of occurrence. Furthermore Weiss *et al.* (1977) showed that the various histological types of epithelial tumours had very similar age distributions, comparable to that shown in Fig. 1.1 for all ovarian cancers. Germ cell tumours and malignant teratomas differed, however, tending to occur at younger ages. The incidence of malignant teratomas peaks at puberty and that of germ cell tumours about a decade later (Walker *et al.* 1984). These rare tumours account for the slight deflection in the age-specific incidence rates of ovarian cancer seen in Fig. 1.1 at ages 20–34 years.

Familial, genetic and ethnic factors

Women whose mother or sister died of ovarian cancer have almost a 20-fold increase in the possibility of developing the disease themselves (Hildreth *et al.* 1981). Nevertheless 95% of women with ovarian cancer have no family history of the condition. Similarly a number of rare conditions, such as the Peutz–Jegher syndrome and various chromosomal anomalies such as Turner's syndrome have been linked with ovarian cancer, but they contribute a small fraction to the burden of ovarian cancer in the community.

As illustrated in Fig. 1.5 the incidence of ovarian cancer varies widely from one country to another. This might be taken to imply that different ethnic groups have a varying susceptibility to ovarian cancer. However, once people of similar ethnic origin living in different countries are compared, as in Fig. 1.6, it becomes clear that the important determinant of risk is place of residence, not ethnic origin. Even for those living in the same country, risks vary according to country of birth. For example, among Jews living in Israel the rate of ovarian cancer is three times higher among those born in Europe or America compared with Asia or Africa (Fig. 1.7).

Hormones, reproduction and ovulation

In the last 10 years a number of studies have reported on the association between ovarian cancer, reproduction and use of hormones (for example, Hildreth *et al.* 1981; Risch *et al.* 1983). Two consistent observations have emerged: pregnancy

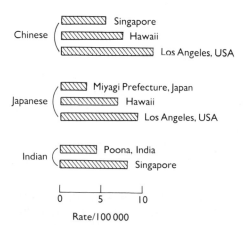

Fig. 1.6. Age-standardized incidence of ovarian cancer in Chinese, Japanese and Indians living in various countries (IARC 1982).

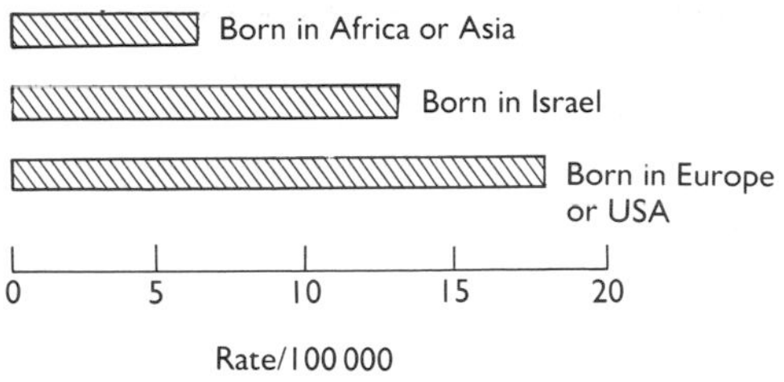

Born in Africa or Asia

Born in Israel

Born in Europe or USA

Fig. 1.7. Age-standardized incidence of ovarian cancer in Jews living in Israel, according to their place of birth (IARC 1982).

Rate/100 000

protects a woman from developing ovarian cancer — the more pregnancies she has, the greater is the protection; and oral contraceptives reduce the risk of ovarian cancer — the longer the Pill is taken the greater is the protection. Late menarche and early menopause also reduce the risk of disease. These observations suggest that any process which suppresses ovulation or reduces the number of ovulations which a woman experiences in her lifetime may protect against ovarian cancer. This supports Fathalla's hypothesis (1971) that 'incessant ovulation' is an important cause of epithelial ovarian cancers.

The increasing incidence of ovarian cancer over time and the geographic and ethnic differences in its incidence can probably be accounted for by variations in the number of children that women have had in the past (Beral *et al.* 1978). The high rates of disease in industrialized countries and in the upper social classes are correlated with the small completed family size in these populations; and the increasing incidence of ovarian cancer in England and Wales during the last decade may be accounted for by the smaller average family size which successive generations of women have been experiencing.

Environment

Perhaps the most interesting recent findings about the aetiology of ovarian cancer are the reported associations with exposure to asbestos or talc. Several studies have reported that women exposed to asbestos at work have increased rates of ovarian cancer (Acheson *et al.* 1982; Wignall & Fox 1982). Although the authors were aware of the problem, it is still unclear whether some of these tumours were truly ovarian cancers or mesotheliomas misclassified as ovarian cancer. Talc may sometimes be contaminated with asbestos and a high proportion of ovarian tumours have been reported to contain talc particles embedded in them (Henderson *et al.* 1971). Cramer *et al.* (1982) reported that women who dust their perineal area or sanitary napkins with talc may be at an increased risk of ovarian cancer. Their findings are worrisome but judgement about their relevance must be reserved until a number of studies specially designed to examine the relationship have been completed.

A variety of other possible causal factors have been suggested — including consumption of a high-fat diet, drinking coffee, exposure to mumps in childhood

and the use of stilboestrol for menopausal symptoms—but the evidence for all
these is weak or contradictory. Pelvic irradiation increases the risk of all cancers
of the genital tract (Smith 1977) and a number of studies have suggested that
hysterectomy may reduce the risk of ovarian cancer although the mechanism for
this is far from clear (Annegers *et al.* 1979; Hildreth *et al.* 1981).

Cancer of the uterine cervix

Contrary to ovarian malignancies, cancer of the uterine cervix is a condition of
the poor. It is more frequent in developing than developed countries and its
incidence is highest in the lower social classes (Figs 1.4 and 1.8). Survival is
moderately high in England and Wales with 54% living for 5 years or longer after
the condition is diagnosed (Toms *et al.* 1981).

The discussion here is mainly concerned with invasive cancer of the cervix.
While *in situ* cervical cancer may progress to invasive disease, there is considerable evidence that it also is a reversible lesion (Walton Report 1976). In England
and Wales in 1984, 8400 women had *in situ* cervix cancer registered (though this
may be an underestimate); it is still a larger number than the 4000 cases of
invasive disease registered. Furthermore the numbers of reported cases of *in situ*
disease is increasing rapidly each year (Draper & Cook 1983). A major factor in
determining the reported incidence of *in situ* cervix cancer is, however, the

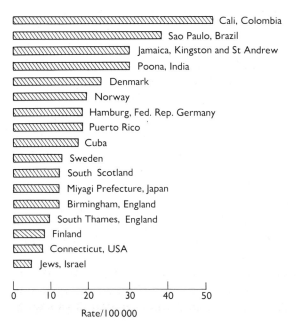

Fig. 1.8. Age-standardized incidence of
cancer of the uterine cervix in selected
countries (IARC 1982).

frequency with which women are screened. Hence the reported incidence rate of *in situ* cervix cancer is an unreliable indicator of the true incidence of disease.

Infection as a cause of cervical cancer

Over the past 20 years there has been growing evidence that cervical cancer is mainly caused by an infectious agent or agents, transmitted sexually. There is a wealth of information indicating that women with cervical cancer are those most likely to acquire a sexually transmitted infection: for example, they have had more sexual partners than other women, more sexually transmitted infections, begun intercourse earlier, and were less likely to use barrier methods of contraception (Beral 1974; Wright *et al.* 1978). It is not only their sexual behaviour which is important, but that of their partners as well; and it is becoming clear that some men may harbour the infectious agent for some time and so be important in transmitting the disease (Buckley *et al.* 1981; Skegg *et al.* 1982). Further evidence for an infectious origin of cervix cancer comes from the observed association between penile cancer in males and cervix cancer in females. Smith *et al.* (1980) found that the wives of men who died of penile cancer were three times more likely than average to die from cervical cancer.

What the infection is and whether more than one agent is involved has yet to be determined. The herpes virus was a favoured contender during the 1970s, but recent evidence suggesting that the papillomavirus may be the culprit is persuasive although still inconclusive (zur Hausen 1982).

Numerous studies of the association between human papillomavirus and cervical cancer have been carried out in the last few years. The findings from more than thirty such studies were reviewed by Bosch & Munoz (1988). Most reports suggested that human papillomavirus type 16, and to a lesser extent type 18, were associated with invasive cervical cancer, whereas types 6 and 11 were associated with condylomas and low-grade cervical intraepithelial neoplasia. Follow-up studies of women with mild intraepithelial neoplasia suggested that women with cervical lesions associated with human papillomavirus types 16 and/or 18 are more likely to progress to advanced disease than are lesions in women with types 6 and/or 11 papillomavirus (Campion *et al.* 1986; Syrjanen *et al.* 1986; Schneider *et al.* 1987). One case-control study, based in Latin America, reported a three-fold increase in risk of cervical cancer associated with papillomavirus types 16/18 (Reeves *et al.* 1987). A workshop held in May 1988 to review the recent data concluded that, while there was substantial consistency in the evidence suggesting that types 16 and 18 might cause cervical cancer, the studies published so far were sufficiently limited to prevent firm conclusions being drawn at this stage (*Lancet*, 1988).

The distribution of cervical cancer in the population including ethnic difference (Fig. 1.9) is probably largely explicable by the distribution of infectious agents. For example, the high rates of disease in Latin American countries shown

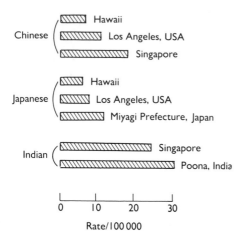

Fig. 1.9. Age-adjusted incidence of cancer of the uterine cervix in Chinese, Japanese and Indians living in various countries (IARC 1982).

in Fig. 1.8 may reflect the sexual activity of males in that society (Skegg *et al*. 1982); the decreasing rate of cervix cancer in older women (Fig. 1.2) may well reflect the increasing use of barrier methods of contraception or of genital hygiene; and the increasing rates of disease at young ages may reflect the recent rise in sexually transmitted disease and abandonment of barrier methods of contraception (Beral 1974).

Reproductive and hormonal factors

It has long been recognized that cervix cancer is more frequent in parous than nulliparous women (Green *et al*. 1988). Initially this was ascribed to the sexual behaviour of parous women. Analyses of data adjusting for number of partners have shown, however, that the association with parity persists and may well be a direct effect of the pregnancy (Brinton *et al*. 1987).

Women taking oral contraceptives have higher rates of cervical cancer than do other women (Vessey *et al*. 1983; Brinton *et al*. 1986a; Beral *et al*. 1988). The longer the duration of oral contraceptive use, the greater the risk. In the Royal College of General Practitioner's follow-up study of 47 000 women, those who had taken the Pill for 10 years or longer had incidence rates of cervical cancer four times that of women who had never taken the Pill (Beral *et al*. 1988). As with the association of cervical cancer and parity, these findings were initially thought to reflect the different sexual behaviour of women who took the Pill and of other women. As the evidence was examined in detail, taking into account the sexual behaviour of the women, it has become clear that oral contraceptives might well influence the rate at which cervical cancer develops. This view is supported by the work of Stern *et al*. (1977) who showed that oral contraceptives hasten the rate at which dysplastic changes on the cervix progress to more severe lesions. Thus although pregnancy and exogenous hormones do not necessarily initiate new tumours, they may well promote the growth of existing ones.

Environmental factors

Numerous studies have found that women who smoke are at an increased risk of cervical cancer; the relationship is so strong that some have concluded that it may well be causal (Brinton et al. 1986b).

There have also been suggestions that the wives of men working in dusty and dirty occupations may be at an increased risk of disease. A systematic survey of deaths from cervical cancer in England and Wales between 1970 and 1972 revealed, however, no consistent association between such occupations in men and their wives' risk of cervical cancer (Primic Zakelj et al. 1984).

Cancer of the uterine body

The vast majority of malignancies of the body of the uterus arise in the endometrium and so the discussion here is largely concerned with endometrial cancer. Survival is even better than for cervical cancer, with 66% living for 5 years or longer after diagnosis (Toms et al. 1981). Incidence rates are especially high in North America and low in developing countries (Fig. 1.10).

Country of residence is clearly an important determinant of the disease, groups of similar ethnic origin living in different countries having very variable incidences of the condition (Fig. 1.11). Its incidence, until recently, has been falling in the UK (Fig. 1.2), but has been reported to be increasing in the USA (Weiss et al. 1979).

Reproduction and hormones

There is considerable evidence that oestrogens, unopposed by the action of progestogens, play a large role in the aetiology of endometrial cancer. It is now generally accepted that menopausal oestrogen therapy increases the risk of endometrial cancer (Editorial 1979). These oestrogen-induced tumours tend to be of low malignant potential, and associated with very good survival rates. The addition of progestogen therapy to the oestrogens has been reported to reduce both the incidence of endometrial hyperplasia and of endometrial carcinoma (Thom et al. 1979). Combined oral contraceptives reduce the risk of endometrial carcinoma whereas sequential ones—which contain some unopposed oestrogen tablets—increase the risk (Henderson et al. 1983).

Pregnancy is a powerful factor in protecting against ovarian cancer, perhaps related to the shedding of the endometrium which occurs at parturition. The more pregnancies a women has the greater her protection from endometrial carcinoma. Infertility is a strong risk factor for the disease, especially in women of childbearing age where it is associated with the Stein—Leventhal syndrome in 20% of cases (Kelsey & Hildreth 1982). As with ovarian cancer, the risk of endometrial cancer is higher with late onset of the menopause.

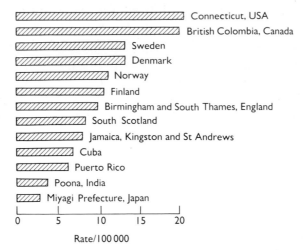

Fig. 1.10. Age-adjusted incidence of cancer of the body of the uterus in selected countries (IARC 1982).

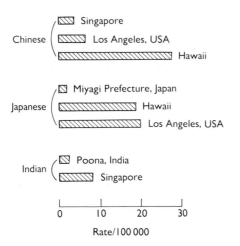

Fig. 1.11. Age-adjusted incidence of cancer of the body of the uterus in Chinese, Japanese and Indians living in various countries (IARC 1982).

Other factors

Obesity is a significant risk factor of endometrial cancer, especially gross obesity. This has been explained by the excessive production of oestrogens by adipose tissue of obese women and their lower levels of sex-hormone binding globulin (MacDonald *et al.* 1978). Hypertension and diabetes have also been associated with endometrial carcinoma, but it is unlikely that these are causal factors.

Vulval cancer

Malignancies of the vulva are relatively rare and have not been studied intensively. Little can be said about their distribution in the population, since until recently national and international statistics did not list these cancers separately, but grouped them with vaginal cancer.

No studies have been carried out to identify possible risk factors for the disease and so its aetiology is unknown. Perhaps the most interesting observation is that vulval carcinoma may be multicentric in origin and associated with cancer in the cervix, vagina or anogenital area (Green *et al.* 1958). Furthermore it is frequently associated with genital warts, which are caused by the papillomavirus. This had led zur Hausen (1982) to suggest that vulval cancer has a viral cause.

Vaginal cancer

Vaginal cancer is even rarer than vulval cancer and had been little studied until the last decade, when an association with *in utero* exposure to diethylstilboestrol was reported for clear cell adenocarcinomas (Herbst *et al.* 1971). Since then there have been many reports of the association, the risk of vaginal cancer being somewhere between one in 700 and one in 7000 for those exposed *in utero*. The earlier in gestational life the exposure and the higher the dose of oestrogens to which the children were exposed, the greater was the incidence of disease (Herbst *et al.* 1977).

Despite the interest in vaginal cancer in young girls, the vast majority of cancers arise in older women as is shown in Fig. 1.1 and are of squamous type; factors contributing to their aetiology have not been studied.

Other malignancies

Other cancers of the female genital tract are very uncommon indeed. As pointed out earlier, choriocarcinoma is extremely rare in England and Wales, but it is a fascinating tumour (see Chapter 12 of this volume).

Conclusions

During the past 20 years we have greatly improved our understanding of the aetiology of diseases of the female genital tract. Ovarian cancer is related to ovulation, although the mechanism of this is not understood; cervical cancer is probably caused by a sexually transmitted infection and endometrial cancer by the action of unopposed oestrogens.

Oral contraceptives affect the development of all three malignancies, increasing the risk of cervical cancer but reducing the risk of ovarian and endometrial cancer. Taken together the excess risk of cervical cancer in Pill users is balanced by the deficit of ovarian and endometrial cancers (Beral *et al.* 1988). Of great relevance to clinical practice is that the distribution of primary cancer sites differs substantially in Pill users and other women: cervical cancer accounts for 75% of invasive genital cancers in women who have taken the Pill but only 31% of such cancers in women who have never taken the Pill. Given that our knowledge has advanced so far, the next step should be aimed at prevention—but how this is achieved is a more difficult question to answer.

Acknowledgements

I thank Helen Edwards for typing the manuscript, and the Office of Population Censuses and Surveys for permission to reproduce Tables 1.1 and 1.2 and Fig. 1.1.

References

Acheson E.D., Gardner M.J., Pippard E.C. & Grime L.P. (1982) Mortality of two groups of women who manufactured gas masks from chrysotile and crocidolite asbestos: a 40-year follow-up. *Br. J. Ind. Med.*, **39**, 344−48.

Annegers J.F., Strom H., Decker D.G., Dockerty M.B. & O'Fallon W.M. (1979) Ovarian cancer: incidence and case-control study. *Cancer*, **43**, 723−29.

Beral V. (1974) Cancer of the cervix: a sexually transmitted infection? *Lancet*, i, 1037−40.

Beral V., Fraser P. & Chilvers C. (1978) Does pregnancy protect against ovarian cancer? *Lancet*, i, 1083−87.

Beral V., Hannaford P. & Kay C. (1988) Oral contraceptives and malignancies of the genital tract: results from the Royal College of General Practitioner's Oral Contraceptive Study. *Lancet*, ii, 1331−5.

Berg J.W. & Baylor S.M. (1973) The epidemiologic pathology of ovarian cancer. *Hum. Path.*, **4**, 537−47.

Bosch F.X. & Munoz N. (1989) Human papillomavirus and cervical neoplasia: critical review of the available epidemiological evidence. *In*: Human Papillomavirus in the etiology of cancer of the uterine cervix. Munoz N. & Jensen O. (eds), IARC Scientific Publications No. 94 Lyon pp. 135−51.

Brinton L.A., Hamman R.F., Huggins G.R., Lehman H.F., Levine R.S., Mallin K. & Fraumeni J.F. (1987) Sexual and reproductive risk factors for invasive squamous cell cervical cancer. *J. Natl. Cancer Inst.*, **79**, 23−30.

Brinton L.A., Huggins G.R., Lehman H.F., Mallin K., Savitz D.A., Trapido E., Rosenthal J. & Hoover R. (1986a) Long-term use of oral contraceptives and risk of invasive cervical cancer. *Int. J. Cancer*, **38**, 339−44.

Brinton L.A., Schairer C., Haenszel W., Stolley P., Lehman H.F., Levine R. & Savitz D.A. (1986b) Cigarette smoking and invasive cervical cancer. *JAMA*, **255**, 3265−69.

Buckley J.D., Harris R.W.C., Doll R., Vessey M.P. & Williams P.T. (1981) Case-control study of the husbands of women with dysplasia or carcinoma of the cervix uteri. *Lancet*, ii, 1010−14.

Campion M.J., McCance D.J., Cuzick J. & Singer A. (1986) Progressive potential of mild cervical atypia: prospective cytological, colposcopic and virological study. *Lancet*, ii, 237−40.

Human papillomavirus and cervical cancer. (1988) *Lancet*, i, 756−57.

Cramer D.W., Welch W.R., Scully R.E. & Wojciechowski D.A. (1982) Ovarian cancer and talc. A case-control study. *Cancer*, **50**, 372−76.

Draper G.J. & Cook G.A. (1983) Changing patterns of cervical cancer rates. *Br. Med. J.*, **287**, 510−12.

Editorial (1979) Oestrogen therapy and endometrial cancer. *Lancet*, i, 1121−22.

Fathalla M.F. (1971) Incessant ovulation—a factor in ovarian neoplasia? *Lancet*, ii, 163.

Franceschi S., Doll R., Gallwey J., La Vecchia C., Peto R. & Spriggs A.I. (1983) Genital warts and cervical neoplasia: an epidemiological study. *Br. J. Cancer*, **48**, 621−28.

Green A., Beral V. & Moser K. (1988) Mortality in women in relation to their childbearing history. *Br. Med. J.*, **296**, 391−94.

Green T.H., Ulfelder H. & Meigo J.V. (1958) Epidermoid carcinoma of the vulva: an analysis of 283 cases. I. Etiology and diagnosis. *Am. J. Obstet. Gynecol.*, **75**, 834.

Henderson B.E., Casagrande J.T., Pike M.C., Mack T., Rosario I. & Duke A. (1983) The epidemiology of endometrial cancer in young women. *Br. J. Cancer*, **47**, 749−56.

Henderson W.J., Joslin C.A.F., Turnbull A.C. & Griffiths K. (1971) Talc and carcinoma of the ovary and cervix. *J. Obstet. Gynaec. Br. Commonwealth*, **78**, 266−72.

Herbst A.L., Cole P., Colton T., Robboy S.J. & Scully R.E. (1977) Age-incidence and risk of diethylstilbestrol-related clear cell adenocarcinoma of the vagina and cervix. *Am. J. Obstet. Gynecol.*, **128**, 43−50.

Herbst A.L., Ulfelder H. & Poskanzer D.C. (1971) Adenocarcinoma of the vagina. *New Engl. J. Med.*, **284**, 878−81.

Hildreth N.G., Kelsey J.L., Li Volsi V.A., Fischer D.B., Holford T.R., Mostow E.D., Schwartz P.E. & White C. (1981) An epidemiologic study of epithelial carcinoma of the ovary. *Am. J. Epidemiol.*, **114**, 398−405.

International Agency for Research on Cancer (1982) *Cancer Incidence in Five Continents*, Volume IV, IARC Scientific Publications, No. 42, Lyon.

Kelsey J.L. & Hildreth N.G. (1982) *Breast and Gynecologic Cancer Epidemiology*. CRC Press Inc, Boca Raton, Florida.

MacDonald P.C., Edman C.D., Hemsell D.L., Porter J.C. & Siiteri P.K. (1978) Effect of obesity on conversion of plasma androstenedione to estrone in postmenopausal women with and without endometrial cancer. *Am. J. Obstet. Gynecol.*, **130**, 448.

Office of Population Censuses and Surveys (1988) *Cancer Statistics: Registrations*. Series MB1 No. 16. HMSO, London.

Office of Populations Censuses and Surveys (1988) *Cancer Statistics: Registrations*. Series MB1 No. 16. HMSO, London.

Primic Zakelj M., Fraser P. & Inskip H. (1984) Cervical cancer and husband's occupation. *Lancet*, **i**, 510.

Reeves W.C., Caussy D., Brinton L.A., Brenes M.M., Montalvan P., Gomez B., de Britton R.C., Morice E., Gaitan E., Loo de Lao S. & Rawls W.E. (1987) Case-control study of human papillomaviruses and cervical cancer in Latin America. *Int. J. Cancer*, **40**, 450−54.

Risch H.A., Weiss N.S., Lyon J.L., Daling J.F. & Liff J.M. (1983) Events of reproductive life and the incidence of epithelial cancer. *Am. J. Epidemiol.*, **117**, 128−39.

Schneider A., Sawada E., Gissmann L. & Schah K. (1987) Human papillomaviruses in women with a history of abnormal papnicolaou smears and their male partners. *Obstet. Gynecol.*, **69**, 554−62.

Skegg D.C.G., Corwin P.A., Paul C. & Doll R. (1982) Importance of the male factor in cancer of the cervix. *Lancet*, **ii**, 581−83.

Smith P.G. (1977) Leukaemia and other cancers following radiation treatment of pelvic disease. *Cancer*, **39**, 1901−5.

Smith P.G., Kinlen L.J., White C.C., Adelstein A.M. & Fox A.J. (1980) Mortality of wives of men dying with cancer of the penis. *Br. J. Cancer*, **41**, 422−28.

Stern E., Forsythe A.B., Youkeles L. & Coffelt C.F. (1977) Steroid contraceptive use and cervical dysplasia; increased risk of progression. *Science*, **196**, 1460−62.

Syrjanen K., Mantyjarvi R., Parkkinen S., Vayrynen M., Saarikoski S., Syrjanen S. & Castren O. (1986) Prospective follow-up in assessment of the biological behaviour of cervical HPV-associated dysplasic lesions. *In*: Peto, R. & Zur Hausen, H. (eds), *Viral Etiology of Cervical Cancer (Banbury Report No. 21)*, Cold Spring Harbor Laboratory, 167−77.

Thom M.H., White P.J., Williams R.M., Sturdee D.W., Paterson M.E.L., Wade-Evans T. & Studd J.W.W. (1979) Prevention and treatment of endometrial disease in climacteric women receiving oestrogen therapy. *Lancet*, **ii**, 455.

Toms J.R., Draper G.J., Stiller C.A., Adelstein A.M., Donnan S.P.B., Fox A.J., Macdonald Davies I.M. & White C.C. (1981) Cancer statistics: incidence and survival and mortality in England and Wales. *Studies in Medical and Population Subjects*, **43**, 69−78.

Vessey M.P., Lawless M., McPherson K. & Yeates D. (1983) Neoplasia of the cervix uteri and contraception: possible adverse effect of the pill. *Lancet*, **ii**, 930−34.

Walker A.H., Ross R.K., Pike M.C. & Henderson B.E. (1984) A possible rising incidence of malignant germ cell tumours in young women. *Br. J. Cancer*, **49**, 669−72.

Walton Report (1976) Cervical cancer screening programs. *Can. Med. Ass. J.*, **114**, 1003−33.

Weiss N.S., Homonchuk T. & Young J.L. (1977) Incidence of the histologic types of ovarian cancer: the US Third National Cancer Survey, 1969–71. *Gynecol. Oncol.*, **5**, 161–67.

Weiss N.S., Szekeley D.R., English D.R. & Schweid A.I. (1979) Endometrial cancer in relation to patterns of menopausal oestrogen use. *JAMA*, **242**, 261–64.

Wignall B.K. & Fox A.J. (1982) Mortality of female gas mask assemblers. *Br. J. Ind. Med.*, **39**, 34–38.

Wright N.H., Vessey M.P., Kenward B., McPherson K. & Doll R. (1978) Neoplasia and dysplasia of the cervix uteri and contraception: a possible protective effect of the diaphragm. *Br. J. Cancer*, **38**, 273–79.

zur Hausen H. (1982) Human genital cancer: synergism between two virus infections or synergism between a virus infection and initiating events. *Lancet*, **ii**, 1370–72.

2

The Pathology of CIN, VAIN and VIN

MALCOLM C. ANDERSON

The pathology of cervical intraepithelial neoplasia

Nomenclature

The epithelial abnormalities of the cervix fall into two main categories. First, there are those changes such as reserve cell hyperplasia, immature and mature squamous metaplasia and the 'congenital transformation zone' which are predominantly physiological and therefore benign conditions; it could be argued that they should not even be called abnormalities. Secondly, there is the group of abnormalities, of which some examples have apparent malignant potential, that has been known for many years as dysplasia and carcinoma *in situ* and, more recently, as cervical intraepithelial neoplasia (CIN).

Dysplasia was first used as a term by Reagan *et al.* (1953) and was an attractive term to apply to the cervix because it was sufficiently vague and non-committal in its implications to fit in with the uncertainties which existed regarding the nature and behaviour of the changes that it was used to describe. These uncertainties are reflected in the definition of the International Committee of Histological Terminology (Editorial 1962) which characterizes dysplasia as 'all other disturbances of differentiation of the squamous epithelium of lesser degree than carcinoma *in situ*', a definition which is too broad to have any meaning or to be of any practical help to the pathologist in making a precise diagnosis. The World Health Organization (Poulsen *et al.* 1975) defines dysplasia as 'a lesion in which part of the thickness of the epithelium is replaced by cells showing varying degrees of atypia', a definition which is more precise but may be no more accurate, because even the mildest types of epithelial neoplasia have cells on the surface which show nuclear atypia. This feature, of course, forms the basis of the cytological diagnosis of these conditions. Dysplasia has usually been divided into mild, moderate and severe degrees (Reagan & Hamonic 1956) although the precise guidelines for these subdivisions have not been defined and this grading has always been highly subjective.

Carcinoma *in situ* requires the whole thickness of the epithelium to be replaced by undifferentiated cells (Editorial 1962; Govan *et al.* 1969), so that the definition is more precise. Even so, the World Health Organization definition (Poulsen *et al.* 1975), 'a lesion in which all or most of the epithelium shows the cellular features of carcinoma', accepts that there may be some differentiation on the surface. Similarly, both Burghardt (1976) and Koss (1978) allow carcinoma *in situ* to show surface differentiation. The distinction between dysplasia and carcinoma *in situ* is therefore a poorly defined one resulting in a situation in which there is both vagueness of diagnostic criteria and subjectivity of interpretation. To illustrate the latter point, Cocker *et al.* (1968) and Bellina *et al.* (1982) demonstrated not only a lack of agreement between pathologists in the diagnosis of epithelial abnormalities but also inconsistency in the diagnosis made by a single pathologist at different times on the same slides. The use of the two terms, dysplasia and carcinoma *in situ*, to describe cervical abnormalities tends to imply that there are two different disease processes and that carcinoma *in situ* is always more serious than dysplasia; some even go so far as to consider carcinoma *in situ* a malignant condition and dysplasia a benign one. This has the effect that some women with carcinoma *in situ* are over-treated and some with dysplasia are either under-treated or the lesion is disregarded altogether. When the uncertainty about the precise histological diagnosis is superimposed upon this attitude to management, it can be appreciated that a very unsatisfactory situation exists, with somewhat arbitrary decisions about management being based upon equally woolly histological opinions.

The evidence which has been accumulating over the last 20 years by light microscopy, electron microscopy (Shingleton *et al.* 1968), autoradiography (Richart 1963), microspectrophotometry (Wilbanks *et al.* 1967), tissue culture (Richart *et al.* 1967) and cytogenetics (Kirkland *et al.* 1967; Spriggs *et al.* 1971) has led to the conclusion that CIN is a continuous spectrum of disease; it is one disease of various degrees rather than a number of separate, although related conditions. This is an infinitely variable spectrum in which each degree of abnormality merges imperceptibly into the next; the differences between the cells and the epithelium in one part of the spectrum compared with another are quantitative rather than qualitative. The theoretical concept of CIN as a continuum is not really reconcilable with the subdivision of the disease at all. However, for the purposes of classification and, more importantly, for the purposes of determination of management, it is customary for CIN to be divided. From a practical point of view, it would seem necessary to divide CIN merely into those which are thought to be at *high risk* and those which appear to be at *low risk* of becoming invasive in the near future. On this basis and bearing in mind its dependence on the use of morphological criteria to predict the biological behaviour of the epithelium, the decision may be made to treat immediately or to delay treatment and observe by cytology, in the hope that regression may take place. This decision will also depend on the methods of treatment which are available. If low morbidity outpatient methods of treatment are used, then there are arguments in favour of treating minor abnormalities and, in these circumstances, the degree of

CIN is of less importance than its distribution. However, despite the concept of CIN as a single disease process and the practical requirement to use two subdivisions, CIN is customarily subdivided into three. CIN 1 is equivalent to mild dysplasia, CIN 2 to moderate dysplasia and CIN 3 includes the lesions which were previously called both severe dysplasia and carcinoma *in situ*. This avoids the unnecessary but sometimes difficult and time-consuming exercise of differentiating between severe dysplasia and carcinoma *in situ* histologically. It will be apparent, or course, that ascribing a particular grade to a CIN is open to all the criticisms of imprecision and subjectivity that have already been made concerning dysplasia and carcinoma *in situ*.

The advantages of the CIN terminology compared with the dual dysplasia/carcinoma *in situ* terminology are as follows:

1 it is in keeping with the concept of a single disease process;
2 it recognizes dysplasia as a neoplastic process, and
3 it is in accord with the modern therapeutic approach to CIN.

The main objection to the use of the CIN terminology is that it regards even the most minor form of dysplasia as neoplastic, perhaps causing over-reaction and excessive treatment for minor, reversible conditions. It must be borne in mind, of course, that most CIN 3 lesions are probably preceded by CIN 1, so that many examples of CIN 1 require treatment eventually. From the point of view of the scientific concept as well as its affect on treatment attitudes, the advantages of the CIN terminology outweigh its disadvantages.

The natural history of CIN

The relationship of one grade of CIN to another and the relationship of CIN to invasive cancer have been exhaustively studied, although rather more is known about the former than the latter. Most of this work was done when the dysplasia/carcinoma *in situ* terminology was used and so it is necessary to revert to these terms for a few paragraphs. Using cytology and colpomicroscopy, but without taking biopsies, Richart & Barron (1969) followed 557 patients who had a cytological diagnosis of cervical dysplasia. The patients left the study and were treated when they developed carcinoma *in situ*. It was found that the medium transit times for the progression of mild dysplasia, moderate dysplasia and severe dysplasia to carcinoma *in situ* were 58, 38 and 12 months, respectively. Only about 6% regressed, a low number which the authors attribute to the fact that biopsies can affect the natural history of intraepithelial neoplasia. On the other hand, Johnson *et al*. (1968) found that 50.4% of women with dysplasia who were followed by cytology and biopsy regressed whereas only 1.4% developed carcinoma *in situ* over the same length of time. The subject was examined by Galvin *et al*. (1955) who found that 53.9% of the mild abnormalities regressed and 16.1% progressed, whereas the reverse was true for the severe abnormalities, with 17.1% regressing and 65.7% progressing to carcinoma *in situ*. Similar results have been reported by many authors, including Hall & Walton (1968) using biopsies and Fox (1967) using cytology.

The second point to consider in the natural history of cervical neoplasia is the all important one of progression from CIN to invasive cancer. The two assumptions that (1) a significant proportion of women who have CIN would eventually develop invasive cancer if left untreated, and (2) most invasive carcinomas are preceded by a demonstrable intraepithelial phase have formed the basis for screening programmes to detect CIN by cytology and its treatment before malignancy can develop. The hope, of course, is that if the disease can be picked up and treated while it is still in the preinvasive phase, then the incidence of cervical cancer and the number of deaths from it will be greatly reduced.

The most widely quoted figures for the rate of progression from CIN to invasive carcinoma are those from two separate series by Petersen & Kottmeier, published over 30 years ago. Kottmeier's results (1953) at first showed that eight out of 59 women with untreated carcinoma *in situ* developed invasive carcinoma, a 13.6% rate of progression. In 1955, however, Kottmeier admitted that only 14 of the cases had acceptable carcinoma *in situ*, of whom eight developed invasive cancer (57%). Later still, Kottmeier (1961) reported 31 patients who had been followed for at least 12 years; 22 of these (71%) developed invasive carcinoma. Petersen (1956) found invasive carcinoma developing in 34 out of 127 patients with epithelial atypia (26%). In a fuller account of the same group of patients (Petersen 1955) it was admitted that only 67 of these patients had recognizable abnormalities at the end of the first year of the study. Two-thirds of the remaining 67 ultimately developed invasive carcinoma. It is a pity that these amended figures of both authors are seldom quoted.

At the other end of the scale are the findings of Green & Donovan (1970), who reported a large number of patients with carcinoma *in situ* diagnosed by cone biopsy. Only one patient eventually developed invasive carcinoma (0.17%). Seventy-five of these women had persistent abnormal smears after the cone biopsy and were followed up for 11 years; Green & Donovan (1970) reported that none of these developed invasive disease. However, in a later publication, McIndoe *et al.* (1984) analysed the eventual outcome of 948 of these women who had carcinoma *in situ* (CIN 3) diagnosed by histology, most having cone biopsies. One hundred and thirty-one continued to have abnormal cytology, indicative of residual disease, but no further treatment was given. After 10 years, McIndoe *et al.* (1984) report that 18% of this group had developed invasive carcinomas and after 20 years the figure had risen to 36%. Of those whose cytology had been normal following the initial treatment, only 1.5% developed invasive carcinoma and 0.8% developed recurrent carcinoma *in situ*. It was concluded that a woman who has an abnormal smear after histological diagnosis of carcinoma *in situ* has a risk of about 25 times the normal of developing invasive carcinoma when compared with a woman with a normal smear. Further, a woman who has apparently been successfully treated for CIN 3 has a relative risk of 3.2%. In a further study, in which Kinlen & Spriggs (1978) traced 52 women who had positive cervical smears but, for one reason or another, had not been biopsied or treated, 19% were found to have developed invasive carcinoma.

All these studies are open to criticism, the most important being the way that the diagnosis was made in the first place. To establish with certainty that a lesion is entirely intraepithelial, the whole cervix must be examined, which means a cone biopsy. It follows that a precise diagnosis cannot be made without treating the disease, so that follow-up for these purposes is pointless. It seems unlikely that the true figure for the rate of progression from CIN to invasive carcinoma can ever be precisely established. In practice this means that every woman with CIN 3 must be treated as if her lesion is one that would progress. A risk factor as low as 20% would justify this treatment.

The length of the preinvasive phase is also of considerable importance and needs to be taken into account when planning screening programmes and determining the management of any patient with CIN. Although one statistical analysis (Barron *et al.* 1978) suggests a span of 3—10 years for the length of the carcinoma *in situ* phase, most cytological (Richart & Barron 1969) and epidemiological (Fidler *et al.* 1968) studies indicate that CIN 3 takes 10 years to develop into invasive carcinoma. The fact that women with CIN are 10—15 years younger than those with invasive carcinoma supports these figures. However, Berkeley *et al.* (1980) and Prendiville *et al.* (1980) have reported the development of invasive carcinomas in young women who have recently had normal cytology. There are several explanations for these occurrences (MacGregor 1982). The most obvious is that some of the smears were false negatives and would have been found to contain malignant cells on review. Others may have been genuine false negatives, in which the tumour did not exfoliate cells and none were present in the smears. However, it is impossible to escape the conclusion that, at least in some of these women, there had been a genuine progression from a normal cervix to invasive carcinoma in the short length of time between the taking of the smear and the carcinoma being diagnosed, as little as 6 months in some examples. It is not clear whether these small number of cases represent a different disease process or whether, as seems likely, they reflect the extreme short end of a natural history span which is very variable. The suggestion that there are two different forms of cervical cancer was first put forward by Ashley (1966), who proposed that one form occurred in young women and had a slow evolution, with its preinvasive phase being readily detected by cytology. The other type, which is less common, is found in older women and develops rapidly, without a detectable precancerous phase. Hakama & Penttinen (1981) have reiterated the same hypothesis with evidence which depends upon the shape of the age-specific incidence curve. This shows two poorly defined peaks at 50 and 70 years. Although it is possible that two different types of cervical carcinoma do exist, the evidence cannot be taken to be conclusive.

The histology of cervical intraepithelial neoplasia

The histologist must determine, first, whether an epithelium shows CIN or not and, secondly, what degree of CIN is present. There are a number of benign and physiological conditions which may mimic CIN and may be mistaken for CIN, so it is important that they are recognized for what they are. Once it is established that an epithelium shows the features of CIN, the degree of the abnormality has to be determined. Ascribing a degree to an example of CIN is not always straightforward, partly because of the number of varying factors which have to be considered and partly because of the degree of subjectivity involved in the interpretation of features which vary in a quantitative rather than a qualitative fashion. As has already been explained, CIN is graded in the hope that the degree of the histological abnormality relates to the prognosis and so can be used as a guide to the management of the patient. This means that purely morphological criteria are being used to predict the biological behaviour of the abnormal epithelium. It must be remembered that the correlation between appearance and behaviour may not always be good, even though this is a principle that is widely used in histopathology. Furthermore there is, on the whole, no way of knowing whether the histological interpretation which has been given to a particular epithelium is correct or not, because no reliable figures are available to correlate the histology of CIN with its real risk of progression to invasive carcinoma. These comments must be borne in mind when reading the following paragraphs.

The features to be taken into account when making a diagnosis of CIN are as follows:

1 Differentiation (maturation, stratification)
(a) present or absent
(b) proportion of the thickness of the epithelium showing differentiation
2 Nuclear abnormalities
(a) nucleus: cytoplasm ratio
(b) hyperchromasia
(c) nuclear pleomorphism and anisokaryosis
3 Mitotic activity
(a) number of mitotic figures
(b) height of mitoses in the epithelium
(c) abnormal configurations

Differentiation, stratification and *maturation* are words which are often used more or less synonymously but differ slightly in their meaning: as the cells differentiate and mature towards the surface, some stratification is nearly always observed. The commonly used definitions of carcinoma *in situ* demand that there is no surface maturation, with complete absence of differentiation and no stratification as the surface is reached (Govan *et al.* 1969). On the other hand, dysplasia shows a variable degree of differentiation, even though this may be difficult to detect with some of the more severe forms. In fact, the presence of surface differentiation or stratification is the only way of distinguishing severe dysplasia from carcinoma *in situ*. This distinction between carcinoma *in situ* and severe dysplasia becomes unnecessary with the adoption of the CIN terminology so that arguments over the presence or absence of surface differentiation are pointless. The proportion of the epithelium showing differentiation is, in fact, of more importance than the presence or absence of differentiation when it comes to the grading of CIN. The degree of CIN is likely to be less in an epithelium in which the cells start to differentiate just a little way above the basement membrane, compared with one in which the epithelium does not show differentiation until the surface is nearly reached. This is a useful criterion, but should be used in conjunction with the other features discussed below; it cannot be taken as the only diagnostic criterion for grading CIN (Ferenczy 1977). The difficulty of the situation is further added to by the fact that CIN develops as a metaplastic process and the metaplasia itself may show no maturation. It is therefore possible to make a diagnosis of a minor degree of CIN, even if there is no maturation, if the nuclear changes are mild enough.

The presence of *nuclear abnormalities* is a very important criterion for the diagnosis of CIN and for attributing a grade to it. Wilbanks *et al.* (1967) first showed that CIN had an aneuploid DNA content; it is probably this feature which accounts for the striking features of variation in size and shape, as well as the nuclear enlargement, hyperchromasia and chromatin clumping. There is very often a good correlation between the degree of nuclear abnormality and the amount of differentiation which is seen; the more severe the nuclear abnormalities the less is the proportion of the epithelium which is differentiated. If this correlation is not observed, then the degree of nuclear abnormality should be taken as the more reliable guide to the degree of abnormality of the epithelium as a whole than the proportion of epithelium showing differentiation.

Mitotic activity in the normal squamous epithelium of the cervix is confined to the parabasal layers (Langley & Crompton 1973). An increased number of mitotic figures is one of the important diagnostic features of CIN and these may be situated at any level in the epithelium. Chi *et al.* (1977) found that the frequency of cells in mitosis occupying positions throughout the whole thickness of the epithelium increased gradually with the degree of CIN. The number of mitotic figures in the superficial one-third of the epithelium increases significantly with increasingly severe CIN. The vertical position in the epithelium at which mitotic figures are found is therefore a very useful criterion to be taken into account when deciding on the degree of CIN.

Abnormal forms of mitotic figures are common in CIN and may account for as many as 15–30% of the total (Kirkland *et al.* 1967). The most frequently encountered of these abnormalities is the 'three-group metaphase' (Fig. 2.1) in which the main mass of the chromosomes is lined up along the metaphase plate at the equator of the cell with small groups of apparently detached chromosomes lying on either side. A variant of this, the 'two-group metaphase', is also seen quite

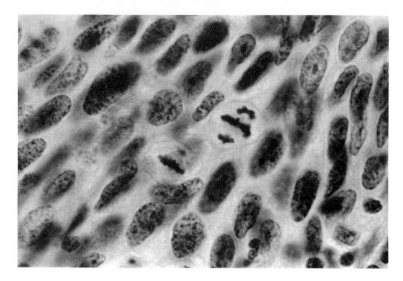

Fig. 2.1. Abnormal mitotic figure; three group metaphase. Most of the chromosomes are lined up along the equatorial plane of the cell, but two groups have separated, one at each end of the cell. When the cell division is complete, the daughter cells will have an abnormal number of chromosomes (H&E×940).

commonly. Less common is the multipolar mitotic figure, either a triaster or a quadraster. Less frequently observed are abnormal anaphase, polyploidy, ring mitoses, V-mitoses and leader mitoses (Langley & Crompton 1973).

The grades of CIN may be characterized in the following way.

CIN 1 (Fig. 2.2)

There is usually maturation in the upper two-thirds of the epithelium. Even so, slight nuclear atypia exists right up to the surface as a reflection of the delay in nuclear maturation. Nuclear abnormalities are most marked in the basal third and are slight. Mitotic figures are also confined to the basal third of the epithelium; they are sparse and abnormal forms are rare.

CIN 2 (Fig. 2.3)

As in CIN 1, nuclear atypia persists to the surface but is rather more marked. Maturation is usually present in the upper half of the epithelium. Mitotic figures are found in the basal half of the epithelium and abnormal configurations may be seen.

CIN 3 (Figs 2.4 and 2.5)

Maturation may be completely absent or confined to the superficial third of the

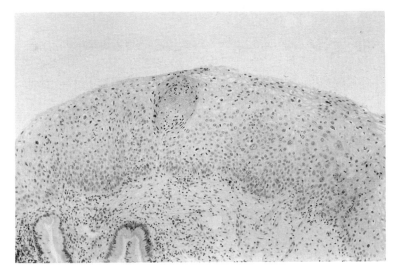

Fig. 2.2. CIN 1 (H&E×110).

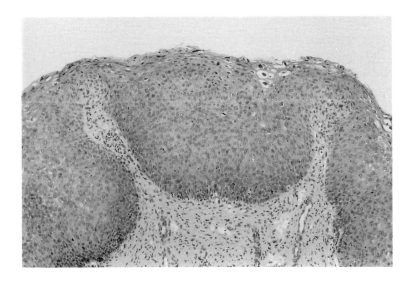

Fig. 2.3. CIN 2 (H&E×110).

epithelium. Marked nuclear abnormalities are seen throughout the whole thickness of the epithelium. Mitotic figures may be abundant and are found at all levels of the epithelium; abnormal mitotic figures are frequent.

Different examples of CIN of the same degree may have different morphological features, so that the preceding lists can be taken as rough guidelines only. Figures 2.4 and 2.5 both show examples of CIN 3 but they are different; Fig. 2.5 shows virtually no differentiation nor maturation with grossly enlarged and

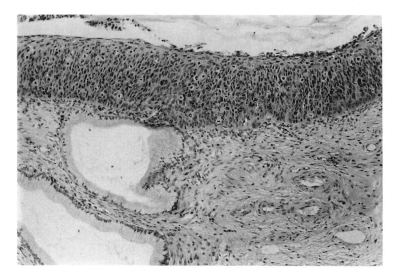

Fig. 2.4. CIN 3: surface differentiation is present and there are numerous mitotic figures, extending up to the top quarter of the epithelium (H&E×110).

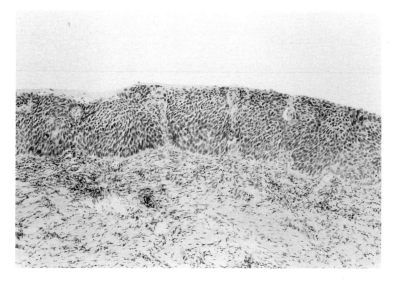

Fig. 2.5. CIN 3: there is no maturation of the epithelium. The nuclei are uniformly enlarged and hyperchromatic but mitotic figures are few (H&E×110).

hyperchromatic nuclei. There are few mitotic figures, however. On the other hand, Fig. 2.4 shows an epithelium with some differentiation and several mitotic figures, a few of which are abnormal. It can be appreciated that the emphasis placed on each diagnostic criterion must vary from one example to another.

Classifications of the histological variants of CIN have been proposed. For example, Poulsen *et al.* (1975) and Buckley *et al.* (1982) divided them into small-cell, non-keratinizing, large-cell, non-keratinizing and keratinizing forms and other classifications have been put forward (Tweeddale & Roddick 1969).

It is very important to remember that CIN affects not only the surface epithelium of the cervix but also the crypts (Fig. 2.6). Anderson & Hartley (1980) studied 343 cervical cone biopsy specimens containing CIN 3 and measured the depth of crypt involvement by the abnormal epithelium. They found that 88.6% showed some involvement of the crypts. The mean depth of the involvement was 1.24 mm and the maximum depth was 5.22 mm with a mean plus three standard deviations of 3.80 mm. This figure embraces 99.7% of the population with CIN 3 and it is this depth of destruction which must be aimed for when CIN is being treated, particularly when local methods of destruction are being employed. When the depth of crypt involvement is correlated with the degree of CIN, it is found that the more severe the CIN, the deeper is the crypt involvement (Abdul-Karim *et al.* 1982). The mean depths of involvement plus three standard deviations were 1.26, 3.06 and 4.80 mm for CIN 1, CIN 2 and CIN 3, respectively. Furthermore,

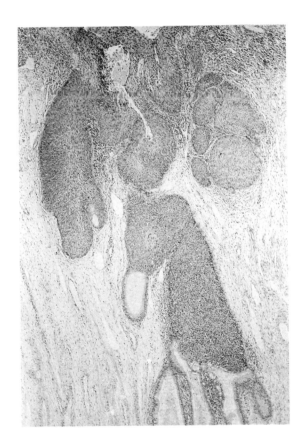

Fig. 2.6. Crypt involvement by CIN. In addition to the surface epithelium, just seen at the top of the photograph, the abnormal epithelium is spreading down the crypts, which can be recognized by the columnar epithelium at their bases (H&E×75).

the same authors found that the more severe forms of CIN cover a larger area on the cervix than the milder forms.

Human papillomavirus infection and the cervix

Human papillomavirus (HPV) produces two types of lesion on the cervix; the well known condyloma acuminatum and a flat lesion. The flat lesion has been referred to by a variety of names, such as a flat condyloma (Meisels *et al.* 1982), noncondylomatous cervical wart virus infection (NCWVI) (Reid *et al.* 1980) and subclinical papillomavirus infection (SPI) (Reid *et al.* 1982). Although these abnormalities are not visible to the naked eye they can be recognized by colposcopy, cytology and histology. The histological and cytological features have been described in detail (Kirkup *et al.* 1982; Meisels *et al.* 1982; Reid *et al.* 1982; Reid *et al.* 1984).

The most constant feature of SPI, both cytologically and histologically, is koilocytotic atypia, which was a term first used by Koss & Durfee (1956). The cell showing koilocytotic atypia has an irregular and hyperchromatic nucleus which exhibits a wrinkled nuclear membrane as the surface of the epithelium is approached. The most prominent feature, however, is the large space around the nucleus with margination of the cytoplasm giving a sharp edge to the halo. The nuclei are usually larger than the nuclei of surrounding, non-ballooned cells (Fig. 2.7). It is important that the normal basket-weave pattern of the intermediate and superficial cells in a normal, well-oestrogenized squamous epithelium is not mistaken for koilocytosis. The nuclei of these normal basket-weave cells are small and regular and the cells in the particular area all look much the same (Fig. 2.8). Koilocytotic atypia is present in the intermediate and superficial layers of the epithelium and is very rarely seen in the parabasal and basal layers; the virus requires cellular maturation for expression of the morphological features of its presence.

The other histological features of SPI are multinucleation, individual cell keratinization (dyskeratosis), parakeratosis, frequent mitotic figures, acanthosis, prominent rete pegs, epithelial pearls and blood vessels surrounded by a little stroma reaching towards the epithelial surface (Kirkup *et al.* 1982; Meisels *et al.* 1982).

There are two ways in which the histological features of CIN and SPI can be associated. CIN and SPI may be present in adjacent areas of epithelium (Fig. 2.9). Secondly, and more importantly, CIN and SPI may be seen together in the same area of epithelium, so that koilocytotic atypia, multinucleation and individual cell keratinization may occur in conjunction with nuclear changes in the basal layer, abnormal mitotic figures and lack of maturation (Fig. 2.10). The diagnosis of the degree of CIN should be made on the appearances of the non-koilocytotic cells.

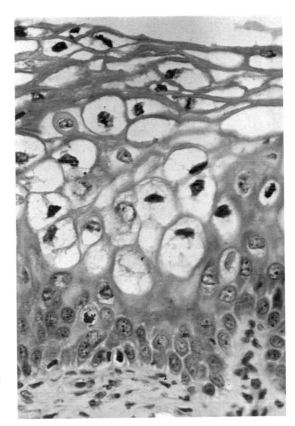

Fig. 2.7. Subclinical papillomavirus infection. Koilocytotic atypia is prominent, the affected cells showing hyperchromasia and irregularity of their nuclei and a marked clear zone, extending to the margin of the cell. One cell at top left shows individual cell keratinization (H&E×620).

This intermingling and juxtapositioning of the features of CIN with those of SPI is common and seems to be becoming commoner; Purola & Savia (1977) found the association in 25% of biopsy specimens, Syrjanen et al. (1981) found 50% in their material and Reid et al. (1984) found the combined appearances in as many as 91% of 80 hysterectomies done for either invasive or preinvasive cervical neoplasia. It is certainly becoming uncommon to find a cervix containing CIN which does not show the features of SPI as well. The frequent finding of this association adds support to the suggestion that infection with HPV plays an important part in the genesis of cervical carcinoma. Reid et al. (1984) suggest that SPI and CIN 3 represent the two extremes of a single neoplastic continuum and it has often been stated that most examples of CIN 1 are merely infections with HPV.

Although a full discussion of the epidemiology and aetiology of cervical cancer is beyond the scope of this chapter, it is appropriate at this point to examine briefly the relationship between human papillomavirus infection and the development of cervical precancer and cancer.

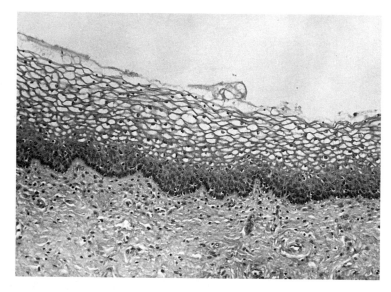

Fig. 2.8. Basket-weave pattern of normal, mature squamous epithelium. Compare with Fig. 2.6. The cells in the upper two-thirds of the epithelium have prominent perinuclear haloes but the nuclei are small and round, becoming pyknotic as the surface is approached (H&E×185).

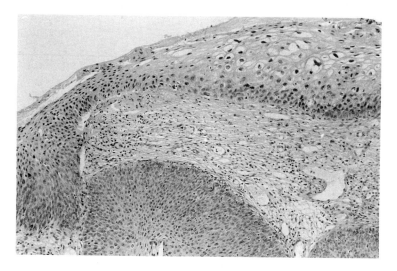

Fig. 2.9. SPI and CIN in adjacent areas of epithelium. The SPI affects the surface epithelium in this example and the CIN mainly the crypts. (H&E×110).

Human papillomavirus infection has been proposed as a possible aetiological agent for cervical cancer since the mid-1970s. In the first reported study (Durst *et al.* 1983) more than 60% of cervical tumours contained HPV-16 DNA. Many subsequent studies have confirmed that a high proportion of cervical tumours

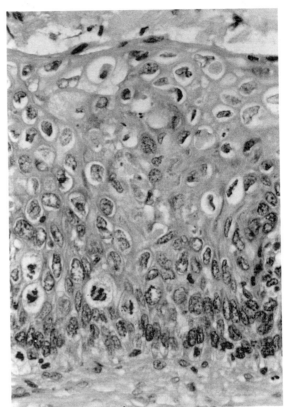

Fig. 2.10. SPI and CIN involving the same area of epithelium. Cells in the upper layers of the epithelium show koilocytotic atypia while there is crowding in the basal layers. Mitotic figures are present, at least one of which is abnormal (H&E×430).

contain HPV-DNA, in particular HPV-16, HPV-18 and HPV-33. Furthermore, the partners of women with condylomata and CIN have a high incidence of penile condylomata and penile intraepithelial neoplasia and the partners of men with penile condylomata have an increased risk of developing CIN (Campion *et al.* 1985; Barrasso *et al.* 1987). HPV therefore appears to be sexually transmitted although this has not been conclusively proved.

The virus cannot be cultured in the laboratory and is classified by a system of viral typing based upon DNA homology rather than serology. Over 60 different HPV types have now been reported and the criteria defined for a new HPV type are that the virus should be related to other HPV-DNA under conditions of low stringency and yet be less than 50% homologous to other HPV-DNA at high stringency (Pfister *et al.* 1986). Although HPV infection is confined to epithelial cells, full viral replication occurs only in cells undergoing final differentiation. The virus persists in the nuclei of infected cells as episomal, circular DNA which is distinct from cellular DNA.

Analysis of the genomes of HPV-16 and HPV-18 shows that the DNA may be divided into three regions, of which the early and late regions are of particular interest. The late proteins form the protein coat of the virus; the L2 protein contains the common papillomavirus antigen which is recognized by many monoclonal antibodies currently available for the immunohistochemical detection of HPV infection (Morin *et al.* 1988). The function of some of the early proteins has been elucidated. In both HPV-16 and HPV-18, the regions and coding of the E6 and E7 proteins have the ability to transform and immortalize cells in culture (Laimins *et al.* 1987), the major ability to transform cells in HPV-16 residing with the E7 protein (Vousden *et al.* 1988).

HPV infection of the cervix may be divided into two subgroups; HPV-6, 11, 31 and 35 are associated with condylomata acuminata and low-grade CIN and only rarely with invasive tumours (Campion *et al.* 1986; Reeves *et al.* 1987). HPV-16, 18 and 33, the so-called 'malignant' HPV, are found in flat condylomata (SPI), high-grade CIN and invasive carcinomas (Scholl *et al.* 1985; Campion *et al.* 1986). These *in vivo* characteristics of the virus are reflected by their *in vitro* activity; HPV-16, 18 and 33 have the ability to transform cells in culture and to co-operate with oncogenes in cellular transformation, whereas HPV-6, 11, 31 and 35 do not (Matlashewski *et al.* 1987). It is also interesting to note that adenocarcinoma of the cervix is associated with HPV infection more frequently than squamous cell carcinoma, possibly suggesting a further level of tissue trophism between HPV-16 and HPV-18 (Wilczynski *et al.* 1988).

The majority of cervical tumours contain a proportion of HPV-DNA that is integrated within the host genome, rather than being episomal. The place at which the episomal HPV-DNA is opened during integration lies within the E1-E2 region; this disrupts the E1-E2 region in cervical tumours, whereas the E6-E7 region is maintained intact (Choo *et al.* 1987; Tidy *et al.* 1988). This results in early gene expression being confined primarily to the E6 and E7 proteins (Shirasawa *et al.* 1988) with loss of E2 expression, which may in turn lead to the altered expression of those proteins which have been demonstrated to possess the ability to transform cells.

The prevalence of HPV infection within the female population is still unknown. A study of over 9000 women in West Germany found evidence of HPV-DNA in approximately 10% of cervical smears (De Villiers *et al.* 1987). However, the methods of detection used were relatively insensitive and since the development of the technique of DNA amplification using the polymerase chain reaction very small quantities of DNA may now be detected (Saiki *et al.* 1988; Young *et al.* 1989). Although early reports using the polymerase chain reaction (PCR) indicated the presence of HPV-DNA in a very high proportion of the normal population (Tidy *et al.* 1989) these results were subsequently retracted as probably being due to accidental contamination. Subsequent investigations have claimed only modest infection rates by HPV-16; Manos *et al.* (1990) found it in no more than 22% of normal cervices. Whatever the prevalence of HPV infection is eventually shown to be, it is likely that infection by HPV is only one step in the multifactorial process giving rise to cervical neoplasia. It may eventually be shown that cervical cancer is caused by several factors, requiring initiation by one agent and promotion by another (zur Hausen 1982). It is even perhaps possible that different aetiologies may be involved in different women.

These indications that infection with HPV may be linked to the development of cervical carcinoma and the very frequent coexistence of the histological features of CIN and SPI together present problems for the histopathologist. On the one hand, it may be felt that the finding of the features of HPV infection in an epithelium showing CIN could mean that the epithelium has increased malignant potential compared with an example of CIN which does not contain HPV. On the other hand, the view might be expressed that, if the features of SPI are found, then all the atypia is the result of infection with HPV and is not an indication of a premalignant condition. The former view may result in over treatment and the latter in under treatment. At the moment it is not known whether the presence of the histological features of SPI in an epithelium which also shows CIN means that the epithelium is more likely to become invasive carcinoma or less likely to do so than a CIN that does not contain HPV. It is recommended that the presence of the HPV is disregarded when treatment is being planned; the woman is treated according to the degree of CIN which is present and the SPI is, for the time being and until the matter is resolved, considered to be an irrelevant, although interesting, finding (Anderson 1982; Kaufman et al. 1984).

Pitfalls in the histological diagnosis of CIN

The difficulties which may be caused in the histological interpretation of an epithelium when there is also HPV infection have already been discussed. There are other benign conditions which can be confused with CIN on occasion. These are: immature metaplasia, the congenital transformation zone and atrophic, postmenopausal epithelium.

IMMATURE SQUAMOUS METAPLASIA

As squamous metaplasia matures it becomes differentiated and stratification of flattened cells occurs towards the surface. However, before this stage is reached, the epithelium may show no differentiation at all, with the cells at the surface being morphologically similar to those at the base of the epithelium. Epithelium which is healing after local destructive treatment (such as laser, diathermy and cryosurgery) may show the same features. This lack of differentiation may lead to an erroneous diagnosis of CIN, unless attention is paid to nuclear detail, when it will be apparent that the nuclei are large but regular, with very few mitotic figures. Nuclei are usually prominent. Metaplasia may, of course, affect the gland crypts.

CONGENITAL TRANSFORMATION ZONE

This is an area of squamous metaplasia which is almost certainly developmental in origin, the metaplastic process commencing *in utero* and continuing into childhood. It may be confused with CIN both colposcopically and histologically. As the process is essentially one of metaplasia, the epithelium shows some of the features of squamous metaplasia. Maturation may not be complete; in fact, it typically shows a disorder of maturation which combines excessive maturation, as exemplified by keratinization, with delayed maturation in the deeper layers of the epithelium. The deeper layers show the same features as a maturing squamous metaplasia; the nuclei are often large but regular, with prominent nucleoli. There is minimal pleomorphism and mitotic figures are infrequent. As maturation appears in the superficial layers it may do so rapidly, in the course of the thickness of three or four cells. A layer of hyperkeratosis or parakeratosis may be present which, when thick, corresponds to the leukoplakia which may be seen colposcopically. Keratinization may be present in one area of a congenital transformation zone and absent from an adjacent area of the same cervix.

One of the most striking features of the congenital transformation zone is the configuration of its lower margin, the epithelial–stromal junction. This is always dentate, presenting an appearance which may resemble the rete ridges of the skin. Sometimes these incursions of the epithelium into the stroma appear to be detached from the overlying epithelium, so that they may give the impression of invasive buds. This impression may be heightened when the centre of the process undergoes differentiation, so that a whorl of keratin is seen in the centre (Fig. 2.11). Attention to the cytological features will show that the congenital transformation zone is not an invasive tumour. It is unusual for there to be any stromal reaction to the congenital transformation zone.

ATROPHIC POSTMENOPAUSAL EPITHELIUM

An epithelium which is not receiving any hormonal stimulus, as is the case after the menopause, is thin and shows no differentiation. The nuclei of the epithelial cells are dark and, as the amount of cytoplasm in the cells is reduced, the nuclear-cytoplasmic ratio may be increased. Furthermore, the nuclei may exhibit some irregularity of shape. This is a picture which can be confused with CIN; indeed, in some instances the distinction may be very difficult. However, the postmenopausal epithelium does not contain mitotic figures and careful attention to the scale of the material, the size of the individual cells and the thinness of the epithelium should make the distinction possible. Nevertheless, this can be one of the most difficult epithelial states to distinguish from CIN, particularly in a small biopsy.

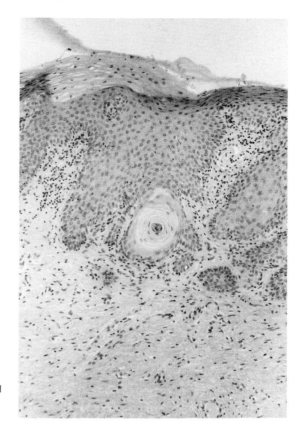

Fig. 2.11. Congenital transformation zone. Maturation in this variety of squamous metaplasia is arrested almost until the surface is reached but there are surface layers of parakeratotic cells. The margin between the epithelium and the stroma is very irregular and a keratin pearl is seen in one of the deepest projections (H&E×185).

The pathology of vaginal intraepithelial neoplasia

Vaginal intraepithelial neoplasia is very much less common than CIN. It may occur in conjunction with CIN or by itself, as indicated below:

1 In continuity with CIN
(a) with cervix present
(b) after hysterectomy
2 Separate from CIN
(a) CIN present
(b) CIN absent

The least uncommon situation in which vaginal intraepithelial neoplasia (VAIN) may be found is in continuity with CIN on the cervix. In these circumstances the VAIN often affects only a small area in the vaginal fornices. Great care must be taken in the colposcopic examination to distinguish between VAIN and a congenital transformation zone extending onto the vagina; there may be important differences in the management of the two lesions. It is of paramount importance that CIN extending onto the vagina is recognized before either conization or hysterectomy is performed; the rule must be that a woman should never be treated for CIN without prior colposcopy. If hysterectomy is performed in a woman who has an unsuspected VAIN associated with a CIN, then it is almost certain that an area of epithelial abnormality will be left at the vault, resulting in a persistent abnormal smear which may give rise to considerable difficulties in diagnosis and treatment which is, at best, eventually a compromise. Although it has been stated that about 4% of women have transformation zones which extend onto the vagina, it is probable that most of these areas of vaginal abnormality are congenital transformation zones and that the true prevalence of CIN extending to an area of VAIN is lower than this figure; Nwabinelli and Monaghan (1990) have shown that 2.5% of 4147 women with CIN have vaginal extension of the lesion.

As indicated, VAIN may be found at sites in the vagina which are separated from the cervix, which may or may not be involved itself. Furthermore, VAIN may be found in the vaginal vault of a woman who had a hysterectomy for CIN several years earlier. The histogenesis of these conditions is not clear; unlike CIN, they cannot arise from an acquired transformation zone, but must develop in the native epithelium of the vagina. It seems a little paradoxical that cervical neoplasia is thought always to develop in the acquired transformation zone and almost never from the original squamous epithelium, whereas vaginal neoplasia, it seems, must originate in the native squamous epithelium. This difference in the histogenesis may account for the much greater frequency of CIN compared to VAIN.

While on the subject of the histogenesis of VAIN, reference must be made to epithelial abnormalities in diethylstilboestrol-exposed individuals. These women often have very large transformation zones, frequently involving the vagina, the most extreme vaginal changes being vaginal adenosis. Lesser alterations result in abnormal epithelium covering a larger or smaller area of cervix or vagina. This greatly expanded transformation zone has, in the past, been a cause of concern because it has been thought that it may be a possible source of origin to CIN, on the basis that the larger the transformation zone, the greater the chance of CIN supervening (Stafl & Mattingly 1974). This fear of an increased risk of CIN and VAIN in DES-exposed women has not been confirmed (Robboy *et al*. 1977). These women can develop CIN, just as individuals who are not exposed to the drug do but the incidence does not appear to be increased; when CIN develops in a DES-exposed girl, it originates in the central, acquired transformation zone, not the vaginal epithelium, which is mainly of congenital transformation zone type.

The histological appearances of VAIN are identical to those of CIN and all the morphological appearances described on the cervix may be seen; it is not necessary to describe them again. The only difference, which is of course very important when considering treatment, is that gland crypts are not present in the vagina (except when there is adenosis). Moreover, VAIN also very often exhibits the morphological features associated with wart virus infection, as described on the cervix.

The pathology of vulval intraepithelial neoplasia

The epithelial changes which occur in the vulva are customarily divided into three categories:
1 dystrophies
2 vulval intraepithelial neoplasia (VIN), and
3 human papillomavirus infection
   The *vulval dystrophies* are a group of chronic dermatoses of unknown aetiology. A classification is shown below (Kaufman *et al.* 1976):
1 Hyperplastic dystrophy
(a) without atypia
(b) with atypia
2 Lichen sclerosus
3 Mixed dystrophy (lichen sclerosus with foci of epithelial hyperplasia)
(a) without atypia
(b) with atypia
   They cover a spectrum of disease, ranging from the hyperplastic dystrophy at one extreme to lichen sclerosus at the other; mixed forms also occur. The microscopy of a hyperplastic dystrophy shows hyperkeratosis, acanthosis, a prominent granular layer, irregular prolongation of the rete ridges and a mixed chronic inflammatory infiltrate in the superficial dermis (Fig. 2.12). This condition has often been referred to as leukoplakia, both clinically and histopathologically. Of interest in a discussion of intraepithelial neoplasia is the finding, in some examples of hyperplastic and mixed dystrophy, of nuclear atypia, increased mitotic activity, nuclear hyperchromasia and irregularity of nuclear size and shape. These changes are confined to the basal layers and maturation of the epidermis takes place rapidly. This atypia is the basis of the overlap between the dystrophies and VIN; if the immature cells extend further into the more superficial layers of the epithelium, then the epithelial abnormality satisfies the diagnostic criteria outlined below for VIN. Lichen sclerosus does not show nuclear atypia; it is characterized histologically by marked thinning of the epidermis, slight, flaky hyperkeratosis and loss of rete ridges. The subepidermal dermis shows striking hyalinization and, deep to this, is a layer of infiltrating chronic inflammatory cells (Fig. 2.13).
   Until fairly recently, the intraepithelial precursors of vulval carcinoma have been called carcinoma *in situ* or Bowen's disease; minor abnormalities have either been ignored or included with the dystrophies. The term 'dysplasia' is also used occasionally to describe vulval abnormalities and adds extra confusion as it

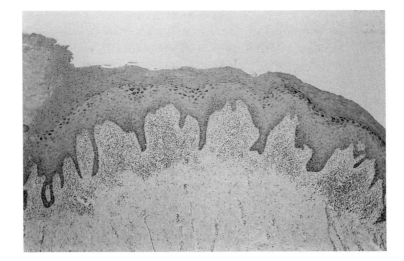

Fig. 2.12. Hyperplastic vulval dystrophy. The epidermis shows parakeratosis and there is a prominent granular layer. The epidermis is thickened with irregular prolongations of the rete ridges. A mixed chronic inflammatory cell infiltrate is present in the superficial dermis (H&E×44).

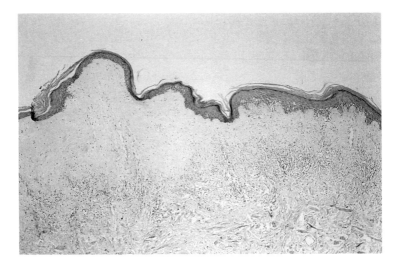

Fig. 2.13. Lichen sclerosus. Flaky hyperkeratosis is present and the epithelium is markedly thinned, with loss of rete ridges and atrophy of the skin appendages. Beneath the epidermis the superficial dermis is hyalinized and oedematous. A chronic inflammatory infiltrate is present in the dermis beneath this pale zone (H&E×44).

may apply both to the range of VIN and also to dystrophies. In the last decade, as the CIN terminology has become more widely accepted, there has been a move towards expressing vulval abnormalities in the same way. The result is that VIN is subdivided into three grades, VIN 1, VIN 2 and VIN 3, the last corresponding to carcinoma *in situ*. On the whole, this classification seems to be less easy to apply to the vulva than to the cervix. There are less of the minor abnormalities in the vulva, perhaps because there are no early diagnostic methods akin to cervical cytology; it is difficult to believe that there are not the same proportions of minor precursors as there are in the cervix.

The histological features of VIN closely parallel those of CIN, the main difference being that VIN tends to show more pronounced differentiation and maturation at the surface and keratinization is common. The distinction between the grades of VIN is made on the same grounds as the similar subdivisions of CIN and examples are shown in Figs 2.14, 2.15 and 2.16. As with CIN, there is a considerable degree of subjectivity in the allocation of a grade to VIN.

The skin appendages may be involved by CIN, although not with the same frequency that the cervical crypts are involved by CIN. The involvement of the pilosebaceous units of the vulva is of great importance when planning the depth of destruction to be achieved when using the laser; if the destruction is too superficial then residual VIN in the skin appendages will result in failure to eradicate the disease. On the other hand, healing is very prolonged if vaporization is carried out to a depth where all the appendages are also destroyed. The depth of involvement of these pilosebaceous units may be as much as 10 mm (Mene & Buckley 1985). The hair follicles of the labia majora are the most frequently affected appendages; it is uncommon to find the sebaceous and sweat glands of the non-hair bearing skin of the vulva involved by intraepithelial neoplasia.

Vulval intraepithelial neoplasia has previously been thought of as a disease affecting women after the menopause. In recent years, however, it is being seen

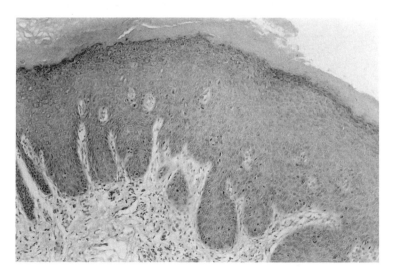

Fig. 2.14. VIN 1. The epidermis is somewhat thickened and there is some hyperkeratosis. Maturation is quite good, but nuclear atypia with mitotic activity is apparent in the basal third of the epithelium (H&E×110).

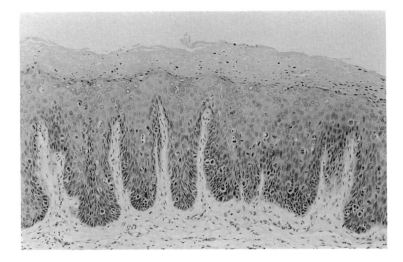

Fig. 2.15. VIN 2. Maturation is, if anything, better than that seen in Fig. 2.14, but the nuclear atypia in the lower half of the epithelium is more marked (H&E×110).

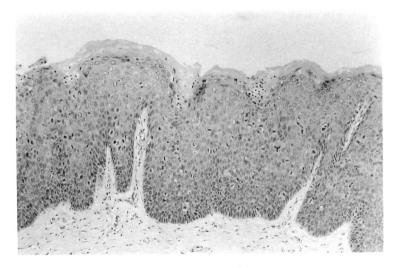

Fig. 2.16. VIN 3. Nuclear atypia is striking and extends almost to the surface of the epithelium. There are numerous mitotic figures, with abnormal configurations (H&E×110).

more and more in younger women (Crum 1987). Coincidentally, the association between VIN and wart virus infection of the vulva is becoming more widely recognized. An association between vulval condylomata acuminata and invasive carcinoma has already been shown (Shafeek *et al*. 1979) but there are two other ways in which wart virus infection and VIN may be found together. First, VIN may show the features of wart virus infection that have already been described; koilocytotic atypia, multinucleation and individual cell keratinization (Fig. 2.17).

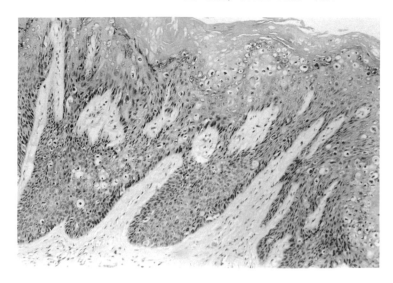

Fig. 2.17. VIN 3 with features of SPI. In addition to nuclear atypia warranting a diagnosis of VIN 3, the superficial layers show individual cell keratinization and koilocytotic atypia (H&E×110).

The presence of the wart virus can be confirmed in this tissue by the use of immunocytochemical stains (Ferenczy *et al*. 1981) and DNA-DNA hybridization (Gupta *et al*. 1985). Using Southern transfer hybridization, it has been shown that 84% of samples from VIN 3 contain HPV and 96% of these were HPV-16 (Buscema *et al*. 1988).

Another, less well proven association has been proposed in the form of a lesion known as Bowenoid dysplasia (Ulbright *et al*. 1982) or Bowenoid papulosis (Wade *et al*. 1978). This condition is characterized in the vulva by multifocal lesions which may be raised and pigmented and mistaken for condylomas. They occur particularly in young women and may appear for the first time during the course of a pregnancy. It has been suggested that these lesions are reversible, have no significant malignant potential and are the result of infection with the wart virus (Berger & Hori 1978); the evidence for this seems dubious. The histological features of Bowenoid dysplasia are, in common with VIN, an arrest of maturation, nuclear enlargement and crowding and numerous mitotic figures. A distinction from VIN is suggested by the 'blandness' of the nuclei, with open, finely stippled chromatin and lack of striking pleomorphism. Multinucleation is frequent, as are abnormal mitotic figures. Nevertheless, there seems to be danger in making distinctions that may not be fully justified, if these result in modifications of treatment protocols, possibly to the detriment of patients whose real VIN may in consequence be under diagnosed and inadequately treated. As in the cervix, it would be sensible to consider any example of VIN as having malignant potential, whether or not it has the coexistent features of Bowenoid papulosis or wart virus infection.

The risk of progression from VIN to invasive carcinoma of the vulva is not known. Many women with invasive carcinoma have adjacent areas of VIN and foci of early invasion may be found in what is predominantly an intraepithelial lesion, both these findings confirming that a relationship exists. It has been assumed that VIN is a premalignant condition so that a certain, although undefined, proportion of women with the disease would develop carcinoma, although it has been felt that this risk is less than in the cervix. Reliable figures are not available; suffice to say that a woman with VIN runs some risk of carcinoma developing, so that treatment is indicated. (As most women with VIN have severe pruritus this, by itself, is reason enough for treatment.) The increasing proportion of young women with VIN has caused increasing concern over excessive treatment for a disease which may have little malignant potential and, although progression to invasive carcinoma has been reported in young women, this seems to be an even less common occurrence than in older women (Crum 1987).

The relationships between the epithelial changes in the vulva are even more difficult to understand than those of the cervix because of the additional group of the dystrophies. Although their malignant potential is recognized, they overlap VIN only when the dystrophies show atypia. Apart from the question of whether HPV infection is causally related to VIN, morphological features of the two are frequently found in the same epithelium, so that they also show a histological overlap. This notion of the overlap of VIN, HPV infection and vulval dystrophies is represented as a Venn diagram in Fig. 2.18. It must be emphasized that this is a highly speculative suggestion but one which seems to approach the reality of the situation. An overlap between wart virus infection and the dystrophies has not, in fact, been adequately demonstrated although wart virus has been found in dystrophies (Karram *et al.* 1988), so this part of the scheme must remain speculative for the time being. Support is given by the statement of Crum (1982) that a diagnosis of VIN should be made irrespective of whether the epithelium also shows the features of dystrophy or HPV infection. The recent interest in vulval epithelial abnormalities which has been stimulated by the wart virus may also result in fuller study of the dystrophies, so that their relationship to the other two conditions may become clearer in time.

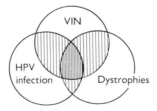

Fig. 2.18. A possible relationship between VIN, wart virus infection and vulval dystrophies.

Multifocal neoplasia of the lower genital tract

It has been apparent for some years that there is a real association between intraepithelial and invasive carcinoma of the cervix, vagina and vulva (Hansen & Collins 1967). More recently, Hammond & Monaghan (1983) have shown that 31% of women with VIN will develop intraepithelial or invasive neoplasia of the cervix, either at the same time or at a later date. Some aspects of the relationship between CIN and VAIN have been discussed above. This phenomenon of multi-focal lower genital tract neoplasia has two important implications. First, it is apparent that any woman who has squamous neoplasia in one area of the lower genital tract is at increased risk of developing the disease in another area. In practice this means that a woman with VIN should be followed assiduously because of this increased risk of the development of CIN or VAIN. It also means, of course, that patients with CIN should have regular vulval inspection, preferably with the colposcope, to recognize vulval abnormalities as soon as they develop. However, the high incidence of CIN and the relatively low incidence of VIN makes it debatable whether this careful follow-up is cost effective in time; most women with VIN will present of their own accord when the disease causes pruritis, as it almost always does.

The second point of interest about the association of VIN, CIN and VAIN is the inference that the association means a common aetiology. There is a consider-able amount of evidence that links infection by HPV with CIN (McCance et al. 1983), although a causal relationship has yet to be proved (see above). Similarly, there is mounting evidence to point to the same action of HPV and the vulva (Kurman et al. 1981) and the vagina. It may be that the virus infection causes a field change throughout the whole of the lower genital tract. As the transformation zone of the cervix is the most susceptible to transformation, CIN is the most common but in the minority the disease appears over the whole field, giving rise to multifocal intraepithelial neoplasia (MIN). The development of MIN, particularly when all areas are affected at the same time, may reflect a degree of immunological incompetence in the individual concerned, or perhaps a more virulent strain of the virus.

References

Abdul-Karim F.W., Fu Y.S., Reagan J.W. & Wentz W.B. (1982) Morphometric study of intraepithelial neoplasia of the uterine cervix. *Obstet. Gynecol.*, **60**, 210–14.

Anderson M C. (1982) In: *Proceedings of the Fourth World Congress for Colposcopy and Cervical Pathology.* Fourth World Congress for Colposcopy and Cervical Pathology, London. p. 57.

Anderson M.C. & Hartley R.B. (1980) Cervical crypt involvement by intraepithelial neoplasia. *Obstet. Gynecol.*, **55**, 546–50.

Ashley D.J.B. (1966) Evidence for the existence of two forms of cervical carcinoma. *J. Obstet. Gynaecol. Br. Commonwealth*, **73**, 382–89.

Barrasso R., De Brux J., Croissant O. & Orth G. (1987) High prevalence of papillomavirus-associated penile intraepithelial neoplasia in sexual partners of women with cervical intraepithelial neoplasia. *New Engl. J. Med.*, **317**, 916—23.

Barron B.A., Cahill M.C. & Richard R.M. (1978) A statistical model of the natural history of cervical neoplastic disease. The duration of carcinoma *in situ*. *Gynecol. Oncol.*, **6**, 196—205.

Bellina J.H., Dunlop W.P. & Riopelle M.A. (1982) Reliability of histopathologic diagnosis of cervical intraepithelial neoplasia. *South. Med. J.*, **75**, 6—8.

Berger B.W. & Hori Y. (1978) Multicentric Bowen's disease of the genitalia. *Arch. Dermatol.*, **114**, 1698—99.

Berkeley A.S., LiVolsi V.A. & Schwartz P.E. (1980) Advanced squamous cell carcinoma of the cervix with recent normal Papanicolaou tests. *Lancet*, **ii**, 375—76.

Buckley C.H., Butler E.P. & Fox H. (1982) Cervical intraepithelial neoplasia. *J. Clin. Pathol.*, **35**, 1—13.

Burghardt E. (1973) Early histological diagnosis of cervical cancer. *In*: Friedman E.A. (ed), *Major Problems in Obstetrics and Gynecology*, Volume 6. Saunders, Philadelphia, London, Toronto.

Burghardt E. (1976) Premalignant conditions of the cervix. *Clin. Obstet. Gynaecol.*, **3**, 257—95.

Buscema J., Naghashfar Z., Sawada E. *et al.* (1988) The predominance of human papillomavirus type 16 in vulvar neoplasia. *Obstet. Gynecol.*, **71**, 601—6.

Campion M.J., McCance D.J., Cuzick J. & Singer A. (1986) Progressive potential of mild cervical atypia: prospective cytological, colposcopic, and virological study. *Lancet*, **ii**, 237—40.

Campion M.J., Singer A., Clarkson P.K. & McCance D.J. (1985) Increased risk of cervical neoplasia in consorts of men with penile condylomata acuminata. *Lancet*, **i**, 943—46.

Chi C.H., Rubio C.A. & Lagerlof B. (1977) The frequency and distribution of mitotic figures in dysplasia and carcinoma *in situ*. *Cancer*, **39**, 1218—23.

Choo K-B., Pan C-C. & Han S-H. (1987) Integration of human papillomavirus type 16 into the cellular DNA of cervical carcinoma: preferential deletion of the E2 gene and invariable retention of the long control region and the E6/E7 open reading frames. *Virology*, **161**, 259—61.

Cocker J., Fox H. & Langley F.A. (1968) Consistency in the histological diagnosis of epithelial abnormalities of the cervix uteri. *J. Clin. Pathol.*, **21**, 67—70.

Crum C.P. (1982) Vulvar in neoplasia: The concept and its application. *Hum. Pathol.*, **13**, 187—89.

Crum C.P. (1987) Vulvar intraepithelial neoplasia. *In*: Wilkinson E.J. (ed), *Pathology of the vulva and vagina*. In: Roth L.M. (ed), *Contemporary Issues in Surgical Pathology*, Vol. 9. Churchill Livingstone, New York. p. 97.

Crum C.P. (1987) Vulvar intraepithelial neoplasia. *In*: Wilkinson E.J. (ed), *Pathology of the vulva and vagina*. In: Roth L.M. (ed), *Contemporary Issues in Surgical Pathology*, Vol. 9. Churchill Livingstone, New York. p. 95.

De Villiers E-M., Wagner D., Schneider A. *et al.* (1987) Human papillomavirus infection in women with and without abnormal cervical cytology. *Lancet*, **ii**, 703—6.

Durst M., Gissman L., Ikenberg H. & zur Hausen H. (1983) A papillomavirus DNA from a cervical carcinoma and its prevalence in cancer biopsy samples from different geographic regions. *Proc. Natl. Acad. Sci. USA*, **80**, 3812—16.

Editorial (1962) International committee of histological definition (1961). *Acta Cytol.*, **6**, 235—36.

Ferenczy A. (1977) Cervical intraepithelial neoplasia. *In*: Blaustein A. (ed), *Pathology of the Female Genital Tract*. Springer-Verlag, New York, Heidelberg, Berlin. p. 146.

Ferenczy A., Braun L. & Shah K.H. (1981) Human papillomavirus (HPV) in condylomatous lesions of the uterine cervix. A comparative ultrastructural and immunohistochemical study. *Am. J. Surg. Pathol.*, **5**, 661—70.

Fidler F.M., Boyes D.A. & Worth A.J. (1968) Cervical cancer detection in British Columbia. *J. Obstet. Gynaecol. Br. Commonwealth*, **75**, 392—404.

Fox C.H. (1967) Biologic behaviour of dysplasia and carcinoma *in situ*. *Am. J. Obstet. Gynecol.*, **99**, 960—74.

Galvin G.A., Jones H.W. & TeLinde R.W. (1955) The significance of basal cell hyperactivity in cervical biopsies. *Am. J. Obstet. Gynecol.* **70**, 808—21.

Govan A.D.T., Haines R.M., Langley F.A., Taylor C.W. & Woodcock A.S. (1969) The histology and cytology of changes in the epithelium of the cervix uteri. *J. Clin. Pathol.*, **22**, 383—95.

Green G.H. & Donovan J.W. (1970) The natural history of cervical carcinoma *in situ*. *J. Obstet. Gynaecol. Br. Commonwealth*, **77**, 1—9.

Gupta J., Gendelman H.E., Naghashfar Z. *et al.* (1985) Specific identification of human papillomavirus type in cervical smears and paraffin sections by *in situ* hybridization with radioactive probes: a preliminary communication. *Int. J. Gynecol. Pathol.*, **4**, 211–18.

Hakama M. & Penttinen J. (1981) Epidemiological evidence for two components of cervical carcinoma. *Br. J. Obstet. Gynaecol.*, **88**, 209–14.

Hall, J.E. & Walton L. (1968) Dysplasia of the cervix: a prospective study of 206 cases. *Am. J. Obstet. Gynecol.*, **100**, 662–71.

Hammond I.G. & Monaghan J.M. (1983) Multicentric carcinoma of the female lower genital tract. *Br. J. Obstet. Gynaecol.*, **90**, 553–56.

Hansen L.H. & Collins C.G. (1967) Multicentric squamous cell carcinoma of the lower female genital tract. *Am. J. Obstet. Gynecol.*, **98**, 982–86.

Johnson L.D., Nickerson R.J., Easterday C.L., Stuart R.S. & Hertig A.T. (1968) Epidemiological evidence for the spectrum of change from dysplasia through carcinoma *in situ* to invasive cancer. *Cancer*, **22**, 901–14.

Karram M., Tabor B., Smotkin D., Wettstein F., Bhatia N. & Micha J. (1988) Detection of human papillomavirus deoxyribonucleic acid from vulvar dystrophies and vulvar intraepithelial neoplastic lesions. *Am. J. Obstet. Gynecol.*, **159**, 22–23.

Kaufman R.H. *et al.* (1976) New nomenclature for vulvar disease. Report of the committee on terminology. *Obstet. Gynecol.*, **47**, 122–24.

Kaufman R.H., Koss L.G., Kurman R.J. *et al.* (1984) Statement of caution in the interpretation of papillomavirus-associated lesions of the epithelium of the uterine cervix. *Hum. Pathol.*, **14**, 202.

Kinlen L.J. & Spriggs A.I. (1978) Women with positive cervical smear but without surgical intervention. *Lancet*, **ii**, 463–65.

Kirkland J.A., Stanley M.A. & Cellier K.M. (1967) Comparative study of histological and chromosomal abnormalities in cervical neoplasia. *Cancer*, **20**, 1934–52.

Kirkup W., Evans A.S., Brough A.K., Davis J.A., O'Loughlin T., Wilkinson G. & Monaghan J.M. (1982) Cervical intraepithelial neoplasia and warty atypia—a study of colposcopic, histologic and cytological characteristics. *Br. J. Obstet. Gynaecol.*, **89**, 571–77.

Koss L.G. (1978) Dysplasia: a real concept or a misnomer? *Obstet. Gynecol.*, **51**, 374–79.

Koss L.G. & Durfee D.R. (1956) Unusual patterns of squamous epithelium of uterine cervix: cytologic-pathologic study of koilocytotic atypia. *Ann. NY Acad. Sci.*, **63**, 1235–61.

Kottmeier H.L. (1953) Cited in Burghardt E. (1973).

Kottmeier H.L. (1955) Cited in Burghardt E. (1973).

Kottmeier H.L. (1961) Évolution et traitment des epitheliomas. *Rev. Fr. Gynecol. Obstet.*, **56**, 821–26.

Kurman R.J., Shah K.H., Lancaster W.D. & Jensen A.B. (1981) Immunoperoxidase localisation of papilloma virus antigens in cervical dysplasia and vulvar condylomas. *Am. J. Obstet. Gynecol.*, **40**, 931–39.

Laimins L.A., Bedell M.A., Jones K.H. & Long J.A. (1987) Transformation of NIH-3T3 and primary rat embryo fibroblasts by human papillomavirus type 16 and type 18. In: Steinberg B.M., Brandsma J.L. & Taichman L.B. (eds), *Cancer Cells*. Cold Spring Harbor, New York. pp. 201–9.

Langley F.A. & Crompton A.C.C. (1973) Epithelial abnormalities of the cervix. *Recent Results in Cancer Research*, **40**, pp. 129–32. Heinemann, London.

McCance D.J., Walker P.G., Dyson J.L., Coleman D.V. & Singer A. (1983) Presence of human papillomavirus DNA sequences in cervical intraepithelial neoplasia. *Br. Med. J.*, **287**, 784–88.

MacGregor J.E. (1982) Rapid onset cancer of the cervix. *Br. Med. J.*, **284**, 441–42.

Manos M., Lee K., Greer C., Waldman J., Kiviat N., Holmes K. & Wheeler C. (1990) Looking for human papillomavirus type 16 by PCR. *Lancet*, **335**, 734.

Matlashewski G., Schneider J., Banks L., Jones N., Murray A. & Crawford L. (1987) Human papillomavirus type 16 DNA co-operates with activated ras in transforming primary cells. *EMBO J.*, **6**, 1741–47.

McIndoe W.A., McLean M.R., Jones R.W., Mullins P.R. (1964) The invasive potential of carcinoma *in situ* of the cervix. *Obstet. Gynecol.*, **64**, 451–8.

Meisels A., Morin C. & Casas-Cordero M. (1982) Human papilloma virus infection of the uterine cervix. *Int. J. Gynecol. Pathol.*, **1**, 75–94.

Mene A. & Buckley C.H. (1985) Involvement of the vulval skin appendages by intraepithelial neoplasia. *Br. J. Obstet. Gynaecol.*, **92**, 634–38.

Morin C., Bouchard C., Fortier M., Levesque R. & Meilsels A. (1988) A colposcopical lesion of the uterine cervix frequently associated with papillomavirus type 16 as detected by *in situ* and Southern blot hybridization: a cytohistological correlation study. *Int. J. Cancer*, **41**, 531–37.

Petersen O. (1955) Precancerous changes of the cervical epithelium. *Acta Radiol.*, Supplement 127, 87 pp.

Petersen O. (1956) Spontaneous course of cervical precancerous conditions. *Am. J. Obstet. Gynecol.*, **72**, 1063–71.

Pfister H., Krubke J., Dietrich W., Iftner T. & Fuchs P.G. (1986) Classification of the papilloma-viruses — mapping the genome. *In*: Evered D. & Clark S. (eds), *Ciba Foundation Symposium*. Wiley, Chichester. pp. 3–22.

Poulsen H.E., Taylor C.W. & Sobin L.H. (1975) Histological typing of female genital tract tumours. *International Histological Classification of Tumours*, No 13. World Health Organization, Geneva. p. 56.

Prendiville W., Guillebaud J., Bamford P., Beilby J. & Steele S.J. (1980) Carcinoma of the cervix with recent normal Papanicolaou tests. *Lancet*, **ii**, 835–54.

Purola E. & Savia E. (1977) Cytology of gynecologic condyloma acuminata. *Acta Cytol.*, **21**, 26–31.

Reagan J.W. & Hamonic J.J. (1956) Dysplasia of the uterine cervix. *Ann. NY Acad. Sci.*, **63**, 1236–44.

Reagan J.W., Seidemand I.L. & Saracusa Y. (1953) The cellular morphology of carcinoma *in situ* and dysplasia or atypical hyperplasia of the uterine cervix. *Cancer*, **6**, 224–35.

Reeves W.C., Caussy D., Brinton L.A. *et al.* (1987) Case-control study of human papillomaviruses and cervical cancer in Latin America. *Int. J. Cancer*, **40**, 450–55.

Reid R., Herschmann B.R., Crum C.P. *et al.* (1984) Genital warts and cervical carcinoma. V. The tissue basis of colposcopic change. *Am. J. Obstet. Gynecol.*, **149**, 293–303.

Reid R., Laverty C.R., Coppleson M., Wiwatwong I. & Hills E. (1980) Non-condylomatous cervical wart virus infection. *Obstet. Gynecol.*, **55**, 476–83.

Reid R., Stanhope C.R., Herschmann B.R. *et al.* (1982) Genital warts and cervical carcinoma. I. Evidence of an association between subclinical papillomavirus infection and cervical malignancy. *Cancer*, **50**, 377–87.

Richart R.M. (1963) A radiographic analysis of cellular proliferation in dysplasia and carcinoma *in situ* of the uterine cervix. *Am. J. Obstet. Gynecol.*, **86**, 925–30.

Richart R.M. & Barron B.A. (1969) A follow-up study of patients with cervical dysplasia. *Am. J. Obstet. Gynecol.*, **105**, 386–93.

Richart R.M., Lerch V. & Barron B.A. (1967) A time-lapse cinematographic study *in vitro* of mitosis in normal human cervical epithelium, dysplasia, and carcinoma *in situ*. *J. Natl. Cancer Inst.*, **39**, 571–7.

Robboy S.J., Keh P.C., Nickerson R.J. *et al.* (1977) Squamous cell dysplasia and carcinoma *in situ* of the cervix and vagina after prenatal exposure to diethylstilbestrol. *Obstet. Gynecol.*, **51**, 528–35.

Saiki R.K., Grelfand D.M., Stoffel S. *et al.* (1988) Primer directed amplification of DNA with a thermostable DNA polymerase. *Science*, **239**, 487–91.

Scholl S.M., Kingsley Pillers E.M., Robinson R.E. & Farrell P.J. (1985) Prevalence of human papilloma-virus type 16 DNA in cervical carcinoma samples in East Anglia. *Int. J. Cancer*, **35**, 215–18.

Shafeek M.A., Osman M.I. & Hussein M.A. (1979) Carcinoma of the vulva arising in condylomata acuminata. *Obstet. Gynecol.*, **54**, 120–23.

Shingleton H.M., Richart R.M., Weiner J. & Spiro D. (1968) Human cervical intraepithelial neoplasia: fine structure of dysplasia and carcinoma *in situ*. *Cancer Res.*, **28**, 695–706.

Shirasawa H., Tomita Y., Kubota K. *et al.* (1988) Transcription differences of the human papillomavirus type 16 genome between precancerous lesions and invasive carcinomas. *J. Virol.*, **62**, 1022–27.

Spriggs A.I., Bowey C.E. & Cowdell R.H. (1971) Chromosomes of precancerous lesions of the cervix uteri. *Cancer*, **27**, 1239–54.

Stafl A. & Mattingly R.F. (1974) Vaginal adenosis: a precancerous lesion? *Am. J. Obstet. Gynecol.*, **120**, 666–77.

Syrjanen K.J., Heinomen U-M. & Kauraniemi T. (1981) Cytologic evidence of the association of condylomatous lesions with dysplastic and neoplastic changes in the uterine cervix. *Acta Cytol.*, **25**, 70–72.

Tidy J., Vousden K.H., Mason P. & Farrell P.F. (1988) A novel deletion within the upstream regulatory region of episomal human papillomavirus type 16. *J. Gen. Virol.* (*in press*).

Tidy J.A., Parry G.C.N., Ward P. *et al.* (1989) High rate of human papillomavirus type 16 infection in cytologically normal cervices. *Lancet*, **i**, 434.

Tweeddale D.N. & Roddick J.W. (1969) Histologic types of squamous cell carcinoma *in situ* of the cervix. *Obstet. Gynecol.*, **33**, 35–40.

Ulbright T.M., Stehman F.B., Roth L.M., Ehrlich C.E. & Ransburg R.C. (1982) Bowenoid dysplasia of the vulva. *Cancer*, **50**, 2910–19.

Vousden K.H., Doniger J., DiPaolo J.A. & Lowy D.R. (1988) The E7 open reading frame of human papillomavirus type 16 encodes a transforming gene. *Oncogene Res.*, **3**, 167–75.

Wade T.R., Kopf A.W. & Ackerman A.B. (1978) Bowenoid papulosis of the penis. *Cancer*, **42**, 1890–903.

Wilbanks G.D., Richart R.M. & Terner J.Y. (1967) DNA content of cervical intraepithelial neoplasia studied by two wave-length Feulgen cytophotometry. *Am. J. Obstet. Gynecol.*, **98**, 792–99.

Wilczynski S.P., Walker J., Shu-Yuan L., Bergen S. & Berman M. (1988) Adenocarcinoma of the cervix associated with human papillomavirus. *Cancer*, **62**, 1331–36.

Young L.S., Bevan I.S., Johnson M.A. *et al.* (1989) The polymerase chain reaction: a new epidemiological tool for investigating cervical human papillomavirus infection. *Br. Med. J.*, **298**, 14–18.

zur Hausen H. (1982) Human genital cancer: synergism between two virus infections or synergism between a virus and initiating events? *Lancet*, **ii**, 1370–72.

3

The Management of CIN, VAIN and VIN

JOE A. JORDAN

In 1886 in London Sir John Williams gave the Harveian Lecture reporting eight cases of cervical cancer, one of which provided the first description of the lesion described today as cervical intraepithelial neoplasia (CIN or carcinoma *in situ*). He stated 'this is the earliest condition of undoubted cancer of the portio vaginalis that I have met with; and it is the earliest condition which is recognisable as cancer. It presented no distinct symptoms, and was discovered accidentally.'

Other reports followed, and the significance of the precancerous state was summarized by Rubin (1910) who commented 'the routine and complete pathological examination of parts or whole of the uterus removed for whatever cause may often furnish the first evidence of a latent carcinoma, and the pathological diagnosis of carcinoma of the uterus in the preclinical stage is possible.' He went on to say 'What shall we regard as metaplastic, non-malignant epithelial changes, and what shall we regard as typical carcinomatous epithelium, or an atypical epithelium that will sooner or later develop into a fully fledged carcinoma? Unless we can decide upon the determining features of the diagnosis of a cancerous epithelium, it is evident that we may never hope to improve prophylactic therapy for carcinoma.'

Thus in 1910, pathologists and clinicians had decided that there was such a condition as preclinical carcinoma and that if this could be detected and treated then this would give infinitely better results than treating established cancer with the methods available to them at that time, namely surgery and radiotherapy. For many years the diagnosis of the existence of the preinvasive lesion was a chance occurrence based on the histological examination of a cervix removed for other reasons. A major breakthrough occurred in 1925 when Hinselmann in Germany described the earliest colposcope, a microscope with which he expected to observe cancer at its very earliest stage either as a small ulcer or a small exophytic lesion invisible to the naked eye.

At about the same time Schiller (1929) described the Schiller iodine test. He had observed that squamous carcinomas of the cervix were conspicuously lacking in large amounts of glycogen, whereas normal squamous epithelium was characterized by an abundance. As a result of this observation he described the test in which an iodine solution containing iodine (2 g), potassium iodide (4 g), and distilled water to 300 ml, was applied to the cervix and upper vagina. Normal squamous epithelial cells containing glycogen stained dark brown whereas columnar epithelium and abnormal epithelium containing little or no glycogen remained unstained. Schiller recommended that all non-staining areas of the portio should be carefully scraped to permit the detection of abnormal epithelium.

In spite of the introduction of colposcopy and the Schiller iodine test it was not until Papanicolaou & Traut (1943) described their technique of exfoliative cytology that clinicians recognized that at last they had an effective and simple way of detecting premalignant lesions of the cervix.

Colposcopy

There are two basic schools of colposcopy, that which practises 'classical or extended colposcopy' and the other using the 'saline technique': many centres use a combination of both.

Classical or extended colposcopy

This is the method which is practised in most centres. The patient is placed in the modified lithotomy position. The cervix and upper vagina are first examined at magnifications of ×6 or ×10 following which excess mucus is removed from the cervix with a dry cotton wool swab and the cervix again inspected. If necessary a cervical smear can be taken at this stage with care being taken not to traumatize the cervix, otherwise this may affect the picture which the colposcopist sees. However, cytology at the first colposcopy visit is not mandatory, as the reason for the visit to the colposcopy clinic is usually because the patient is already known to have an abnormal smear. Acetic acid (3% or 5%) is applied by cotton wool swab. This removes the mucus and causes some swelling of epithelium, particularly columnar epithelium and abnormal epithelium, the latter appearing as a thick white epithelium (aceto-white epithelium). Aceto-white epithelium is usually easier to distinguish from normal epithelium because of a sharp line of demarcation between the two. The Schiller iodine test may then be used. Most experienced colposcopists do not use the Schiller test but all beginning colposcopists should, because from time to time it will alert the colposcopist to the presence of abnormal epithelium which may otherwise have remained undetected by the acetic acid test alone.

The saline technique

This method was devised by Koller and developed by Kolstad both working from the Norwegian Radium Hospital in Oslo. After exposing the cervix, mucus is gently removed with a cotton wool swab and the cervix moistened with physiological saline. This allows the subepithelial angioarchitecture to be studied in great detail. To see the capillaries most clearly the colposcopist must use a green filter and high magnification: in this way the red capillaries appear darker and stand out more clearly. The technique depends entirely on the visualization of various vessel patterns and although it is a more difficult technique to master it allows the colposcopist to predict the underlying histological pattern with greater accuracy.

Diagnostic criteria for colposcopy

In its simplest form colposcopy is the recognition of aceto-white epithelium but since benign conditions. can produce aceto-white epithelium the colposcopist must be aware of other features which suggest underlying abnormality. These are as follows:

1   The subepithelial vascular pattern
2   Intercapillary distance
3   Colour tone differences at the junction of normal and abnormal tissue
4   Surface pattern
5   Sharp line of demarcation between different types of epithelium

   Of these criteria the most important are the vascular pattern and intercapillary distance. The commonly observed vascular patterns are as follows.

Punctation (Fig. 3.1)

Punctation is an easily recognized vessel pattern in which the vessels are arranged in a prominent punctate fashion usually within a well demarcated area. In Fig. 3.1 it can be seen that the vessels on the left are more widely spaced than the vessels on the right indicating that the epithelium on the left side of the lesion is CIN III while that on the right, with the vessels more closely packed together, is CIN I–II. Note the sharp line of demarcation between normal and abnormal epithelium.

Mosaic (Fig. 3.2)

The capillaries here are arranged parallel to the surface in a characteristic mosaic or 'crazy paving' pattern. In Fig. 3.2 the mosaic pattern represents carcinoma *in situ*.

Atypical vessels (Fig. 3.3)

These are readily recognized and will always raise the suspicion of invasive carcinoma. Typically they are irregular in size, shape and course and the inter-capillary distance is significantly greater than that which is found in normal epithelium.

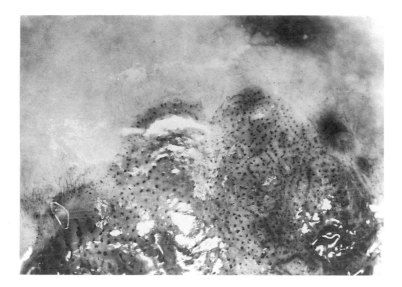

Fig. 3.1. Punctation: the punctate pattern is formed by the tips of subepithelial capillaries as they grow towards the surface. The wider the space between the vessels, the more advanced the stage of CIN. This photograph represents CIN III on the left and CIN I–II on the right.

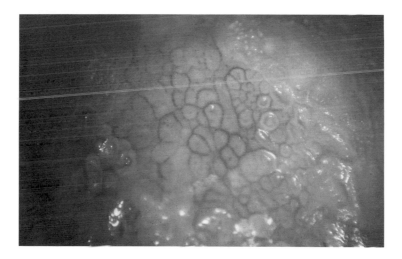

Fig. 3.2. Mosaic: the mosaic pattern is also formed by subepithelial capillaries, but in this case they run parallel to the surface. As with punctation, the larger the distance between the vessels, the more advanced the degree of CIN. This photograph represents CIN III — on each side of the mosaic pattern are HPV changes.

Cervical intraepithelial neoplasia (CIN)

Cytology is now accepted as the most cost effective way in which CIN can be recognized. Most authorities agree that the introduction of a comprehensive

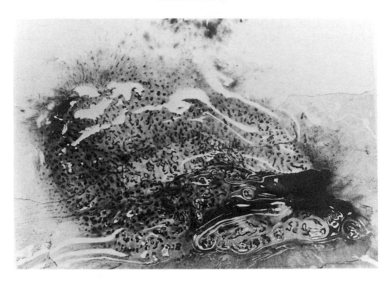

Fig. 3.3. Atypical vessels: in this instance, the vessels run parallel to the surface but are totally irregular in size, shape and course. This photograph represents microinvasive disease.

cytology screening programme has resulted in a significant reduction in morbidity and mortality from the disease, whereas mortality rates in countries that do not use cytology to a great extent have changed very little. Following cervical cytology the clinician is faced with the problem of how to deal with the patient who is found to have an abnormal smear. In 1982 the Royal College of Obstetricians and Gynaecologists stated 'ideally, no patient with CIN should be treated unless there has been prior colposcopic assessment. If colposcopy is not available in a particular hospital then the patient should be referred to someone who can perform a colposcopic assessment following which proper treatment can be planned' (Jordan et al. 1982). Although colposcopy was first described by Hinselmann in 1925 it was almost 30 years before it was adopted by the English-speaking nations. It is now used throughout the world and for detailed accounts of the technique the reader is referred to the following texts; Coppleson et al. (1971); Kolstad & Stafl (1972); Jordan & Singer (1976); Cartier (1977).

In centres which do not practice colposcopy the clinician is severely disadvantaged in his choice of treatment because he is unable to identify either the site of origin of the abnormal cytology or the underlying histological pattern, be it inflammatory, premalignant or malignant. If there is clinical evidence of invasive carcinoma then the management is clear but in the majority of patients with abnormal cytology the cervix will look perfectly normal. When the cytology is positive or persistently suspicious then a cone biopsy aided by the use of Schiller's iodine test is obligatory. If the cone is to be therapeutic as well as diagnostic then the surgeon must remove all of the endocervical canal knowing that in most instances this will be an unnecessarily radical procedure. Even though it is planned to proceed to hysterectomy, a cone biopsy should first be performed for diagnostic purposes so that occult invasive carcinoma can be excluded.

If colposcopy is available the management becomes more simple and will consist of either surgical excision (cone biopsy, local excision, diathermy loop excision or hysterectomy) or local ablation (cryocautery, radical diathermy, cold coagulation, or laser vaporization).

Surgical excision of CIN

Cone biopsy

The aim of the cone biopsy should be 2-fold. First it should be diagnostic, and secondly, if properly planned, it should be therapeutic.

Reporting in 1960 McLaren stated that since 1952 he had been experimenting with deep ring biopsy and conization as a means of curing carcinoma *in situ* but that at the time of his report only half of his patients could be left without subsequent hysterectomy. In 1967 he concluded that a large cone biopsy appeared to be therapeutic in 93% of cases; soon afterwards, colposcopy was introduced and consequently colposcopically directed cone biopsies tended to be smaller, had fewer complications, but were equally therapeutic (Jordan 1972, 1976) (Fig. 3.4).

In the absence of colposcopy Schiller's test should be used and the line of incision on the ectocervix made outside the Schiller positive area with the upper limits of excision being the internal os or a point immediately caudal to it. This is a rather crude technique as the lesion may be extremely small whereas Schiller's test outlines the entire transformation zone. Colposcopy offers a great advantage in accurately determining how large or small the cone biopsy should be.

Ideally the size and shape of the cone biopsy should be governed by the colposcopic findings (Fig. 3.4). If normal columnar epithelium can be seen above the lesion then it can be assumed that there is no abnormality at a higher level and under these circumstances it is unnecessary to remove any of the endocervical canal. It is desirable to leave as much of the endocervical canal as possible for several reasons;

(a) the amount of tissue removed is reduced and control of haemorrhage is rarely a problem except when a large amount of ectocervix has to be removed;

(b) the endocervical canal, so important for fertility, is retained in a form which although slightly reduced in length will function normally and

(c) the internal os is left intact. In nulliparous patients or patients desirous of further children these are obviously important factors to be considered.

Reference to Fig. 3.4 will show that if the lesion is small and completely visible it can be removed by either a small cone or ring biopsy (Fig. 3.4a) or by

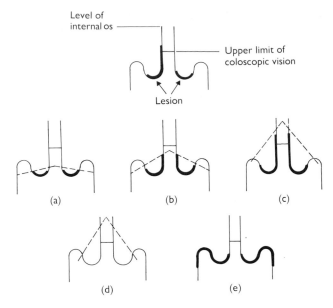

Level of
internal os

Upper limit of
coloscopic vision

Lesion

(a)   (b)   (c)

(d)   (e)

Fig. 3.4.   Types of cone biopsy based on colposcopic findings (from Jordan 1976).

a cone biopsy which removes the lower third of the endocervical canal (Fig.
3.4b). If the lesion extends beyond the limit of colposcopic vision then the
whole of the endocervical canal must be sacrificed (Fig. 3.4c). Occasionally a
patient with positive cytology will show no colposcopic abnormality on the
ectocervix or lower endocervical canal; if the cytologist confirms that the abnormal
cells are squamous in origin then a cone biopsy is indicated. Under these
circumstances the cone biopsy should remove any visible transformation zone
together with the entire length of the endocervical canal (Fig. 3.4d).

Finally, in a small proportion of patients colposcopy will show that the lesion
involves the upper vagina in which case the treatment must be modified (Fig.
3.4e); in such cases where the lesion involves most of the ectocervix in addition
to parts of the vagina, surgery would involve excision of the abnormal vaginal
epithelium with amputation of the cervix or alternatively a hysterectomy with a
cuff of vagina.

Recently the introduction of the Hamou hysteroscope has allowed further
evaluation of the endocervical canal and by this means it is possible for the
surgeon to see how far up the endocervical canal the lesion extends and, therefore,
modify the length of his cone biopsy accordingly (Soutter et al. 1984).

The results of treatment of a properly planned therapeutic cone biopsy are
excellent but regular cytologic follow-up is obligatory. The development of subsequent invasive carcinoma is extremely rare. Coppleson (1981) reviewed the
world literature and of 5442 reported cases of patients treated by conization or
amputation of cervix only 18 subsequently developed invasive carcinoma, an

incidence of 0.3%. Lest this be thought unacceptable he also compared the incidence of invasive carcinoma following treatment of CIN by hysterectomy: he reviewed 8998 cases reported in the world literature and found that 38 subsequently developed invasive carcinoma, an incidence of 0.4%.

Local excision

Occasionally colposcopy reveals that the lesion is extremely small and can be removed by one or more punch biopsies or by excision under general anaesthesia. This approach is only of practical value if the lesion is first seen and identified by a competent colposcopist.

Diathermy loop excision

This is a relatively new technique which may well become the treatment of choice for the outpatient management of women with premalignant disease of the cervix. It is based on an idea of Rene Cartier who described the technique of removing cervical tissue for biopsy using a small diathermy loop. The technique was subsequently modified by Prendeville (1989) using a larger loop. The principle of the technique is that cervical epithelium can be excised on an outpatient basis using local anaesthesia and a vasoconstrictor. The advantages of the technique can be summarized as follows.
1   The whole of the specimen can be sent for histological assessment. This eliminates the problem occasionally faced by the colposcopist, particularly inexperienced colposcopists, of relying on a single punch or multiple punch biopsies to eliminate invasive disease prior to destructive methods.
2   The procedure can be carried out on an outpatient basis using local anaesthesia.
3   When a deeper cone biopsy is required the loop can be used to remove the larger cone under general anaesthesia.
4   The histological specimen is processed as a cone biopsy: the amount of tissue damage is minimal and perfectly acceptable to the pathologist.
5   The cost of the machine is relatively cheap and many operating theatres already have a diathermy machine which would be suitable for this type of procedure. The only expenditure would therefore be that of the diathermy loops.

Hysterectomy

Since conization is clearly an excellent treatment for premalignant disease of the cervix it follows that hysterectomy is an over treatment for the majority of such patients. However, it may be the treatment of choice in some circumstances such as:
1   If, following conization, there is evidence of residual epithelial abnormality as

shown by positive cytology and/or colposcopy; even so such residual lesions can often be treated successfully by local excision, by repeat conization or by local destruction.

2 If the lesion involves the upper vagina. In this case conization will obviously be inadequate treatment and hysterectomy with removal of the upper part of the vagina may be necessary. An alternative to this may be laser destruction of the entire lesion or, alternatively, laser destruction of the vaginal part of the lesion followed by either cone biopsy or hysterectomy.

3 If there is a coexisting indication for hysterectomy such as fibroids, menorrhagia or prolapse. Even so the possibility of occult invasive carcinoma must be remembered and it should be histologically excluded by colposcopically directed punch or wedge biopsies or by a cone biopsy. Hysterectomy without prior histological exclusion of invasive carcinoma can rarely be justified.

4 Occasionally, for technical reasons, a cone biopsy may be extremely difficult in which case the safest and easiest way to remove a cervical lesion may be by primary hysterectomy.

Local destruction of CIN

Most patients with premalignant disease of the cervix can be safely treated by local ablation provided that the following criteria are strictly met:

1 The patient is seen and assessed by a competent colposcopist. It is difficult to qualify the expression 'competent colposcopist' but the key to the success or failure of destructive methods of treatment lies in very careful colposcopic assessment. It is not possible for a gynaecologist to become a competent colposcopist by simply attending a 2- or 3-day colposcopy training course or by attending a colposcopy clinic for a few sessions. One or both of these programmes will teach the basic rudiments of colposcopy but only after the colposcopist has seen many patients over a period of months and correlated his findings very carefully with a cytologist and a pathologist can he begin to call himself an expert.

2 The colposcopist is able to see the lesion in its entirety.

3 By colposcopically directed biopsy or biopsies the colposcopist can satisfy himself that there is no invasive carcinoma.

4 There is no suspicion, colposcopically or cytologically, of abnormal columnar cells.

5 The ablation is carried out by the colposcopist.

6 There is good cytology and/or colposcopy follow-up.

Several locally ablative methods are available; cryosurgery, electrocautery, electrodiathermy, cold coagulation, and the CO_2 laser. The principle of each of these methods is the same, namely to destroy selective areas of cervical epithelium which will then be replaced by normal squamous epithelium.

Cryosurgery

Cryosurgery has the advantage that it can be performed with minimal or no discomfort as an outpatient procedure. The cervix should be exposed with the widest speculum which the patient will accept, following which it is cleaned with acetic acid and the extent of the disease determined colposcopically. The gynaecologist then chooses the appropriate tip and applies it to the cervix. It is important that the operator allows enough time for the tissue to freeze to a depth of about 4 mm; this usually takes 2 to 3 min. The probe is then defrosted and the cervix inspected to ensure that the ice ball has extended beyond the limits of the lesion. With large lesions, more than one application may be necessary. Some operators use a freeze—thaw—re-freeze technique.

In selected cases skilled operators undoubtedly achieve good results (Crisp *et al*. 1970; Townsend & Ostergard 1971; Creasman *et al*. 1973; Kaufman *et al*. 1973; Di Saia *et al*. 1975; Richart *et al*. 1980). Townsend (1981) claimed an overall success rate with a single freeze—thaw technique of 88%. This of course does not mean that cryocautery failed in 12% of cases treated because re-treatment of the majority of failures at a second cryosurgery session increased the cure rate to 95%. He did, however, point out that the success rate depended to a large extent on the size of the lesion. Small lesions were more likely to be cured with a single treatment but when the lesion covered most of the ectocervix regardless of histologic diagnosis, there was a primary failure rate approaching 50%.

Some cases of invasive carcinoma following cryotherapy have been described (Sevin *et al*. 1979) but a review of these cases has shown that the problem is largely due to inadequate colposcopic assessment rather than the technique itself. If the patient is assessed carefully as described above, invasive carcinoma will be an uncommon occurrence but whatever method is used, be it local destruction or surgical excision, the occasional invasive carcinoma is inevitable.

Electrocautery

This technique can be performed in the outpatient clinic but is more likely to be unsuccessful because it is not possible to destroy tissue in this way beyond a depth of 2 or 3 mm: to do so would induce too much pain. However, in small areas of colposcopically localized areas of abnormality, particularly CIN 1 or CIN 2 it has proved effective (Richart & Sciarra 1968; Odell *et al*. 1971; Wilbanks *et al*. 1973).

Radical electrocoagulation diathermy

Electrocoagulation diathermy has been shown to be an extremely effective way of treating all grades of CIN (Chanen & Hollyock 1971; Hollyock & Chanen 1976;

Chanen & Rome 1983). A major disadvantage of the technique is that it requires general anaesthesia but Chanen & Rome (1983) feel that this is justified. Of 2504 patients presenting in their clinic with histologically proven CIN or preclinical invasive cancer 74.4% were suitable for treatment with electrocoagulation diathermy and of these 98.3% were cured with a single treatment. They concluded that 'a single application of electrocoagulation diathermy is a safe and effective means of treating most patients with pre-malignant disease of the cervix regardless of its extent or severity. The risk of subsequent invasive cancer in these patients has been virtually eliminated.'

The technique is simple and requires no more than a needle and ball electrode. The cervix is first dilated to a number 6 or 7 Hegar's dilator, the lesion reviewed colposcopically and if necessary further biopsies taken, and the cervix then stained with Schiller's iodine. A needle electrode is inserted to a depth of approximately 1 cm and multiple insertions are made into the whole transformation zone, the lesion and into the columnar epithelium in the lower part of the endocervical canal. Following this the ball electrode is used and by a process of fulguration and coagulation the whole surface area, already subjected to the needle electrode, is systematically diathermied (Chanen 1981).

Cold coagulation

The Semm 'cold' coagulator is being used in some centres to treat CIN. Duncan (1982) described how 296 patients had been treated with an overall cure rate of 94.3%.

The procedure is carried out in the outpatient department without anaesthesia. A thermosound, rather like the cryotherapy probe, is applied to the cervical surface for 20 seconds and rapidly heated to a temperature of 100°C. The whole of the transformation zone is destroyed, usually in five slightly overlapping areas, including the lower endocervix, and the usual treatment time is approximately 100 seconds.

The technique is simple and relatively cheap. Most patients experience pelvic cramping lasting for the duration of treatment. Rarely does the treatment have to be abandoned but occasionally local anaesthesia may be necessary. The technique is obviously worthy of further study and assessment.

Carbon dioxide laser

The word 'laser' is an acronym derived from the first letters of the words Light Amplification by Stimulated Emission of Radiation. The laser converts energy such as heat, light or electricity into radiant energy at a specific wavelength. The actual wavelength is determined by the type of laser. For example, the CO_2 laser, the laser most widely used in gynaecology, produces energy at a wavelength of 10.6 μm which is in the infra-red portion of the spectrum, where it is invisible to the naked eye. This energy, by a system of mirrors and lenses, can be focused to a specific spot, usually about 1.7 mm in diameter, and at its focal point it releases an enormous amount of energy. Any tissue at the focal point of the laser is then vaporized. The laser itself is attached to a colposcope and at all times the area to be destroyed is under direct vision of the person performing the laser surgery. Manipulation of the beam is simple and any experienced colposcopist can be taught how to use the laser in a very short period of time. Patients are selected for treatment as described above. In most instances the patient can be treated in the outpatient department without any form of analgesia or anaesthesia although occasionally a paracervical block or even general anaesthesia may be necessary. No preoperative preparation of the vagina is necessary.

Those using laser surgery for the first time may well be disappointed with their results, but failures occur because the operator has failed to destroy tissue to an adequate depth. The surgeon must recognize that CIN may extend beneath the surface into the crypts or clefts and this must be taken into consideration when any destructive treatment is used. The laser surgeon should, therefore, aim to destroy tissue to a depth of 5–7 mm (Mylotte & Jordan 1981; Jordan *et al.* 1985). A histological study by Anderson & Hartley (1980) showed that 99.7% of lesions extended less than 4 mm below the surface but since it is almost impossible to gauge depth of destruction to exactly 4 mm a depth of 5–7 mm should be the depth to aim for. With proper patient selection and an adequate depth of destruction, cure rates in excess of 95% can be expected (Wright *et al.* 1983, 1984; Jordan *et al.* 1985).

When the laser was first introduced it was used only to vaporize CIN but more recently Dorsey & Diggs (1979) and Wright *et al.* (1984) have described how it can be used to remove a cone of tissue in patients who would otherwise have cold knife conization. They performed the operation under general anaesthesia and claimed that the patient could be discharged home the same day. Haemorrhage was controlled by lateral haemostatic sutures and the use of vasopressin. Using a small spot size with a power density from 1000 to 27 500 W per cm^2 the cone can be rapidly cut. Conization is perhaps the wrong word to use for this type of tissue removal because the authors stressed that a cylinder of tissue should be removed rather than the traditional cone. The upper part of the specimen was cut with a scalpel and any bleeding controlled by reducing the power density and increasing the spot size of the laser. In cases where there is a large surface area involvement of the ectocervix together with the lesion extending into the endocervical canal the operator can modify this technique so that the peripheral part of the lesion is vaporized and the endocervical part of the lesion is removed as described above ('top hat' technique).

Management of cervical human papillomavirus (HPV) infection

Management of the patient with abnormal cervical cytology has been complicated by the diagnosis of HPV infection since Meisels *et al.* (1977) first postulated that HPV infection of the cervix might be a precursor of cervical cancer. Since that

time many types of HPV have been identified. HPV types 6 and 11 are associated
with benign exophytic growths or warts, usually on the cervix, vagina, vulva and
perianal areas (Gissman *et al.* 1983). Others however such as HPV 16 (Durst *et al.*
1983) and HPV 18 (Boshart *et al.* 1984) are associated with flat aceto-white lesions
which are thought by some to be a precursor of cervical cancer especially when
found in the transformation zone. HPV types 31, 33, 35, 39, 42, 45, 49, 52b and 53
have also been discovered in cervical epithelium, but are very uncommon.

Following the discovery of this link between HPV and cervical malignancy it
was understandable that clinicians should feel obliged to detect and treat HPV
infection. The problem, however, has been compounded by the discovery of
HPV 16 in the cervical epithelium of normal women in 70% (Young *et al.* 1989)
and 84% (Tidy *et al.* 1989) of cases. Furthermore, Munoz *et al.* (1988) on reviewing
published epidemiological evidence stated that while experimental data suggested
an oncogenic potential for HPV the epidemiological evidence implicating it as a
cause of cervical neoplasia was still rather limited.

From a purely clinical point of view there is acceptance that HPV seems to be
involved in the chain of events leading to the development of cervical malignancy,
but the significance of its role, and the effect of its presence on treatment,
remains open to debate. For example Woodman *et al.* (1986) studied a group of 45
women referred to a colposcopy clinic with cytological abnormality and found to
have no more than infection with HPV: 26 underwent spontaneous regression
over a period of 28 months. On the other hand Campion *et al.* (1986) studied 100
women with cytological and colposcopical evidence of cervical intraepithelial
neoplasia grade I and reported that regression over 2 years occurred in only 7,
whereas the lesion progressed to cervical intraepithelial neoplasia grade 3 in 26.

If a decision is taken to treat HPV there is no guarantee that any treatment
will be 100% successful, a problem highlighted by Ferenczy *et al.* (1985), who
showed that destruction of genital warts was often followed by further overt
disease at adjoining sites because removal of the lesion did not eradicate all
subclinical infection.

Exophytic warts on the vulva should be treated and most gynaecologists
accept that small exophytic warts can be treated fairly easily by using topical
agents or some method of destruction. On the other hand, in those women who
have a mass of exophytic warts involving the vulva, perineum and perianal
areas, laser vaporization undoubtedly produces the best results: even so the
patient should be warned that local recurrences are common but can usually be
dealt with on an outpatient basis.

Should exophytic warts on the cervix and vagina be treated? Some would say
'yes' because they are a source of infection. Others say 'not necessarily', because
even if the warts are removed by laser or diathermy reinfection from the vaginal
reservoir of HPV is extremely common: furthermore, very extensive warts such
as those which occur in patients who are immunosuppressed are usually impossible to eradicate. If very extensive warts cannot be treated it would seem a waste
of time to treat small exophytic warts.

By comparison, subclinical HPV infection of the cervix and vagina is easy to treat if it is not too extensive, but if it involves the whole cervix or vagina then treatment becomes more difficult. It is possible to remove very extensive areas by laser vaporization but there is a definite morbidity attached to the procedure and reinfection is common. Chemical stripping with 5FU has also been described but patients do not tolerate it well and the results are disappointing.

As a compromise the gynaecologist may elect to treat HPV of the cervix and vagina only if it is associated with CIN, in which case it is the CIN which has prompted the treatment, and not the HPV.

Until such time as the true sequence of events is clear, there will be difference of opinion as to whether or not to treat minor degrees of CIN with HPV and until the problem is resolved many women, especially young women, will suffer the anxiety of referral to a colposcopy clinic and may even be subjected to treatment which will eventually be shown to have been unnecessary (Jordan 1988).

References

Anderson M.C. & Hartley R.B. (1980) Cervical crypt involvement by intraepithelial neoplasia. *Obstet. Gynecol.*, **55**, 546–50.

Boshart M., Gissman L., Ikenberg H., Kleinheinz A., Scheurlen W. & zur Hausen H. (1984) A new type of papilloma virus DNA, its presence in genital biopsies and in cell lines derived from cervical cancer. *EMBO J.*, **3**, 1151–57.

Campion M.J., McCance D.J., Cuzick J. & Singer A. (1986) Progressive potential of mild cervical atypia: prospective cytological, colposcopic and virological study. *Lancet*, **ii**, 237–40.

Cartier R. (1977) *Practical Colposcopy*. Karger, London. p. 100.

Chanen W. (1981) Radical electrocoagulation. Diathermy. *In*: Coppleson M. (ed.), *Gynecologic Oncology*. Churchill Livingstone, London. pp. 821–25.

Chanen W. & Hollyock V.E. (1971) Colposcopy and electrocoagulation diathermy for cervical dysplasia and carcinoma *in situ*. *Obstet. Gynecol.*, **37**, 623–28.

Chanen W. & Rome R.M. (1983) Electrocoagulation diathermy for cervical dysplasia and carcinoma *in situ*: a 15 year survey. *Obstet. Gynecol.*, **61**, 673–79.

Coppleson M. (1981) CIN: Clinical features and management. *In*: Coppleson M. (ed.), *Gynecologic Oncology*. Churchill Livingstone, London pp. 408–33.

Coppleson M., Pixley E. & Reid B.L. (1971) *Colposcopy. A Scientific and Practical Approach to the Cervix in Health and Disease*. C.C. Thomas, Springfield, Illinois.

Creasman E.T., Weed Jr J.G., Curry S.L., Johnston W.W. & Parker R.T. (1973) Efficacy of cryosurgical treatment of severe intraepithelial neoplasia. *Obstet. Gynecol.*, **41**, 501–6.

Crisp W.E., Smith M.S., Asadourian L.A. & Warrenburg C.B. (1970) Cryosurgical treatment of pre-malignant disease of the uterine cervix. *Am. J. Obstet. Gynecol.*, **107**, 737–42.

Di Saia P.J., Morrow C.P. & Townsend D.E. (1975) *Synopsis of Gynecologic Oncology*. Wiley, New York.

Dorsey J.M. & Diggs E.S. (1979) Microsurgical conization of the cervix by CO_2 laser. *Obstet. Gynecol.*, **54**, 565.

Duncan I.D. (1982) Treatment of CIN by destruction—'Cold coagulator'. *In*: Jordan J.A., Sharp F. & Singer A. (eds), *Preclinical Carcinoma of the Cervix*. Royal College of Obstetricians and Gynaecologists, London. pp. 197–202.

Durst M., Gissmann L., Ikenberg H. & zur Hausen H. (1983) A papillomavirus DNA from a cervical carcinoma and its prevalence in cancer biopsies from different geographic regions. *Proc. Natl. Acad. Sci. USA*, **60**, 3812–15.

Ferenczy A., Mitao M., Nagai N., Silverstein S.J. & Crum C.P. (1985) Latent papillomavirus and recurring genital warts. *New Engl. J. Med.*, **313**, 784–88.

Gissman L., Wolnik L., Ikenberg H., Koldovsky U., Schurch H.G. & zur Hausen H. (1983) Human papillomavirus types 6 and 11 DNA sequences in genital and laryngeal papillomas and in some cervical cancers. *Proc. Natl. Acad. Sci. USA*, **80**, 560–63.

Hinselmann H. (1925) Verbesserung der Inspektionsmoglichkeit von Vulva, Vagina and Portio. *Munchener Medizinische Wochenschrift*, **77**, 1733.

Hollyock, V.E. & Chanen, W. (1976) Electrocoagulation diathermy for the treatment of cervical dysplasia and carcinoma *in situ*. *Obstet. Gynecol.*, **47**, 196.

Jordan J.A. (1972) Colposcopy in gynaecological practice. *In*: Jakob C.A. & Franco M.A. *Proceedings of the First World Congress of Colposcopy and Cervical Pathology*. Molachino Establecimiento, Grapio, Rosano, Argentina. pp. 131–37.

Jordan J.A. (1976) The diagnosis and management of premalignant conditions of the cervix. *Clin. Obstet. Gynaecol.*, **3**, 2, 295–315.

Jordan J.A. (1988) Minor degrees of cervical intraepithelial neoplasia. *Br. Med. J.*, **297**, 6.

Jordan J.A., Sharp F. & Singer A. (1982) *Preclinical Neoplasia of the Cervix. Proceedings of the Ninth Study Group of the Royal College of Obstetricians and Gynaecologists*. Royal College of Obstetricians and Gynaecologists, London. p. 299.

Jordan J.A. & Singer A. (1976) *The Cervix*. W.B. Saunders, London.

Jordan J.A., Woodman C.B.J., Mylotte M.J., Emens J.M., Williams D.R., MacAlary M. & Wade-Evans T. (1985) The treatment of cervical intraepithelial neoplasia by laser vaporisation. *Br. J. Obstet. Gynaecol.*, **92**, 394–98.

Kaufman R.H., Strama T., Norton P.K. & Conner J.J. (1973) Cryosurgical treatment of cervical intraepithelial neoplasia. *Obstet. Gynecol.*, **42**, 881–86.

Koller O. (1963) *The Vascular Patterns of the Uterine Cervix*. Scandinavian University Books, London.

Kolstad P. (1964) *Vascularisation, Oxygen Tension and Radiocurability in Cancer of the Cervix*. Scandinavian University Books, London.

Kolstad P. & Stafl A. (1972) *Atlas of Colposcopy*. Universitetsforlaget, Oslo.

Kunschner A., Kanbour A.I. & David B. (1978) Early vulvar carcinoma. *Am. J. Obstet. Gynecol.*, **132**, 599.

McLaren H.C. (1960) The treatment of carcinoma *in situ*. *Extrait de Acta Union Internationale Contre le Cancer*, **16**, 385.

McLaren H.C. (1967) Conservative management of cervical precancer. *J. Obstet. Gynaecol. Br. Commonwealth*, **74**, 487–92.

Meisels A., Fortin R. & Roy M. (1977) Condylomatous lesions of the cervix. II. Cytologic, colposcopic and histopathologic study. *Acta Cytol.*, **21**; 379–90.

Munoz N., Bosch X. & Kaldor J.M. (1988) Does human papillomavirus cause cervical cancer? The state of the epidemiological evidence. *Br. J. Cancer*, **57**, 1–5.

Mylotte M.J. & Jordan J.A. (1981) Laser treatment of cervical intraepithelial neoplasia, *Rev. Fr. Gynecol. Obstet.*, **5**, 353–6.

Odell L.D., Rimker K. & Hagerty C. (1971) Electrocautery for cervical neoplasia. *J. Reprod. Med.*, **6**, 143–46.

Papanicolaou G. & Traut H.F. (1943) *The Diagnosis of Uterine Cancer by the Vaginal Smear*. Commonwealth Fund, New York.

Prendeville W., Cullimore J. & Norman S. (1989) Large loop excision of transformation zone (LLETZ): a new method of management for women with cervical intraepithelial neoplasia. *Br. J. Obstet. Gynaecol.*, **96**, 1054–60.

Richart R.M. & Sciarra J.J. (1968) Treatment of cervical dysplasia by outpatient electrocauterisation. *Am. J. Obstet. Gynecol.*, **101**, 200–5.

Richart R.M., Townsend D.E., Crisp W., De Petrillo A., Ferenczy A., Johnson G., Lickrish G., Roy M. & Villasanta U. (1980) An analysis of long term follow up results in patients with CIN treated by cryotherapy. *Am. J. Obstet. Gynecol.*, **137**, 823–26.

Rubin I.C. (1910) The pathological diagnosis of incipient carcinoma of the uterus. *Am. J. Obstet. Gynecol.*, **62**, 668–76.

Rutledge F. & Sinclair M. (1968) Treatment of intraepithelial carcinoma of the vulva by skin excision and graft. *Am. J. Obstet. Gynecol.*, **102**, 806.

Schiller W. (1929) Jodpinselung und Abschabung des Portioepithels. *Zentralblatt fur Gynakologie*, **53**, 1056–64.

Sevin B., Ford J.H., Girtanner R.D., Hoskins W.J., Ng A.B.P., Nordquist S.R.B. & Averette H.E. (1979) Invasive cancer of the cervix after cryosurgery. *Obstet. Gynecol.*, **45**, 456.

Soutter W.P., Fenton D.W., Gudgeon P. & Sharp F. (1984) Quantitative microcolpohysteroscopic assessment of the extent of endocervical involvement by cervical intraepithelial neoplasia. *Br. J. Obstet. Gynaecol.*, **91**, 7, 712 15.

Tidy J.A., Parry G.C.N., Ward P., Coleman D.V., Peto J., Malcolm A.D.B. & Farrel P.J. (1989) High rate of HPV 16 infection in cytologically normal cervices. *Lancet*, **i**, 434.

Townsend D.E. (1981) Cryosurgery in gynecologic oncology. *In*: Coppleson M. (ed.), *Gynecologic Oncology*. Churchill Livingstone, London. pp. 809−15.

Townsend D.E. & Ostergard D.R. (1971) Cryocauterisation for preinvasive cervical neoplasia. *J. Reprod. Med.*, **6**, 171−76.

Wilbanks G.D., Creasman W.T., Kaurfman L.A. & Parker R.T. (1973) Treatment of cervical dysplasia with electrocautery and tetracycline suppositories. *Am. J. Obstet. Gynecol.*, **117**, 160−63.

Williams Sir John (1886) Cancer of the uterus. *Harveian Lectures for 1886*. H K Lewis, London.

Woodman C.B.J., Byrne P., Fung S., Wade-Evans T. & Jordan J.A. (1986) Human papillomavirus infection of the cervix−a self limiting disease? *Colposcopy and Gynaecological Laser Surgery*, **2**, 9−13.

Wright V C., Davies E. & Riopelle M.A. (1983) Laser surgery for cervical intraepithelial neoplasia: Principles and results. *Am. J. Obstet. Gynecol.*, **145**, 181.

Wright V.C., Riopelle M.A., Rubinstein E., Rylander E. & Joelsson I. (1984) CO_2 laser and cervical intraepithelial neoplasia. *Acta Obstet. Gynecol. Scand.*, Supplement **125**.

Young L.S., Bevan I.S., Johnson M.A., Blomfield P., Bromidge T., Maitland N.J. & Woodman C.B.J. (1989) The polymerase chain reaction: a new epidemiological tool for investigating cervical human papillomavirus infection. *Br. Med. J.*, **298**, 14−18.

4

Cervical Cancer: The Surgical Management of Early Stage Disease

JOHN H. SHEPHERD

The cervix is an internal genital organ that is eminently assessable by careful clinical examination. Screening procedures, or early investigation of abnormal symptoms that concern the patient enough to seek medical advice, should lead to the prompt detection of clinical cancer or an asymptomatic precancer. Invasive cancer remains predominantly a disease of the over 45-year age group although there has been a suggestion that the incidence in younger women is changing. This may be related to a change in the natural history of the disease and biology of the tumour, perhaps associated with the human papillomavirus (HPV). Approximately 4000 new cases of invasive cervical carcinoma occur in England and Wales annually, whereas in America there are about 16 000 cases each year (American Cancer Society 1984). The most recent office of population and census survey figures indicate 4043 cases of cervix cancer registered in 1984 (OPCS 1984). The number of deaths recorded was 2207 (OPCS 1986). These figures in total are reasonably static except that there appears to be a trend in the younger age groups (below 35) for an increase in incidence of the tumour but not a disproportionate rise in the death rate.

Approximately half of the overall number of cases present at an early stage (Falk *et al*. 1982). It is hoped that with effective screening programmes and earlier diagnosis, this percentage will increase at the expense of the more advanced disease and eventually the majority of patients may present at a preinvasive stage. Nevertheless, at present it is an alarming fact that 50% of those patients with invasive disease will die within 5 years of diagnosis and the disease will be implicated in their death to some degree. Widespread use of cytological screening may result in early detection of an otherwise debilitating and deeply invasive tumour leading to a more favourable cure rate.

Correct clinical assessment at the time of presentation allows an individualization of treatment of all early stage tumours so that either radiotherapy, surgery or a combination of both may be used in the treatment of this disease. Five-year survival rates of between 75 and 90% are quoted for whichever modality is chosen (Brady 1979; Perez *et al*. 1987) but no consistent advantage of any single method is apparent as regards cure. The side effects and complications of the treatment may, however, weigh heavily in favour of one method or another.

Natural history and pathology

The aetiology and risk factors associated with this disease are numerous and have been discussed in Chapter 1. The invasive potential of carcinoma of the cervix is now generally accepted (Peterson 1955; Boyes *et al*. 1982; McIndoe *et al*. 1984). There can be little doubt that the majority of cervical cancers pass through a premalignant phase before becoming truly invasive over 5–10 years. Many of the more minor lesions regress and resolve spontaneously (McGregor & Taper 1978) although some may subsequently recur (Stern 1969).

Cervical screening has had a beneficial impact on the mortality and incidence of invasive cancer as shown in data from British Columbia (Walton 1982). Those Nordic countries with a screening programme have reduced mortality by 50% but those with no organized programme by only 10% (Laara *et al*. 1987).

The exact role that HPV plays is uncertain but the determination of which particular lesions do progress may be governed by the presence or absence of certain sub-types of HPV.

Despite the fact that cervical cancer mortality in England and Wales is decreasing, an analysis of the incidence rate for 1950–83 indicated an increase in cervical cancer in young women since 1970 (Beral & Booth 1986). Further concern was raised regarding the change in character of cervical cancer in young women in Australia (Elliott *et al*. 1989) suggesting that the clinical and pathological behaviour of cervical cancer changed between the years of 1953 and 1986. However, it would appear that the death rate is reasonably stable below the age of 50 if one looks at figures for 1978–87. The original predicted increase has not been confirmed except for a continuing rise in the age group between the ages of 35 and 39 (Villard *et al*. 1989). Thus, recent data would indicate that although there has been an increase in cervical deaths in young women over the past 15 years, the most recent data is more reassuring in that these rates appear to be stabilizing with the increased impact of cervical screening and treatment of cervical intraepithelial neoplasia. It would also appear that cervical cancer does not progress more rapidly in younger women (Robertson *et al*. 1988). The majority of tumours are squamous originating within the transformation zone with approximately 10% of lesions being adenocarcinomas. This figure may increase in prevalence in the future because of a decreasing overall incidence of squamous cell carcinoma as a result of improving early detection and treatment of preinvasive lesions. Mixed carcinomas of both squamous and glandular origin occasionally occur. Both types of tissue are invasive as in the adenosquamous tumours, but adenoacanthomas are basically malignant adenocarcinomas with benign squamous metaplasia coexisting. These terms are being discarded in favour of more descriptive pathological terminology although they do convey a specific meaning to a particular lesion.

Squamous cell tumours may be graded according to differentiation and this appears also to be correlated with the outcome (Reagan & Wentz 1967). The commonest tumours are keratinizing squamous cell carcinomas with an overall 5-year survival of 45%. Large cell non-keratinizing cell carcinomas have a better prognosis (5-year survival of 77.5%) whereas small cell carcinomas fare far worse (17%). The mean age of patients with squamous cell carcinoma of the cervix is similar to the mean age of patients with adenocarcinoma (50 years) (Shingleton *et al.* 1981; Berek 1984). However, in younger women with cervical cancer a much higher percentage of cases may be adenocarcinoma (Gallup & Abell 1977; Tamimi & Figge 1982). Indeed, in the first two decades of life, more than three-quarters of cervical cancers reported will be adenocarcinomas (Pollack & Taylor 1947). There is also a suggestion that during pregnancy, a large proportion (62%) of patients will have adeno- or adenosquamous carcinomas (Cherry & Gluckman 1961) although this has not been confirmed in other series (Hacker *et al.* 1982). Under the age of 35, 26% of patients with cervical cancer appear to have adenocarcinomas (Berkowitz *et al.* 1979). Similarly, in another series, half the patients with adeno-squamous carcinomas were under the age of 40 (Gallup *et al.* 1985).

There are a variety of different histological patterns of adenocarcinoma. The commonest is a malignancy arising from the endocervical glands which may have coexisting squamous metaplasia or squamous cell malignancy also (adeno-squamous). 'Glassy cell' carcinoma also occurs, especially in young women, and is said to be highly malignant during pregnancy (Cherry & Gluckmann 1961; Littman *et al.* 1976) although other series have not confirmed this (Shingleton *et al.* 1981). Clear cell carcinoma is found in adolescent girls and young women half as often on the cervix as in the vagina and related to diethylstilboestrol exposure. Such tumours arise from the Müllerian or paramesonephric structures.

Benign and malignant tumours can arise from the mesonephric (Wolffian) duct as it passes through the lateral cervical wall. Papillary adenoma has been described (Mackles *et al.* 1958) but is very rare. Adenocarcinoma is commoner but again rare (McGee *et al.* 1962). It is important to establish that the carcinoma is confined to the lateral cervical stroma (Rosen & Dolan 1975).

Adenoid cystic carcinoma of the cervix occurs predominantly in postmeno-pausal elderly black women (Gallagher *et al.* 1971). The histology resembles an adenoid cystic carcinoma of the salivary gland, breast or lung and it may be associated with CIN or invasive carcinoma of the adjacent mucosa (Lowe & Hudson 1988).

Adenoma malignum has recently been described (McKelvey & Goodlin 1963; Michael *et al.* 1984). They are rare, representing only 1% of cervical adenocarci-nomas (Kaminski & Norris 1983). They are mostly slow growing; if they are treated adequately at an early stage they have a good prognosis to early stage cervical cancer or adenocarcinoma. Despite their quite innocuous histological appearance, they can, however, act in a highly malignant manner once spread has occurred beyond the cervix with a subsequent poor prognosis (Kaku & Enjoji 1983).

Carcinoid tumours of the cervix arise from the argyrophil cells of the normal endocervical canal (Yamasaki *et al*. 1984). Their prognosis is poor (Silva *et al*. 1984). Some of these tumours secrete adrenocorticotrophic hormone (Jones *et al*. 1976) and insulin (Kiang *et al*. 1973).

Other rare types of carcinoma of the cervix include gestational choriocarcinoma which when it involves the cervix alone is extremely unusual. Malignant melanoma is also extremely rare and identical to the disease elsewhere in the body (Krishnamoorthy *et al*. 1986). Primary cervical sarcoma can arise as a malignant change in a benign neoplasm or *de novo*. This usually occurs after the age of 50 years (Abell & Ramirez 1973). Embryonal rhabdomyosarcoma on the other hand is a rare tumour of the cervix arising in children and adolescents. This is sometimes called botryoid rhabdomyosarcoma.

Malignant lymphoma arising in the cervix is less common than the involvement of the cervix by systemic lymphoma (Lathrop 1967). Both Hodgkins and non-Hodgkins lymphomas may occur. Other tumours described include Wilms's tumour (Bell *et al*. 1985) and yolk sac tumour (Copeland *et al*. 1985)' as well as alveolar soft part sarcoma (Flint *et al*. 1985).

Spread of cervical carcinoma occurs predominantly by either direct extension into adjacent structures or lymphatic permeation. Rarely, blood-borne metastases may occur. Thus, the tumour may invade into the vaginal mucosa extending microscopically beyond visible and palpable disease or into the myometrium of the lower uterine segment and corpus, particularly if the lesion arises in the endocervical canal. It may spread into the cervical stroma and beyond into the paracervical and parametrial tissue, eventually reaching the pelvic side walls. This may result in ureteric obstruction and consequent hydronephrosis from lateral extension, and invasion of either the bladder or rectum from anterior and posterior spread. If lymphatic spaces are invaded then the paracervical lymphatics will lead to the most commonly involved pelvic lymph nodes as described by Hendrikson (Hendrikson 1949). Primarily the lymphatic channels drain to paracervical and parametrial or ureteric nodes and then from there to obturator, internal iliac or external iliac nodes. Rarely, sacral nodes may develop metastases. From these primary groups, the common iliac nodes are involved and subsequently the para-aortic nodes. On occasions, the inguinal nodes may be involved either by retrograde spread from the external iliac group, or metastasis via the round ligaments. Haematogenous spread less commonly occurs to the liver or bony skeleton including the vertebral column, the pelvis or long bones. Metastases to the skin, lungs and brain are rare.

Clinical staging

Invasive carcinoma of the cervix by definition involves tumour that has broken through the basement membrane. The depth of invasion will determine the likelihood of spread beyond the cervix. Staging is assessed according to clinical examination findings in association with ancillary investigations. This may be inaccurate as subsequent surgical examination may reveal further extension of disease that was impalpable or not visualized preoperatively. Alternatively, induration and nodularity in the pelvis assumed to be of malignant origin may in fact be benign and a consequence of inflammatory or endometriotic disease. There is an over-staging of cervical cancer of up to 40% (Zander *et al*. 1981). This is an inevitable result of accepting nonoperative staging for international classification. However, as the majority of patients with cervical cancer are treated by radiotherapy, there is little alternative. Hopefully, improvement in noninvasive techniques such as computerized axial tomography or nuclear magnetic resonance will help to improve the accuracy of staging.

The International Federation of Obstetrics and Gynaecology (FIGO) classification was modified in 1985 omitting the term 'occult'. At the same time, microinvasive carcinoma, which involves invasion to a depth of less than 5 mm, has been subdivided into two categories (stage Ia1 and Ia2). The diagnosis of microinvasion should be based on microscopic examination of removed tissue, preferably by a cone biopsy which must include the whole lesion. Such tumours include minimal microscopically evident stromal invasion as well as small cancerous tumours of a measurable size. Microscopic minute foci of invasion are included in stage Ia1, whereas larger lesions to a depth of invasion of less than 5 mm from the base of the epithelium with a second dimension indicating horizontal spread not exceeding 7 mm are included in stage Ia2. Larger lesions are staged as Ib.

The full definition of clinical staging in carcinoma of the cervix uteris as defined by FIGO 1985 is outlined in Table 4.1.

Presentation

The majority of patients presenting with an invasive cancer will have either had post-coital bleeding, intermenstrual bleeding, menorrhagia or a foul discharge that has led them to seek advice from a gynaecologist. A certain number will be detected on routine screening and cytology. These patients should be assessed with a directed biopsy or a wedge biopsy taken under anaesthesia. On occasions a cone biopsy would be necessary to make the diagnosis. Other symptoms including backache, referred pain to the leg, leg oedema, haematuria or an alteration in bowel habit may indicate more advanced disease. The general malaise, weight loss and anaemia associated with many cancers is a late manifestation in patients with cervical cancer.

Investigations

Further investigations are essential to fully assess the patient and her disease before deciding upon the choice of therapy. Apart from the standard haemato-

Table 4.1. Staging of cervical cancer, FIGO 1985

Stage 0	Carcinoma *in situ*, intraepithelial carcinoma. Cases of stage 0 should not be included in any therapeutic statistics for invasive carcinoma
Stage I	The carcinoma is strictly confined to the cervix (extension to the corpus should be disregarded)
Stage Ia	Preclinical carcinoma of the cervix, that is those diagnosed only by microscopy
Stage Ia1	Minimal microscopically evident stromal invasion
Stage Ia2	Lesions detected microscopically that can be measured. The upper limit of the measurement should not show a depth of invasion more than 5 mm taken from the base of the epithelium, either surface or glandular, from which it originates. A second dimension, the horizontal spread, must not exceed 7 mm. Larger lesions should be staged as stage Ib
Stage Ib	Lesions of greater dimensions than stage Ia2 whether seen clinically or not. Preformed space involvement should not alter the staging but should be specifically recorded so as to determine whether it should affect treatment decision in the future
Stage II	The carcinoma extends beyond the cervix, but has not extended on to the pelvic wall. The carcinoma involves the vagina, but not as far as the lower third
Stage IIa	No obvious parametrial involvement
Stage IIb	Obvious parametrial involvement
Stage III	The carcinoma has extended on to the pelvic wall. On rectal examination there is no cancer-free space between the tumour and the pelvic wall. The tumour involves the lower third of the vagina. All cases with a hydronephrosis or non-functioning kidney should be included, unless they are known to be due to other causes
Stage IIIa	No extension on to the pelvic wall, but involvement of the lower third of the vagina
Stage IIIb	Extension on to the pelvic wall or hydronephrosis on non functioning kidney
Stage IV	The carcinoma has extended beyond the true pelvis or has clinically involved the mucosa of the bladder or rectum
Stage IVa	Spread of the growth to adjacent organs
Stage IVb	Spread to distant organs

logical and biochemical evaluation, a chest X-ray is required to exclude pulmonary metastases or other disease. An intravenous urogram is vital to assess renal function and exclude uropathy and ureteric obstruction. A lymphangiogram can be of great value when performed in a centre that is familiar with this investigation

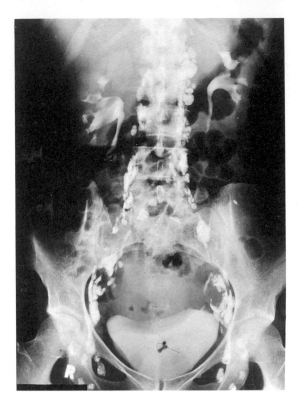

Fig. 4.1. Lymphangiogram showing a filling defect and metastatic disease in the left common iliac nodes.

(Fig. 4.1) (Smales *et al*. 1986). It is essential to take delayed films and follow these up after therapy to be able to assess change in the nodal appearance. Although microscopic disease cannot be excluded, with experience small metastases may be detected and changes in the filling pattern of nodes may occur over a fortnight. Larger disease may be located by the use of computerized axial tomography (CT) but lymph nodes must be 1−2 cm in diameter before CT scans are of value. Traditionally, the patient is examined under an anaesthetic and a cystoscopy performed as well as a biopsy of the cervix taken with a subsequent uterine curettage. However, and the yield of positive cystoscopy findings in the presence of a normal intravenous urogram with early stage disease is virtually nil.

Treatment: a choice between surgery and radiotherapy

Traditionally there may be a choice in treatment with early stage disease (stage Ib or IIa) between either surgery or radiotherapy. Although younger fitter patients are often selected as being suitable for surgery, it may be that certain older and sometimes fragile patients would suffer less with a single anaesthetic and a radical hysterectomy than by 6 weeks of radiotherapy and one or two anaesthetics for intra-cavity applications. Almost identical survival rates are obtained by surgical and radiation treatment for stage Ib carcinoma of the cervix. Large collected series show a 5-year survival of 83.4% following radical surgery and 85.5% with radiotherapy (Delgado 1978). Five-year survival figures are very similar of between 70 and 90% following both radiotherapy and surgery used as primary treatment (Roddick & Greenelaw 1971; Newton 1975; Perez *et al.* 1980). For many years radiotherapy has been the primary treatment of choice in this country mainly due to the surgical skills of gynaecologists lapsing but there has been a resurgence of late, following a trend in the United States to continue and reintroduce radical hysterectomy as a surgically curative procedure. Apart from survival, however, there are other advantages for patients undergoing surgery with early or small primary tumours. Even though radiation therapy can be administered to almost all patients, serious bladder or bowel damage may occur in between 2 and 6% resulting in chronic long term problems. Radiation cystitis or proctitis may occur periodically for years after therapy. Bladder or rectal fistulae following radiotherapy are difficult to repair in view of the inevitable endarteritis that occurs with radiation, reducing the blood supply to the pelvic tissues and thus compromising tissue healing. Sexual dysfunction can occur which is more problematic following radiotherapy, resulting in a rigid and stenosed vagina.

Primary surgical treatment allows a thorough exploratory laparotomy to be performed, thus determining the exact extent of the tumour and so avoiding inaccurate staging. In the young, and this of course is a variable age depending on the age and experience of the operator, the ovaries can be conserved, providing that there is no significant ovarian pathology or pelvic infection. This will prevent the long and short term effects of hormone deprivation. At the same time although a cuff of the vagina is removed this organ is not compromised and will certainly stretch to the size required for satisfactory coitus. Metastases to the ovaries are very rare with early stage cervical lesions and are said to occur in less than 0.5% (Baltzer *et al.* 1981). A re-exploration rate of 7.6% has been reported (Webb 1975) with ovarian pathology occurring in the future. The current practice is to conserve the ovaries in women aged 35 or less although individualization of patients may extend this to 40 years. When bilateral salpingo-oophorectomy is performed there is no reason for hormone replacement therapy to be withheld and indeed such therapy should be encouraged. Nevertheless, there is evidence to show that certain cervical tumours do have oestrogen and progesterone receptors but the exact significance of these is not yet apparent (Soutter *et al.* 1983).

Removal of the tumour also offers a psychological advantage to the patient in that the cancer has been extirpated. At the same time a functional and pliable vagina remains if irradiation is avoided. The complications of surgery, apart from those which can follow any surgical procedure such as postoperative chest infection, pulmonary emboli and possible wound infection, in the main centre around urological problems. An overall fistula or ureteric stricture rate of 1−2% is quoted (Webb & Symmonds 1979a,b; Benedet *et al.* 1980; Zander *et al.* 1981) although higher figures have been reported (Morley & Seski 1976; Langley *et al.*

1980) of up to 5%. In order to minimize complications it is important to maintain an adequate number of radical hysterectomy procedures performed in a single unit. Not only will this enable training of surgical and nursing staff, who may become readily familiar with the operative and postoperative management of such patients, but it will maintain one's own level of experience and skill with such delicate procedures.

A most important factor is knowing how to select patients for a surgical approach (Rutledge & Seski 1979). Primary surgical treatment should not be attempted when the lesion is so large that it precludes tumour-free margins, because if these are less than 1 cm, recurrence within 12−18 months of the operation will occur. The likelihood of adequate resection, therefore, must be of prime consideration before embarking on radical operations as a primary treatment. Although one can deliver postoperative irradiation therapy to patients with an apparently inadequate surgical excision either due to the tumour margins being close, or lymph node involvement being present, the normal anatomy is inevitably altered with adhesions forming so that the mobility of the small bowel and the lower abdomen is compromised. There is in fact no evidence to show that survival is improved by postoperative radiotherapy even though extended fields and higher dosages may be used after surgical removal of cancerous lymph nodes (Morrow *et al*. 1980; Fuller *et al*. 1982). Indeed the increased morbidity and mortality from such complications is quite marked (Rutledge *et al*. 1976).

Preoperative preparation

Preparation of the abdomen, perineum and vagina should be performed in the usual way with antiseptic toileting and douches. It is the author's preference to administer broad spectrum prophylactic antibiotics for 48 h postoperatively having commenced at induction of anaesthesia or with the premedication. The bowel should be emptied by suitable aperients and an enema the night before surgery. This will not only avoid a grossly loaded colon obstructing adequate surgical access to the pelvis, but also prevent severe constipation problems occurring immediately postoperatively. Any medical disorders such as diabetes, hypertension and anaemia, should be corrected as necessary prior to surgery. Preoperative mobilization and physiotherapy is of course vital, and the use of compression elastic stockings advisable. Prophylactic anticoagulation with subcutaneous heparin commencing with the premedication is advisable for any lengthy pelvic procedure to reduce the incidence of deep vein thrombosis and pulmonary embolism.

It is the author's current practice to explore the abdomen of patients with invasive carcinoma through a vertical lower midline incision that may be extended around the umbilicus as necessary. Although it is perfectly acceptable to perform hysterectomy and even radical hysterectomy via a Pfannensteil or low transverse incision, it is not safe or practical to perform para-aortic lymph node biopsies via this approach.

One of the main reasons for surgical treatment is so that an exploratory laparotomy may be carried out. Thorough and full assessment of the upper abdomen and retroperitoneal regions is only possible via such a vertical incision. Access to the pelvis and pelvic side walls for a lymphadenectomy, however, is just as efficient through the lower transverse incision.

Wertheim's radical hysterectomy: historical perspective

In 1878 Freund in Germany described a technique of total hysterectomy to treat cases of cervical cancer. The procedure carried an operative mortality of 50%. At the same time McGraw (1879) strongly recommended total hysterectomy for the treatment of this disease. Six years later it was demonstrated that it was possible to perform a pelvic lymphadenectomy with excision of the broad ligament while performing a hysterectomy in autopsy material (Ries 1895). In 1898 Wertheim from Vienna first performed a radical procedure removing pelvic lymph nodes as well as the parametrium in continuity with a total hysterectomy for cervical cancer (Wertheim 1900). His first 270 cases were reported in 1905 (Wertheim 1905) but a high surgical mortality as well as urinary and bowel fistula complication rate was associated. This meant that the developing use of radium and deep X-ray treatment gradually became more acceptable as an alternative therapy.

While surgical techniques were being explored, Roentgen discovered X-ray properties in 1895. Pierre and Marie Curie in 1898 first described radium which could be later used for the treatment of malignant disease. Margaret Cleeves in 1903 first used this for treating cervical cancer and then once the element had been prepared by Madame Curie in 1910 at the Sorbonne in Paris, its use became more widespread both in Europe and America. Three main centres developed their own techniques for administering radium between 1920 and 1940. These were the Radium Hemmet in Stockholm, the Curie Foundation in Paris and the Christie Hospital in Manchester, England. Meanwhile, Victor Bonney in London continued with the surgical approach and contended that radical abdominal hysterectomy performed in a slightly different way to that originally described by Wertheim should continue as the primary method of treatment for this disease (Bonney 1941). His practice with continued assessment and review of radical surgery (Bonney 1949) rightly earned him the position as the father of British pelvic surgery.

At a similar time, J.V. Meigs in Boston was becoming disenchanted with the results of irradiation therapy and its developing complications and side effects. He advised routine removal of all the pelvic lymph nodes and thus modified Wertheim's operation which had only sampled enlarged and palpable nodes (Meigs 1944). Although he demonstrated a 5-year survival of 75% for stage I and 54% for stage II disease, the postoperative fistula rate was in terms of 9% (Meigs 1951).

The ureter and complications resulting from radical surgery performed on tissues surrounding it, continued to be the *bête noir* of the pelvic surgeon.

However, a 12.5% complication rate including 8.5% incidence of ureterovaginal fistulae and a 4% incidence of ureteric stricture has been more than halved by continuous bladder drainage for 6 weeks postoperatively and by suspending the ureters to the obliterated hypogastric arteries (Green *et al*. 1962). Novak has suggested placing the dissected pelvic ureter on the peritoneal aspect of the pelvic peritoneum thus preserving the lateral mesentery to the terminal ureter. This may reduce the incidence of fistulae to 1–2% (Novak 1963).

These techniques coupled with current procedures including closed retroperitoneal suction drainage of the pelvic side walls, as well as closure of the vaginal vault, limit the incidence of pelvic cellulitis. Although the frequency of urinary tract fistulae is markedly increased after radical surgery following pelvic irradiation, the present incidence of such a complication with primary surgery is less than 2% in those centres undertaking radical pelvic surgery frequently (Webb & Symmonds 1979a,b; Benedet *et al*. 1980; Zander *et al*. 1981).

While this abdominal route was being advocated in Europe, radical vaginal hysterectomy was also being developed (Schauta 1902). The major drawback of this procedure is that excision of the paracervical tissues does not treat the entire tumour field at risk. Thus, if it is used for treating stage Ib lesions there is a failure rate of approximately 15% immediately, particularly in those patients who have metastatic tumour to the pelvic lymph nodes. Although less than half of these patients will be cured whatever the method of treatment chosen, the argument in favour of this local radical surgery must remain highly questionable. Nevertheless, in certain select patients it offers a useful alternative while at the same time gives a low incidence of ureteric fistulae and bladder dysfunction (Barclay & Roman-Lopez 1975). The author's preference is to reserve this particular procedure for patients who have a microinvasive tumour with a degree of uterine prolapse and who themselves would be better treated without an abdominal incision. Such patients might be obese with chronic chest conditions and possibly diabetes. Under these circumstances, the procedure is facilitated by a Schuhardt incision with subsequent mobilization of the upper third of the vagina. This is then closed and used for traction to facilitate dissection of the cervix, paracervical tissue and parametrial tissue. The ureters must be carefully palpated and this may be aided by preoperative ureteric catheterization in order to help identify these structures.

Pelvic lymphadenectomy may not be performed by this approach but an extraperitoneal lymphadenectomy as described by Mitra (1938) may be proceeded with following the hysterectomy.

Radical abdominal hysterectomy: surgical techniques

Having opened the abdomen a thorough exploration is made. Particular attention is paid to the liver, para-aortic nodes, kidneys, and ureters. The subdiaphragmatic spaces as well as the paracolic gutters, spleen, and appendix are inspected. Attention is then drawn to the pelvis where the size of the uterus and cervix is noted. The mobility of the organ is assessed and any extension of disease beyond the cervix into the parametria and paracervical tissue is noted. The ovaries and fallopian tubes are inspected as well as the bladder and rectum. The pelvic side walls are carefully palpated to see if there is any obvious lymph node involvement. If the nodes are negative to palpation, the surgeon is correct 94% of the time (Welander *et al*. 1981). If the nodes, however, are suspicious clinically then the accuracy of this assessment is 59%.

PARA-AORTIC NODE ASSESSMENT

The posterior abdominal wall is displayed and the peritoneum overlying the bifurcation of the aorta incised. The para-aortic nodes must then be palpated and any enlarged or suspicious nodes may be selectively excised for a frozen section assessment. Should these prove positive, then clearly the procedure should be abandoned as the poor survival rate does not justify the morbidity of radical surgery. The incision in the posterior part of the perineum should then be closed and the pelvic resection proceeded with.

PELVIC NODE ASSESSMENT

The round ligaments are grasped and divided approximately midway between the uterus and lateral pelvic wall. The anterior leaf of the broad ligament is then incised both proximally and distally thus exposing the pelvic side walls. The lymph nodes may then be palpated along the external iliac artery distally and then proximally at the bifurcation of the common iliac and from there to the bifurcation of the aorta. Positive common iliac nodes are an ominous finding associated with 5-year survival of only 25% (Martimbeau *et al*. 1982) thus questioning the value of continuing with the procedure should these nodes be grossly involved. Positive nodes below the common iliac were associated with a 60% cure rate in the same report. Thus, it is reasonable to continue with the procedure in the presence of isolated metastases to either the external or internal iliac nodes or even the obturator region. Because of the higher recurrence rate that occurs when pelvic nodes are positive one might argue that the procedure should be terminated if more than one group of nodes were to be involved or if bilaterally involved nodes are encountered. However, although postoperative radiotherapy is not generally associated with an improvement in the survival there is evidence to show that complete and total pelvic lymphadenectomy in the presence of positive nodes accompanied with a radical hysterectomy followed by whole pelvic radiotherapy may be beneficial. Such patients may have a 71% 5-year survival as compared with a 45% survival in patients who only have node sampling followed by radiotherapy (Heller *et al*. 1981).

PELVIC NODE DISSECTION

Having decided that the procedure should continue, a complete and comprehensive pelvic lymphadenectomy is performed removing the external iliac, internal iliac, obturator and common iliac lymph nodes (Fig. 4.2). The dissection thus proceeds from the femoral ring, just proximal to which a small tributary of the external iliac vein crosses the artery. This is the superficial circumflex iliac vein and marks the limit of the dissection. The genito-femoral nerve is identified and carefully preserved. The external iliac vessels should be carefully mobilized and inspected posteriorly to ensure that there are no further nodes hidden from view along the pelvic side wall. The sheath of lymph node tissue in the obturator fossa is carefully mobilized and attention paid to the obturatory nerve. Occasionally an aberrant obturator vein may be present and one should avoid severing this if at all possible. Inter-iliac nodes may be present and these are removed in continuity with the hypogastric or internal iliac lymph nodes. If this vessel is to be ligated as part of the procedure this may be performed at this stage. Common iliac lymph nodes are removed in a similar fashion, care being paid to avoid damaging the adjacent veins throughout, especially in this region where the vena cava commences on the right side.

CONSERVATION OF OVARIES?

A decision must be made as to whether the ovaries are to be conserved or not. The infundibulopelvic ligaments are ligated and divided in the usual way if they are to be removed and these included in the *en bloc* specimen. Should ovarian

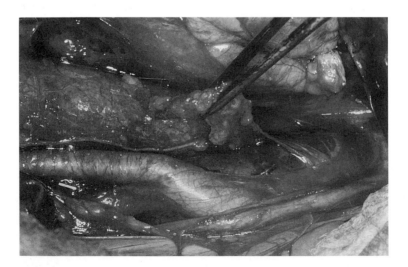

Fig. 4.2.   Pelvic side wall during lymphadenectomy showing the ureter crossing the bifurcation of the common iliac artery.

conservation be decided upon then the ovarian ligament is divided and the ovaries mobilized on their pedicle from the infundibulopelvic ligament. These may be elevated to the pelvic brim and preserved intraperitoneally once the peritoneum is closed at the termination of the procedure. The fallopian tubes are removed in continuity with the broad ligament and the parametrial tissue. The author's policy is to remove the ovaries in patients aged 35 years and over. There is little merit in conserving a single ovary.

URETERIC DISSECTION

The ureter is carefully identified on the medial leaf of the broad ligament and this is mobilized and separated from the peritoneum. A medium-sized soft rubber drain may be placed around the ureter for identification and gentle traction to facilitate separation for the peri-ureteric fascia and lymph nodes as well as the peritoneum. This is divided proximal to the cardinal ligament where the ureter enters a tunnel formed by the condensation of fascia spreading from the uterus laterally to the pelvic side wall. This tissue is situated between the paravesical space distally and the pararectal space posteriorly. Having identified and divided this fascia the uterine artery is exposed crossing the ureter at this point. This is divided and ligated laterally close to its origin from the anterior division of the internal iliac artery or on occasions the superior vesical artery prior to this division. This block of fascial tissue containing the uterine pedicle and peri-ureteric lymphatics is drawn medially and the fascia forming the ureteric tunnel defined. This tunnel is exposed and deroofed, releasing the ureter allowing direct visualization of the cardinal ligaments. The cardinal ligament is thus incised and the majority included in the specimen. A full Wertheim's radical abdominal hysterectomy includes excision of the cardinal ligaments in continuity with the parametrial and paracervical tissue from the lateral extreme close to the pelvic side wall. This is as opposed to a modified Wertheim's hysterectomy which does not require such extensive mobilization of the ureter and excision of the lateral ligaments.

SEPARATION OF THE BLADDER FROM VAGINA

The ureter is traced and dissected free distally towards the trigone. The uretero–vesical junction is visualized as it is separated from the vagina. At the same time the vesico–cervical fascia is excised and the bladder mobilized anteriorly using an open swab or Lahey dab. Two to three centimetres of vagina may be removed and indeed more if necessary in order to enable a good surgical margin of resection to be obtained (Fig. 4.3). More may be required if the tumour is stage IIa with extension of tumour on to the vaginal fornix.

Having mobilized the vagina anteriorly attention is then paid to the uterosacral ligaments posteriorly. The peritoneum overlying these ligaments is divided thus

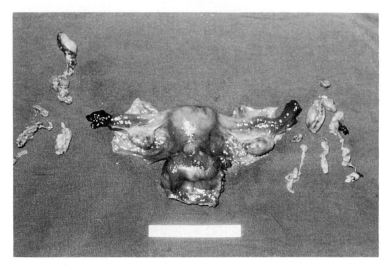

Fig. 4.3.   Radical abdominal hysterectomy specimen. Note adequate parametrial and paracervical tissue clearance as well as a 3 cm cuff of vagina.

incising across the pouch of Douglas. An arch may be identified by elevating the uterus and clearing the fascia from the uterosacral ligaments using a swab on a stick. Denonvilliers's fascia is opened and the rectovaginal septum displayed. The uterosacral ligaments are then clamped and divided allowing the dissection to continue distally. Large curved clamps may be placed immediately beneath the cervix across the vagina in order to obtain more traction and facilitate visualization of the vaginal length that is being removed. The vagina is then transected having held the angles in separate clamps. The specimen is removed (Fig. 4.4) and the pelvis and empty pouch of Douglas are inspected for haemostasis. The vaginal vault is then closed using interrupted figure of eight sutures once the angles have been transfixed.

SUSPENSION OF THE URETERS

The rubber retraction drains are removed from around the ureters and the distal third of these structures is then hitched using 3.0 chromic catgut to the obliterated portion of the hypogastric artery. This in itself is not always obliterated and may in fact continue as the superior vesical artery. This procedure, using two or three separate interrupted sutures through the serosal aspect of the ureteric fascia, will elevate the ureter out of the pelvis and away from inevitable collection of serosanguinous fluid that may pool there. It will also allow a secondary blood supply to form.

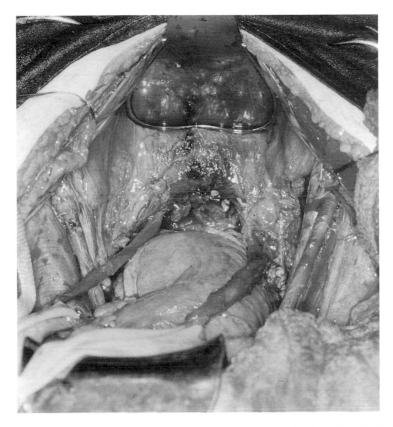

Fig. 4.4. Empty pelvis having closed the vagina prior to reperitonealization. Note both the ureters running over the recto-sigmoid colon in this view.

PERITONEAL CLOSURE

The pelvic peritoneum is closed thus leaving the major pedicles extraperitoneal and covering the pelvic floor so preventing the small bowel from adhering to any raw surfaces. If insufficient peritoneum is available then the recto-sigmoid may be utilized in order to reduce the depth of the pelvis and pouch of Douglas. Should this not be possible, especially in cases that have had preoperative radiotherapy, then the omentum may be mobilized and transplanted into the pelvis. This is most easily achieved by dividing the infracolic omentum and separating it from the hepatic flexure once the two leaves of omentum within their vascular plane have been identified. Approximately half the length of omentum is then laid across the pelvis and secured with interrupted catgut sutures. The small bowel may then be placed across this in anatomical position in such a way as to prevent excessive adhesion formation and subsequent post-operative obstruction.

ABDOMINAL CLOSURE

The abdomen is then closed as for any laparotomy. The author's preference is to use a single layer of a strong monofilament material such as polypropylene. When closed in continuity this is associated with a low dehiscence or incisional hernia rate (Shepherd *et al.* 1982). This layer may then be covered using a continuous fine plain catgut suture to the superficial fascia and the skin closed using either interrupted sutures or fine stainless steel staples.

Surgical staging of cervical cancer

In order to gain a complete assessment about the stage of a particular tumour, it is essential to have adequate information regarding the extent of spread. Although large lymph node metastases may be detected by a CT scan of the pelvis and abdomen, as well as by lymphangiography, in general lymph node disease needs to be greater than 1 cm in diameter for it to be detected. A case can be made for surgical staging even in advanced disease in order to gain precise information about the para-aortic nodes. Fifty percent of all patients with cervical cancer have spread into the parametrium on presentation; these patients will be treated mainly by radiotherapy. Treatment failure will occur, however, unless all the lymph nodes that are involved are included in the field of treatment. In stage I, the incidence of positive aortic nodes varies from 5.6% (Lagasse *et al.* 1980) to 7% (Sudarsanem *et al.* 1978). Stage II disease will increase with positive para-aortic node involvement in about 17% of patients, and in stage III, the incidence is about 28%.

Pretreatment surgical staging has its proponents, claiming that the operation is relatively safe. The argument against this is that complications due to radiotherapy are increased due to postoperative adhesions, especially those that may prevent free movement of the gastrointestinal tract. Also the commencement of radiotherapy treatment is delayed. Providing the dose of radiation given to the para-aortic nodes if these are positive, does not exceed 5000 centigray, the long term morbidity is acceptable particularly if an extraperitoneal approach for the lymphadenectomy is used. Laterally placed incisions do allow an adequate retroperitoneal approach to the para-aortic lymph node area. At the same time, the abdominal contents may be reflected so that sampling of the pelvic nodes may be carried out. Alternatively, a midline incision allows a transabdominal approach for selective lymphadenectomy. At present, however, surgical operative staging has failed to realize its aim of improving survival although it does provide invaluable information on the biological behaviour of the disease and incidence of lymph nodes peripherally (Hacker 1988). The relatively high incidence of positive aortic lymph nodes in patients with advanced cervical cancer may argue in favour of prophylactic extended field radiotherapy without operative staging. This question has been addressed both in the radiation therapy oncology group

(Rotman *et al.* 1986) and the EORTC studies (Haie *et al.* 1988) and neither have shown any significant improvement in survival. However, the EORTC study did demonstrate significant reduction in the frequency of para-aortic metastases and distant metastases without focal recurrence in a group receiving extended field radiation.

Nevertheless, by improving techniques with CT scanning and lymphangiography and perhaps combining the two, a major laparotomy may be avoided. When competition for theatre time with current restriction on bed availability is a determining factor for which patients may be operated upon urgently, it may be better to plan therapy, avoiding this rather radical way of staging the disease. Delay with surgery would only lead to further delay with the commencement of therapy. Nevertheless, it is clear that clinical staging is notoriously inaccurate with a poor correlation between clinical stage and subsequent surgical findings (Lapolla *et al.* 1986). Similarly, occult advanced carcinoma may occur at an early stage and this would explain further treatment failure with unassessable disease being present at the time of primary treatment be it radiotherapy or surgery (Ward *et al.* 1985).

Postoperative care

Closed suction drainage is used to drain the pelvic side walls and the pelvis. Medium sized 'portovac' or 'redivac' drains are inserted after closing the pelvic peritoneum through separate incisions in the left and right iliac fossae so that the catheter tubing may be placed into the obturator fossa. These drains are then sutured to the skin using black silk to prevent inadvertent early removal. It is important that these drains should be kept patent by 'milking' the tube 6-hourly otherwise a clot may form and thus block the tubes. These drains initially yield up to 500 cc within the first 24 h of a sero-sanguinous and lymphatic drainage and this gradually decreases. However, on the fifth or sixth day there may be a sudden increase and so it is worthwhile maintaining this drainage for 7 to 10 days until it has decreased sufficiently. This prevents lymphocyst formation: it is, however, important not to continue drainage for too long as this provides a route of infection.

A catheter is left in the bladder for 10 to 14 days for continuous bladder drainage. This not only prevents retention of urine and over distension of the bladder but also avoids the distal third of the ureter and bladder base being surrounded by any fluid collection which may be present within the pelvis. As sympathetic denervation is inevitable with a radical hysterectomy procedure, this period of bladder drainage reduces the dysfunction that may occur. Bladder physiology is grossly altered by dissection of the lateral ligaments (Forney 1980) but satisfactory bladder control may be obtained with the help of suitable postoperative pelvic floor exercises and physiotherapy. Recatheterization is rarely required but on occasions especially in post radiotherapy cases, it may be necessary for up to 6 weeks.

The average operating time is approximately 2½ h and estimated blood loss between 1000 and 1250 cc. The patient is transfused a suitable volume as replacement and also given plasma expanders using colloid as indicated. It is essential to maintain a good postoperative urine output and so postoperative fluid replacement with crystalloid solutions continues. A urine output of approximately 30–40 cc per hour is maintained by careful manipulation and maintenance of the haemodynamic status. A central venous pressure line is useful for this and should be inserted prior to the procedure. The use of diuretics should be avoided as the usual cause of oliguria is hypovolaemia, which itself should be corrected.

If a para-aortic lymphadenectomy has been performed then nasogastric suction using a Ryles tube should be continued so as to minimize the effects of a paralytic ileus that might ensue from any paravertebral haematoma or fluid collection. This may usually be removed after 48 h. The patient is mobilized the day following surgery and may certainly sit out of bed and have routine chest and passive leg physiotherapy. Low dose anticoagulation continues until full mobilization in order to reduce the risk of deep vein thrombosis. Despite this there is still an 8% pulmonary embolus rate although the incidence of fatal pulmonary embolism is reduced.

The patient is usually discharged home on or around the fourteenth day to continue her convalescence accordingly.

Complications of surgery

The main complications associated with radical pelvic surgery are haemorrhage and sepsis. Haemorrhage may occur during the pelvic lymphadenectomy especially following radiotherapy when the pelvic veins are encountered. Dissection of the bladder from the vagina and mobilization of the trigone may also lead to profuse bleeding from large veins or sinuses. Ligation of the hypogastric (internal iliac) artery may reduce this loss but is not routinely necessary or effective.

Prolonged operating time may increase the incidence of postoperative complications especially infection, either pelvic sepsis or pneumonia. The incidence of pelvic thrombosis also increases with undue pressure on the pelvic veins or calves. For this reason, early mobilization as well as the use of stockings to compress the superficial veins or preoperative intermittent calf compression by pneumatic boots may be employed. This is in addition to prophylactic anticoagulation using subcuticular heparin.

The atonic bladder may be a problem in approximately 3% of patients (Green 1966; Langley *et al.* 1980). The latter advised suprapubic drainage and the former urethral catheterization for 6 weeks. As this complication rate is similar in both reports the occurrence of bladder atony therefore may be assumed to be due to bladder denervation and not to the method of postoperative bladder drainage.

Although this incidence may be decreased by a lesser procedure avoiding excessive excision of the lateral ligaments and thus sympathetic nerve destruction (Forney 1980; Lowe *et al.* 1981) this would not be suitable for radical extirpation of an invasive tumour.

Ureteric fistula was formerly the most feared complication of this operation. As already discussed, it is now relatively uncommon with current operative techniques and surgical practice, being in terms of 1–2% (Shepherd & Crowther 1988). Urinary infection may occur in approximately 10% of patients and is more common when urethral catheters are used. Once prophylactic parenteral antibiotics have been stopped after 48 h, then catheter antiseptic prophylaxis is employed using a sulphonamide. A broader spectrum of antibiotics may be used as indicated from urine cultures. A postoperative intravenous urogram will show transient ureteric dilatation above the pelvic brim associated with a dilatation of the renal pelvis but these changes usually return to normal within 3 months.

Febrile morbidity is low, occurring in 10–20% of patients, and the major causes of this are pulmonary atelectasis, urinary tract infections, wound infections or haematoma, pelvic cellulitis, pelvic or deep venous thrombosis and a pelvic abscess.

Pelvic lymphocysts may form with an incidence of between 1 and 29% being quoted (Dodd *et al.* 1970; Kaser *el al.* 1973). Although they develop relatively infrequently, up to 70% of those developing lymphocysts will have poorly differentiated tumours (Ilancheran & Monaghan 1988). This may be the first indication of recurrent disease. Careful attention to detail creating lymphostasis as well as haemostasis when performing the lymphadenectomy and also suction drainage of the pelvic side wall, can minimize this risk. Most lymphocysts will resolve but should they not decrease in size, or become symptomatic then simple aspiration with a needle may be carried out as necessary. On occasions, transperitoneal marsupialization of the lymphocyst or drainage may become necessary especially if ureteric compression occurs.

Damage may occur to the obturator nerve either by severing during dissection of the obturator nodes or pressure from traction causing temporary neurotmesis. If severed it should be resutured so that it may regenerate, otherwise weakness in adduction of the thigh may result (although this is not a major disability). Femoral nerve compression can result in a neuropathy from self-retaining retractors, with pressure exerted on the ilio-psoas muscle. Similarly, peroneal nerve compression may result from the pressure on the neck of the fibula if the patient is placed in the lithotomy position for the procedure (although this is not the usual practice).

Follow up

Having been discharged home, the patient is reviewed for follow up postoperatively 4 to 6 weeks later and then 3-monthly for 2 years. Visits are then decreased to 6-monthly and then annually as indicated. Should recurrence occur, this will usually manifest within 12 months and the majority of patients will die within the next 2 years (Calame 1969). Diagnosis of recurrent cervical carcinoma can present a dilemma but it is essential to discover this early if such patients are to be saved (Shepherd *et al.* 1982). Although clinical examination in conjunction with chest X-rays and intravenous urograms are essential for follow up and certainly cost effective (Photopulos *et al.* 1977) the use of computerized axial tomography with fine needle aspiration cytology is proving an invaluable technique (Nordqvist *et al.* 1979). Regrettably, vault smears and even punch biopsies of the surface epithelium of the vagina are associated with a significant false negative rate but deeper needle biopsies using the 'Tru-cut' needle may detect central recurrence at an earlier stage (Shepherd *et al.* 1981).

Results of surgery

The 5-year survival and therefore prognosis is dependent on the presence or absence of certain factors. Clearly survival is dependent upon an adequate surgical excision with wide margins of clearance around the tumour. This is a basic surgical principle. Hence, an adequate vaginal cuff as well as paracervical and parametrial excision is necessary. Deep stromal involvement of the cervix is sinister. The deeper the tumour invades the stroma, the more likely it is to involve lymphatic spaces with subsequent micrometastases to lymph nodes. A large tumour volume is not surprisingly associated with a poor prognosis (Burghardt & Pichel 1980).

Survival rates of 76–87% have been achieved in stage Ib (Morley & Seski 1976; Kovacic *et al.* 1980). This survival drops to 48.5% if between one and four positive pelvic nodes are present and to 19% if five or more nodes are involved (Hsu *et al.* 1972). Although certain reports have found that bilaterally involved pelvic nodes may also halve survival from in terms of 50 to 25% (Pilleron *et al.* 1974) this does not agree with other reports which in contrast ascribe no significance to bilaterality of pelvic node metastases (Webb & Symmonds 1979a; Martimbeau *et al.* 1982).

Age is being repeatedly questioned as a prognostic factor. There is now little evidence to show that patients beneath the age of 40 fare far worse than those over this age.

Comparison of results with radiotherapy and combined treatment

Results obtained by surgery are very similar to those treated by radiotherapy. Currently accepted 5-year survival figures for early stage disease range between 78% (Kottmeier 1964) and 83.5% (Fletcher 1971).

An impressive comparative study reported by Morley (Morley & Seski 1976) showed a 5-year cure rate of 87% with radical surgery as compared with a similar survival (83.4%) with primary radiation therapy. The role, however, of combined radiotherapy and surgery in the treatment of cervical carcinoma, remains controversial. There is little evidence to show that such combination treatment improves the survival rate when compared with either a full radical course of radiation therapy to the pelvis or radical surgery alone (Talbert et al. 1965; Shingleton & Palumbo 1968).

Combination therapy

At face value it would appear that combining radiotherapy with surgery might afford a lesser morbidity in that less radical treatment of either modality may be administered. However, this is not the case and radiotherapy administered either before radical surgery or after extensive radical hysterectomy and subsequent possible adhesion formation may give rise to an increased incidence of fistula due to radionecrosis and endarteritis. This is a continuing problem which can occur for many years after treatment. There appears to be little advantage with survival (Perez et al. 1980; Shingleton & Orr 1983). It has been argued that with a bulky tumour measuring more than 5 cm in diameter, preoperative radiotherapy to the whole pelvis can shrink the tumour size and then allow a less radical extended hysterectomy to be performed (Van Nagell et al. 1979). The theoretical advantage of this approach is that malignant tumour cells may continue to be viable within a large bulky cervical tumour. However, this is not always the case and other retrospective studies have shown that postoperative radiotherapy given when surgically proven positive nodes are present does not necessarily improve survival (Rutledge et al. 1976; Fuller et al. 1982; Martimbeau et al. 1982). Certainly the morbidity can be increased due to postoperative adhesions and the alteration in surgical anatomy (Rutledge et al. 1976). Few randomized studies comparing preoperative radiotherapy and surgery or irradiation alone in the treatment of stage Ib and IIa carcinoma of the cervix have been carried out. Those studies that have been completed however indicate essentially the same survival rates and incidence of complications for radiotherapy alone or in combination with radical hysterectomy (Perez et al. 1987). There are those proponents of radiotherapy who have found a better survival with patients treated by combination treatment (Einhorn et al. 1985). This is in contrast to other treatment combinations combining radiotherapy with surgery (Surwit et al. 1976).

Most authorities would maintain that there does not appear to be a significant advantage to the combined therapy for stages Ib or IIa cervical cancer. However, the combination approach for women with a bulky barrel-shaped endocervical tumour may well still be applicable although whether radiotherapy is given pre- or postoperatively is a matter for debate and perhaps individual preference depending on the unit concerned.

Prognostic factors

The prognosis of a malignant disease is influenced by a variety of factors and will depend on the time and therefore stage at which the tumour is discovered. Pure clinical methods cannot determine a tumour's growth characteristics or predict its tendency to metastasize (Burghardt *et al*. 1987). Morphological analysis indicates that the single most important prognostic factor is tumour size in terms of absolute tumour area and the tumour/cervix quotient as a measure of volumetric density (Haas 1988). The larger the primary tumour, the higher the incidence of positive lymph nodes. Thus, if significant prognostic factors are ranked statistically, the following would be the most significant: (1) tumour/cervix quotient; (2) number of positive lymph node groups; (3) infiltration of the tissue layer containing the large vessels; (4) exophytic growth; (5) parametrial invasion; (6) lymph node involvement, and (7) number of mitoses.

Overall tumour size in terms of volume is more predictive of the outcome than a measurement of diameter which has been used in the past. Nevertheless, once the tumour reaches the diameter of 4 cm the incidence of positive pelvic lymph nodes increases in stage Ib from 15 to 39% and the survival drops from a mean of 84% to 56% (Piver & Chung 1975; Fuller *et al*. 1989). Recurrence in tumours larger than 2 cm in diameter is considerably greater than in those of less than this size (Van Nagell *et al*. 1977).

Conditions requiring special consideration

Large barrel-shaped endocervical lesions

These present a special problem as primary radical surgery is unlikely to effect a cure due to the bulk of tumour. Preoperative whole pelvic radiotherapy followed by a single intracavitary application has therefore been recommended prior to conservative hysterectomy (Fletcher 1979). However, recurrence following this combined irradiation and more conservative hysterectomy approach is more likely to occur in distant sites and not within the radiation field (Nelson *et al*. 1975). A more reasonable approach is therefore to assess each individual case on the merits afforded it. If the response is good with the tumour bulk shrinking clinically, then radiotherapy may be completed avoiding surgery. However, if there is any evidence of residual tumour after whole pelvic radiotherapy has been completed on either endocervical curettage or 'Tru-cut' biopsy of the cervix itself, then clearly hysterectomy is required. The risk of complications in such a patient is increased over that of patients treated with irradiation alone and a fistula rate of 8.6% has been reported under these circumstances (O'Quinn *et al.* 1980).

Adenocarcinoma of the cervix

Cervical adenocarcinoma is less common than squamous cell carcinoma. The reported incidence is between 5 and 10% (Anderson & Fraser 1976; Hurt *et al.* 1977) and there is a suggestion that the relative proportion of adenocarcinoma is increasing (Davis & Moon 1975). Survival rates in stage Ib are as would be expected, significantly worse for those poorly differentiated tumours and for those with involved pelvic lymph nodes. Stage for stage, when compared with squamous cell carcinoma, there appears to be no difference in age at presentation, node metastases or survival (Ireland *et al.* 1984). Results of treatment by either surgery or radiotherapy are much the same. Bulky stage Ib lesions are more suitable for treatment by radiotherapy (Shingleton *et al.* 1981) whereas an acceptable alternative would be whole pelvic radiotherapy followed by a conservative hysterectomy (Nelson *et al.* 1975). It is important when making the diagnosis to assess whether the disease is truly a primary arising in the cervix or an extension of a tumour from the endometrial cavity. Stage for stage, however, it is not unreasonable to treat the patients in much the same way as a squamous cell tumour.

Clear cell adenocarcinoma of the cervix and vagina

Young women and teenagers with clear cell adenocarcinoma should also be treated by radical hysterectomy and lymphadenectomy with vaginectomy (Herbst *et al.* 1979). Wide excision is not enough but on occasions total pelvic exenteration may be necessary with extensive disease (Hill & Galante 1981). Surgery does avoid the complications in the long term of radiotherapy and, as yet, chemotherapy has not been shown to be effective.

Cervical stump carcinoma

This may arise when invasive carcinoma develops in a patient who has previously been treated with a subtotal hysterectomy for a benign condition. This problem is becoming less common but it may present special difficulties both for surgical and radiotherapy techniques. In general, however, the problem may be treated either by a radical cervicectomy in conjunction with a bilateral pelvic lymphadenectomy or by special intracavitary applicators and after-loading equipment for radiotherapy. Alternatively, a low vaginal cone technique in conjunction with whole pelvic radiotherapy may be employed.

Treatment following cone biopsy

Traditionally following conization of the cervix, further surgery is performed either within 48 h or after 6 weeks to minimize the increased risk from pelvic infection. However, recent evidence suggests that this interval prior to radical hysterectomy is not an important factor causing postoperative morbidity (Webb & Symmonds 1979b; Orr *et al.* 1982). Thus, if invasive disease is present, once the patient has recovered from the initial cone biopsy, radical hysterectomy may be proceeded with as soon as it is appropriate.

Unexpected diagnosis at simple hysterectomy

Occasionally the pathology report will indicate invasive carcinoma as a surprising and unexpected diagnosis after hysterectomy has been performed for some other benign pathology and reason. A decision then needs to be taken depending on the depth of invasion as to whether further treatment is required. If a true stage Ib lesion is in fact suspected the choice lies between 'blind' postoperative radiotherapy: intracavity caesium with or without whole pelvic radiotherapy or further surgery. The latter in younger fit women should be considered, although it can be difficult, exacting surgery endangering the bladder, ureters and rectum. This involves completing the radical hysterectomy by performing a radical parametrectomy and upper colpectomy with bilateral pelvic lymphadenectomy and selective para-aortic sampling. The colpectomy is best approached as a combined abdomino—perineal (transvaginal) procedure.

Cervical cancer during pregnancy

These two conditions provide a difficult therapeutic dilemma for not only the gynaecologist but also the patient. The sense of joy and pleasure at being told initially that she is pregnant is then totally shattered by the disastrous news that she has cancer. The pregnancy itself does not appear to alter the course or prognosis significantly but vaginal delivery is absolutely contraindicated. Not only can the disease disseminate through larger cervical venous sinuses and dilated lymphatic spaces, but also can be transmitted down the vagina to result in metastatic disease in the lower third, for example in episiotomy sites. In the first and second trimester the patient should be treated as in a non-pregnant stage, stage for stage, but as foetal viability is approached, then an elective caesarian section followed by the appropriate therapy is indicated. With an early stage tumour, a Wertheim's hysterectomy following delivery of the foetus by a classical caesarian section is the most appropriate method of treatment especially in the young and fit person. As in the non-pregnant state, ovarian conservation may be performed and the long term side effects of radiotherapy can be avoided. The procedure may be more hazardous than when undertaken in the non-pregnant state due to the increased vascularity but fortunately the tissue planes may often be more easily demarcated with an increase in tissue oedema. However, the procedure should only be performed by those familiar with radical surgery and not by the casual obstetric surgeon.

Lymph node metastases

Tumours greater than 2 or 3 cm in diameter which extend into the myometrium or more than two-thirds of the way through the cervix are associated with a high risk of lymph node metastases (Piver & Chung 1975) and also with a lymphatic or vascular space invasion (Gauthier et al. 1985). The recurrence rate is also greater (Ward et al. 1985).

Lymphatic or vascular space involvement significantly decreases survival (Barber et al. 1978) as does lymph node involvement (Lagasse et al. 1974). While microinvasive carcinoma (less than 3 mm of invasion) has reported lymph node incidence of less than 2%, stage Ib has an average of 17% involvement (Hoskins 1988). Series differ with figures varying from 9% (Artman et al. 1987) to 31% (Burghardt et al. 1987). However, once stage III is reached, 50% of lymph nodes may be involved in the pelvis (Shingleton et al. 1983). Para-aortic node involvement varies from 6% in stage Ib to 40% in advanced disease.

Histological grade has an influence on the incidence of nodal metastases with 9% of well differentiated tumours and 25% of poorly differentiated tumours metastasizing to lymph nodes (Fuller et al 1988). Similarly, recurrence in well differentiated tumours may occur in between 10 and 22%, whereas between 28 and 31% of poorly differentiated tumours will recur (Burke et al. 1987).

The question of age affecting the prognosis remains debatable as an independent variable when compared to grade. Kyriakos et al 1971 and Berkowitz et al. 1979 have reported no difference in the rate of recurrence or survival in patients with cervical cancer on the basis of age. However Prempree et al. 1983 reported an increased incidence of more poorly differentiated tumours in patients under the age of 35. The general feeling is that the age of the patient at diagnosis does not appear to be a risk factor and it may be that much of the influence either way is due to anecdotal impressions.

Adjuvant therapy in node positive patients

It would appear that 20 to 25% of patients with early stages of disease will relapse after primary therapy. The majority of these patients will present with recurrent disease either centrally or on the pelvic side walls. The two most important factors which may account for this recurrence within the pelvis are the tumour volume and the presence of lymphatic metastases at the time of primary therapy. Thus, local cure will depend on eradicating macroscopic disease in the cervix as well as occult disease in the vaginal fornices and macroscopic or microscopic metastases in the pelvic lymph nodes and lymphatics. If the cervical tumour is large radiotherapy may fail to eradicate the disease completely. Such large tumours may be relatively radio-resistant. However, there is evidence to show that radiotherapy is capable of sterilizing involved pelvic lymph nodes if adequate dosimetry is achieved (Lagasse *et al.* 1974). Adequate surgery will preclude central recurrence providing the margins of resection are clear of tumour, but the survival of patients with positive lymph nodes is only between 50 and 60%, even with pelvic lymphadenectomy and postoperative external beam therapy (Rutledge *et al.* 1965).

The prognostic factors that are important in cervical cancer are clearly tumour volume, depth of invasion, lymphatic and blood vessel invasion, tumour type and grade, as well as patient age. Lymph node involvement is certainly the most well recognized adverse prognostic factor. These patients have a potential for systemic rather than local and confined disease. With current accepted and conventional management at least 40% of these patients with positive lymph nodes detected at primary surgery will relapse after their initial treatment. There is, therefore, a need for systemic adjuvant therapy.

Phase II trials in recurrent cervical cancer have shown that the most active single agents in this disease are ifosfamide and cisplatinum. These both show response rates of approximately 40%. The most active combination regimes have been those that contain bleomycin and cisplatinum. The results are now becoming available to show that the combination of bleomycin, ifosfamide and cisplatinum (BIP) can produce objective response rates of up to 70% in patients with recurrent disease, and therefore a study has now been commenced to assess this in an adjuvant setting in patients with positive lymph nodes detected at surgery. Other drug combinations being utilized include platinum, methotrexate and bleomycin (PMB) and the morbidity with regard to hair loss and patient acceptability from the latter regime may be more acceptable than the former.

There is clearly a need for full evaluation of such adjuvant therapy and current trials will compare the value of chemotherapy plus radiotherapy versus radiotherapy alone in patients found to have positive lymph nodes at the time of Wertheim's radical hysterectomy.

Conclusion

Cervical cancer remains a disease which may be treated adequately and effectively in the early stage by either radical radiotherapy to the whole pelvis or radical surgery depending on the facilities available in a particular unit. With improving surgical techniques and supportive therapy the advantages of surgical treatment

Table 4.2. Advantages and disadvantages of surgery and radiotherapy

Advantages Radiotherapy as applied to all patients	Surgery
May be given as an outpatient and survival rates are similar to surgery	Psychological effect of extirpation of the primary tumour Conservation of ovaries in the young Coincidental adnexal masses or pyosalpinges with infected adnexal may be removed Accurate surgical staging A more pliable although shortened vagina remains
Disadvantages Radiotherapy	Surgery
Vaginal stenosis with consequent dryness and rigidity with a lack of sensation Urinary tract complications. Haemorrhagic cystitis, urinary frequency and a contracted bladder, chronic haematuria, ureteric stricture, fistulae (uretero−vaginal and vesico−vaginal) Bowel complications. Chronic diarrhoea, flatulence, procto-colitis, rectal stricture, malabsorption from the terminal ileum. Fistula (entero−vaginal and recto−vaginal) Avascular necrosis of the femoral head Pyometria from cervical stenosis Ovarian ablation with consequent enforced menopause Risk of secondary malignancy	Complications from a prolonged operation (anaesthetic complications and haemorrhage) Infection in the chest, wound, urinary tract and pelvis Urological complications. Atonic bladder, frequency, reduced bladder capacity, and fistula (uretero−vaginal and vesico−vaginal) Lymphocyst formation with subsequent lymphoedema Obturator nerve damage during lymphadenectomy Paralytic ileus Thromboembolism Sexual dysfunction from shortened vagina Patient may still require postoperative radio/chemotherapy depending on the final findings at the laparotomy

especially in younger women with small lesions are obvious. The results of either modality are similar but careful consideration must be given to the possible side effects and complications in both short and long term on an individual basis (Table 4.2).

The dilemma arises, however, when patients with apparently localized disease are found to have spread beyond the cervix, be it macroscopic or microscopic in nature. These patients with poor prognostic criteria do not appear to have an increased chance of survival with combined therapy of surgery and radiotherapy. Consideration must therefore be given to adjunctive chemotherapy. The presently accepted regimes, however, have a low incidence of response in cervical cancer associated with a high morbidity rate. Nevertheless, if this group of patients with a poor prognosis is to be cured then this would have to be by a combination of either surgery and radiotherapy in conjunction with a suitable chemotherapeutic regimen. Such studies are in progress.

Finally it must be remembered that about one-third of patients will have recurrent disease (or residual and therefore progressive disease) and this figure increases to approximately two-thirds when the lymph nodes are positive and involved (Potish *et al.* 1985). Sixty percent of patients who develop recurrence will do so within the first year and a further 25% within the second year (Van Nagell *et al.* 1979; Krebs *et al.* 1982). The faster the recurrence, the worse the prognosis and 80% of these patients will die within 2 years of detection of the recurrence. Once recurrence has been detected following surgery then consideration must be given to radiotherapy treatment initially (see Chapter 17) with or without chemotherapy. Certain patients might be suitable for exenterative procedures if they have central mobile disease and radiotherapy has failed (see Chapter 5).

References

Abell M.R. & Ramirez J.A. (1973) Sarcomas and carcinosarcomas of the uterine cervix. *Cancer*, **31**, 1176–92.

ACOG (1977) Classification and staging of malignant tumours of the female pelvis. ACOG. *Tech. Bull.*, **47**.

American Cancer Society (1984) *Cancer Facts and Figures 1984*. American Cancer Society, New York.

Anderson M.C. & Fraser A.C. (1976) Adenocarcinoma of the uterine cervix. A clinical and pathological appraisal. *Br. J. Obstet. Gynaecol.*, **83** (4), 20–35.

Artman L.E., Hoskins W.J. & Bibro M.C. (1987) Radical lymphadenectomy and pelvic lymphadenectomy for stage IB carcinoma of the cervix: 21 years experience. *Gynecol. Oncol.*, **2**, 8–13.

Baltzer J., Lowe K.J., Koepcke W. & Zander J. (1981) Formation of metastases in the ovaries in operated squamous cell carcinoma of the cervix uteri. *Geburtshulfe Und Fraven Leilkunde*, **41**, 672–73.

Barber H.R.K., Sommers S.C., Rotterdam H. & Kwon T. (1978) Vascular invasion as a prognostic factor in Stage IB cancer of the cervix. *Obstet. Gynecol.*, **52**, 343–48.

Barclay D.A. & Roman-Lopez J.J. (1975) Bladder dysfunction after Schauta hysterectomy. *Am. J. Obstet. Gynecol.*, **123**, 519.

Bell D.A., Shimm D.S. & Gang D.L. (1985) Wilm's tumour of the endocervix. *Arch. Pathol. Lab. Med.*, **14**, 543–44.

Benedet J.L., Turko M., Boyes D.A. *et al.* (1980) Radical hysterectomy in the treatment of cervical cancer. *Am. J. Obstet. Gynecol.*, **137**, 254–62.

Beral V. & Booth M. (1986) Predictions of cervical cancer incidence and mortality in England and Wales. *Lancet*, **i**, 495.

Berek J.S., Hacker N. & Fu Y.S. (1984) Adenocarcinoma of the uterine cervix. Histological variables associated with lymph node metastasis and survival. *Obstet. Gynecol.*, **65**, 46.

Berkowitz R.S., Ehrmann R.L., Lavizzo-Mourey R. & Knapp R.C. (1979) Invasive cervical carcinoma in young women. *Gynaecol. Oncol.*, **8**, 311–16.

Bonney V. (1941) The results of 55 cases of Wertheim's operation for carcinoma of the cervix. *J. Obstet. Gynaecol. Brit. Emp.*, **48**, 421–35.

Bonney V. (1949) Wertheim's operation in retrospect. *Lancet*, **i**, 637–63.

Boyes D.A., Morrison B., Knox E.G., Draper G.J. & Miller A.B. (1982) A cohort study of cervical cancer screening in British Columbia. *Clin. Invest. Med.*, **5**, 1–29.

Brady L.W. (1979) Surgery or radiation therapy for stage I and IIA carcinoma of the cervix. *Int. J. Radiation Oncol. Biol. Phys.*, 1877—87.

Burghardt E., Bickel H. & Haas J. (1987) Prognostic factors and optional treatment of stages IB—IIB cervical cancer. *Am. J. Obstet. Gynecol.*, **156**, 988—96.

Burghardt E., Bickel H., Haas J. & Lahousen M. (1987) Prognostic factors and operative treatment of stages IB to IIB of cervical cancer. *Am. J. Obstet. Gynecol.*, **157**, 988—96.

Burke T.W., Hoskins W.J. & Heller P.B. (1987) Clinical patterns of tumour recurrence after radical hysterectomy in stage IB carcinoma of the cervix. *Obstet. Gynecol.*, **69**, 382—85.

Calame R.J. (1969) Recurrent carcinoma of the cervix. *Am. J. Obstet. Gynecol.*, **105**, 380—85.

Cherry C.P. & Gluckmann A. (1961) Histology of carcinoma of the uterine cervix and survival rates in pregnant and non-pregnant patients. *Surg. Gynaecol. Oncol.*, **113**, 763—76.

Copeland L.J., Sneige N., Ordonez N.G., Hancock K.C., Gershenson D.M., Saul P.B. & Kavanagh J. (1985) Endodermal sinus tumour of the vagina and cervix. *Cancer*, **55**, 2558—65.

Davis J.R. & Moon L.B. (1975) Increased incidence of adenocarcinoma of the uterine cervix. *Obstet. Gynecol.*, **45**, 79—83.

Delgado G. (1978) Stage IB squamous cancer of the cervix, the choice of treatment. *Obstet. Gynecol. Surg.*, **33**, 174—83.

Dodd G.D., Rutledge R. & Wallace S. (1970) Post-operative pelvic lymphocysts. *Am. J. Roentgenol.*, **108**, 312—23.

Einhorn N., Patek E. & Sjoberg B. (1985) Outcome of different treatment modalities in cervix carcinoma, stage IB and IIA. *Cancer*, **55**, 949—55.

Elliott P.M., Tattersall M.II., Coppleson M., Russell P., Wong F., Coares A.S., Soliman H.J., Bannatyne P.M., Atkinson K.H. & Murray J.C. (1989) Changing character of cervical cancer in young women. *Br. Med. J.*, **298**, 288—90.

Falk V., Lundgren N., Quarfordt L. *et al.* (1982) Primary surgical treatment stage I of the uterine cervix. *Acta Obstet. Gynecol. Scand.* **61**, 481—86.

Fletcher G.H. (1971) Cancer of the uterine cervix. *Am. J. Roentgenol. Radium Ther. Nucl. Med.*, **111**, 225—42.

Fletcher G.H. (1979) Predominant parameters in the planning of radiation therapy of carcinoma of the cervix. *Bull. Cancer.*, **66**, 561—72.

Flint A., Gikas P.W. & Roberts J.A. (1985) Alveolar soft part sarcoma of the uterine cervix. *Gynecol. Oncol.*, **22**, 263—67.

Forney J.P. (1980) The effect of radical hysterectomy on bladder physiology. *Am. J. Obstet. Gynecol.*, **138**, 374—82.

Freund W.A. (1878) Eine neue Methode der Exstirpation des ganzen Uterus. *Samml. Klin Vort. No.* **133** (Gynak No. 41: 911), Leipzig.

Fuller A.F., Elliott N. *et al.* (1982) Lymph node metastases from carcinoma of the cervix, stage IB and IIA. Implications for prognosis and treatment. *Gynecol. Oncol.*, **13**, 165—74.

Fuller A.F., Elliott N. & Kosloff C. (1989) Determinants of increased risk of recurrence in patients undergoing radical hysterectomy for a Stage IB and IIA carcinoma of the cervix. *Gynecol. Oncol. (in press)* **33**, 34—9.

Fuller A.F., Elliott N., Kosloff C. & Lewis J.L. (1982) Lymph node metastases from carcinoma of the cervix. Stage IB and IIA; implications for prognosis and treatment. *Gynecol. Oncol.*, **13**, 165—74.

Gallagher II.S., Simpson C.B. & Ayala A.G. (1971) Adenoid cystic carcinoma of the uterine cervix; report of four cases. *Cancer*, **27**, 1398—402.

Gallup D.G. & Abell M.R. (1977) Invasive adenocarcinoma of the uterine cervix. *Obstet. Gynecol.*, **49**, 596—603.

Gallup D.G., Harper R.H. & Stock R.J. (1985) Poor prognosis in patients with adenosquamous cell carcinoma of the cervix. *Obstet. Gynecol.*, **65**, 416—22.

Gauthier P., Gore I, Shingleton, H.M., Soong, S.J., Orr J.W. & Hatch K.D. (1985) Identification of histopathologic risk groups in Stage IB squamous cell carcinoma of the cervix. *Obstet. Gynecol.*, **66**, 569—74.

Gray L.A., Peterson G.K. & Barnes M.C. (1964) Combined irradiation and surgical treatment for cancer of the cervix uteri. *Proc. Natl. Cancer Conf.*, **5**, 229—39.

Green T.H. (1966) Ureteral suspension for prevention of ureteral complications following radical Wertheim's hysterectomy. *Obstet. Gynecol.*, **28**, 1—11.

Green T.H. Jr, Meigs J.V., Ulfelder H. *et al.* (1962) Urologic complications of radical Wertheim's hysterectomy: incidence, etiology, management and prevention. *Obstet. Gynecol.*, **20**, 293–303.

Haas J. (1988) Tumormetric measurements and morphometry in cervical cancer in operative treatment. *In*: Burghardt, E. & Monaghan J.M. (eds), *Clinical Obstetrics and Gynaecology*. Ballières.

Hacker N.F. (1988) Clinical and operative staging of cervical cancer in operative treatment of cervical cancer. *In*: Burghardt E. & Monaghan J.M. (eds), *Clinical Obstetrics and Gynaecology*. Ballière Tindall, London pp. 747–59.

Hacker N.F., Berek J. & Lagasse L.D. (1982) Carcinoma of the cervix associated with pregnancy. *Obstet. Gynecol.*, **59**, 735.

Haie C., Pejovic M.H. & Gerbaulet A. (1988) Is prophylactic para-aortic irradiation worthwhile in the treatment of advanced cervical carcinoma? The results of a controlled clinical trial of the EORTC radiotherapy group. *Rad. Oncol.*, **11**, 101.

Heller P.B., Lee R.B. & Lomas M.H. *et al.* (1981) Lymph node positivity in cervical cancer. *Gynecol. Oncol.*, **12**, 328–35.

Hendriksen E. (1949) The lymphatic spread of carcinoma of the cervix and the body of the uterus. A study of 420 necropsies. *Am. J. Obstet. Gynecol.*, **58**, 924–42.

Herbst A.L., Norusis M.J., Rosenow P.J., Welch W.R. & Scully R.E. (1979) An analysis of 346 cases with clear cell adenocarcinoma of the vagina and cervix with emphasis on recurrence and survival. *Gynecol. Oncol.*, **7**, 111–22.

Hill E.C. & Galante M. (1981) Radical surgery in the management of clear cell adenocarcinoma of the cervix and vagina in young women. *Am. J. Obstet. Gynecol.*, **140**, 221–26.

Hoskins W.J. (1988) Prognostic factors in stages IB and IIA in operative treatment of cervical cancer. *In*: Burghardt E. & Monaghan J.M. (eds), *Clin. Obstet. Gynaecol.*, Ballière Tindall, London, 817–28.

Hsu C.T., Chang Y.S. & Su S.C. (1972) Prognosis of uterine cervical cancer with extensive lymph node metastases. *Am. J. Obstet. Gynecol.*, **114**, 954–62.

Hurt W.G., Silverberg S.G. & Frable W.J. *et al.* (1977) Adenocarcinoma of the cervix. Histopathologic and clinical features. *Am. J. Obstet. Gynecol.*, **129**, 304–15.

Ireland D., Hardiman P. & Monaghan J.M. (1984) Adenocarcinoma of the uterine cervix: A study of 73 cases. *Obstet. Gynecol.*, **65**, 82–85.

Jones H.W., Plymate S., Glucks F.P., Miles F.A. & Green J.F. (1976) Small cell non keratinising carcinoma of the cervix associated with ACTH production. *Cancer*, **38**, 1629–35.

Kaku T. & Enjoji M. (1983) Extremely well differentiated adeno carcinoma (adenoma malignum) of the cervix. *Int. J. Gynecol. Path.*, **2**, 28–41.

Kaminski P. & Norris H. (1983) Minimal deviation of carcinoma (adenoma malignum) of the cervix. *Int. J. Gynecol. Path.*, **2**, 141–52.

Kaser O., Ikle F.A. & Hirsch H.A. (1973) *Atlas der gynakologischen operationen unter berucksich-tigung. Gynak-dogisch-Urologischer Eingriffe 3*. Aufluaer Thieme Stuttgart.

Kiang D.T., Bauer G.E. & Kennedy B.T. (1973) Immuno-assayable incidence in carcinoma of the cervix associated with hypoglaecemia. *Cancer*, **31**, 801–05.

Kottmeier, H.L. (1964) Complications following radiation therapy in carcinoma of the cervix and their treatment. *Am. J. Obstet. Gynecol.*, **88**, 854–66.

Kovacic J., Omahen A. & Tomazevic T. *et al.* (1980) The treatment of invasive carcinoma of the cervix at the department of Gynaecology and Obstetrics in Ljubljana. *Eur. J. Gynecol. Oncol.*, **1** (2), 65–71.

Krebs H.B., Helmkamp B.F., Sevin B.U., Poliakoff S.R., Nadji M. & Averette H.E. (1982) Recurrent cancer of the cervix following radical hysterectomy and pelvic node dissection. *Obstet. Gynecol.*, **59**, 422–27.

Krishnamoorthy A., Desai A. & Simanowitz M. (1986) Primary malignant melanoma of the cervix. *Br. J. Obstet. Gynaecol.*, **93**, 84–86.

Kyriakos M., Kempson R.L. & Perez C.A. (1971) Carcinoma of the cervix in young women. *Obstet. Gynecol.*, **38**, 930–44.

Laara E., Day N.E. & Harama M. (1987) Trends in mortality of cervical cancer in the Nordic countries in association with organised screening programme. *Lancet*, 247–49.

Lagasse L.D., Creasman W. & Shingleton H.M. (1980) Results and complications of operative staging in cervical cancer; experience of a Gynaecological Oncology Group. *Gynecol. Oncol.*, **9**, 90.

Lagasse L.D., Smith M.L., Moore J.G., Morton D.G., Jacobs M., Johnson G.H. & Watring, W.G. (1974) The effect of radiation therapy on pelvic lymph node involvement in Stage I carcinoma of the cervix. *Am. J. Obstet. Gynecol.*, **119**, 328–34.

Langley I.I., Moore D.W. & Tarnasky J.W. et al. (1980) Radical hysterectomy and pelvic lymph node dissection. Gynecol. Oncol., 9, 37−42.

Lapolla J., Schlaerth J.B., Gaddis O. & Morrow C.P. (1986) The influence of surgical staging on the evaluation of treatment of patients with cervical carcinoma. Gynecol. Oncol., 24, 194.

Lathrop J.C. (1967) Malignant pelvic lymphomas. Obstet. Gynecol., 30, 137−45.

Littman P., Clements P.B., Henriksen B., Wang C.C., Robboy S.J., Taft P.D., Ulfelder H. & Scully R.E. (1976) Glassy cell carcinoma of the cervix. Cancer, 37, 2238−46.

Lowe D. & Hudson C.N. (1988) Rare tumours of the cervix. In: Williams C.J., Krikorian J.G., Green M.R. & Raghaven D. (eds), Textbook of Uncommon Cancer. pp. 167−82.

Lowe J.A., Mauger G.H. & Carmichael J.A. (1981) The effect of Wertheim's hysterectomy upon bladder and urethral function. Am. J. Obstet. Gynecol., 139, 826−34.

McGee C.T., Cromer D.W. & Green R.R. (1962) Mesonephric carcinoma of the cervix. Differentiation from endocervical adenocarcinoma. Am. J. Obstet. Gynecol. 84, 358−66.

McGregor J.E. & Taper S. (1978) Uterine cervical cytology in young women. Lancet, i, 1029−31.

McIndoe W.A., McLean M.R., Jones R.W. & Mullins P.R. (1984) The invasive potential of carcinoma in situ of the cervix. Obstet. Gynecol., 64, 451−58.

McKelvey J.L. & Goodlin R.R. (1963) Adenoma malignum of the cervix. A cancer of deeply innocent histological pattern. Cancer, 16, 549−57.

Mackles A., Wolfe S.A. & Neigus I. (1958) Benign and malignant mesonephric lesions of the cervix. Cancer, ii, 292−305.

Martimbeau P.W., Kjorstad K.E. & Iversen T. (1982) Stage IB carcinoma of the cervix, the Norwegian Radium Hospital: Results of treatment and major complications. II. Results when pelvic nodes are involved. Obstet. Gynecol., 60 (2), 215−18.

Meigs J.V. (1944) Radical hysterectomy with bilateral pelvic node dissection. Report on 100 cases operated on 5 years or more. Am. J. Obstet. Gynecol., 62, 854−66.

Michael H., Grawe L. & Kraus F.T. (1984) Minimal deviation of endocervical adenocarcinoma. Clinical and histological features, immunohistochemical staining for carcino-embryonal antigen and differentiation from confusing benign lesions. Int. J. Gynecol. Path., 3, 261−76.

Mitra S. (1938) Surgical treatment of carcinoma cervicis uteri by radical vaginal method. J. Obstet. Gynaecol. Brit. Emp., 48, 1003−12.

Morley G.W. & Seski J.C. (1976) Radical pelvic surgery versus radiation therapy for Stage I carcinoma of the cervix (exclusive of microcarcinoma). Am. J. Obstet. Gynecol., 126, 785−98.

Morrow C.P. et al. (1980) Is pelvic radiation beneficial in the post-operative management of Stage IB squamous cell carcinoma of the cervix with pelvic lymph node metastases treated by radical hysterectomy and pelvic lymphadenectomy? Gynecol. Oncol., 10, 105−10.

Nelson A.J., Fletcher G.H. & Wharton J.T. (1975) Indications for adjunctive conservative extra-fascial hysterectomy in selected cases of carcinoma of the uterine cervix. Am. J. Roentgenol. Radium Ther. Nucl. Med., 123, 91−99.

Newton M. (1975) Radical hysterectomy or radiotherapy for Stage I cervical cancer. A prospective comparison with 5 and 10 year follow up. Am J Obstet. Gynecol., 123, 535−42.

Nordquist S.R.B., Sevin B.U., Nadji M. et al. (1979) Fine needle aspiration cytology in gynaecologic oncology. Obstet. Gynecol., 84, 719−24.

Novak F. (1963) Procedure for the reduction of the number of uretovaginal fistulae after Wertheim's operation. Proc. Roy. Soc. Med., 56, 881−84.

OPCS (1983) Cancer Statistics 1978. HMSO, London, MB1 No. 10.

OPCS (1984) Cancer Statistics Registration, England and Wales. HMSO, London. MB1 No. 16.

OPCS (1986) Mortality statistics; Cause, England and Wales. HMSO, London. DH2 No. 13.

O'Quinn A.G., Fletcher G.H. & Wharton T. (1980) Guidelines for conservative hysterectomy after irradiation. Gynecol. Oncol., 9, 68−79.

Orr J.W. Jr, Shingleton H.M. & Hatch K.D. et al. (1982) Correlation of perioperative morbidity and conization − radical hysterectomy interval. Obstet. Gynecol., 59 (6), 726−31.

Perez C.A., Camel H.M., Kao M.S. & Askin F. (1980) Randomized study of pre-operative radiation and surgery or irradiation alone in the treatment of Stage IB and IIA carcinoma of the uterine cervix; preliminary analysis of failure and complications. Cancer, 45, 2759−68.

Perez C.A., Camel H.M., Kao M.S. & Kederman S. (1987) Randomized study of radiation and surgery or radiation alone in the treatment of stage IB and IIa carcinoma of the uterine cervix. Final Report. Gynecol. Oncol., 27 (2), 129−40.

Peterson O. (1955) Precancerous changes of the cervical epithelium. *Acta Radiol.*, **127** (Suppl.) 74–87.

Photopulos G.J., Shirley R.E.L. & Ausbacher R. (1977) Evaluation of conventional diagnostic tests for detection of recurrent carcinoma of the cervix. *Am. J. Obstet. Gynecol.*, **129**, 533–35.

Pilleron J.P., Durand T.C. & Hamelin J.P. (1974) Prognostic value of node metastases in cancer of the uterine cervix. *Am. J. Obstet. Gynecol.*, **119**, 458–62.

Piver M.S. & Chung W.S. (1975) Prognostic significance of cervical lesion size and pelvic node metastases in cervical carcinoma. *Obstet. Gynecol.*, **46**, 507–10.

Pollack R.S. & Taylor H.C. (1947) Cancer of the cervix in the first two decades of life. *Am. J. Obstet. Gynecol.*, **53**, 135.

Potish R.A., Twiggs L.B., Okagaki T., Prem K.A. & Adcock L.L. (1985) Therapeutic implications and the natural history of advanced cervical cancer as defined by pre-treatment surgical staging. *Cancer*, **56**, 956–60.

Prempree T., Patanaphan V. & Sewchand W. (1983) Influence of patients age and tumour grade on the prognosis of carcinoma of the cervix. *Cancer*, **51**, 1764–71.

Reagan J.W. & Wentz W.B. (1967) Genesis of carcinoma of the cervix. *Clin. Obstet. Gynaecol.*, **10**, 883–921.

Ries E. (1895) Eine neue operations methode des uterus-carcinoma. *Z. Geburtsh. Gynak.*, **32**, 266.

Robertson J.H., Woodend B., Crozier E.H. & Hudson J. (1988) Risk of cervical cancer associated with mild dyskaryosis. *Br. Med. J.*, **279**, 18–21.

Roddick J.W. & Greenelaw R.H. (1971) Treatment of cervical cancer. A randomized study of operation and radiation. *Am. J. Obstet. Gynecol.*, **109**, 754–64.

Rosen Y. & Dolan T.E. (1975) Carcinoma of the cervix with cylindromatous features believed to arise in the mesonephric duct. *Cancer*, **36**, 1739–47.

Rotman M., John M. & Chai K. (1986) Prophylactic irradiation of the para-aortic lymph node chain in carcinoma of the cervix. Irradiation Therapy Oncology Group Study update. *Int. J. Rad. Oncol.*, **12**, 94.

Rutledge F.N., Fletcher G.H. & McDonald E.J. (1965) Pelvic lymphadenectomy as an adjunct to radiation therapy in the treatment of cancer of the cervix. *Am. J. Roentgen.*, **93**, 607.

Rutledge F.N. & Seski J. (1979) More or less radical surgery. *Int. J. Rad. Oncol. Biol. Phys.*, **5**, 1881–84.

Rutledge F.N., Wharton J.T. & Fletcher G.H. (1976) Clinical studies with adjunctive surgery and irradiation therapy in the treatment of carcinoma of the cervix. *Cancer*, **38**, 596–602.

Schauta F. (1902) Die operation des Gebarmutterkrebses mittels des Schuchardt'schen Paravaginat-schnittes. *Montasschr. Geburtsh. in Gynak.*, **15**, 133–52.

Sevin B.U., Remos R., Lichtinger M., Girtanner R.E. & Averette H.E. (1984) Antibiotic prevention of infections complicating radical abdominal hysterectomy. *Obstet. Gynecol.*, **64**, 539–45.

Shepherd J.H., Cavanagh D., Riggs D. *et al.* (1982) Abdominal wound closures using a nonabsorbable single layer technique. *Obstet. Gynecol.*, **61** (2), 248–52.

Shepherd J.H., Cavanagh D., Ruffulo E. & Praphat H. (1981) The value of needle biopsy in the diagnosis of gynaecologic cancer. *Gynecol. Oncol.*, **11**, 309–20.

Shepherd J.H. & Crowther M.E. (1986) Complications of gynaecological cancer surgery; a review. *J. Roy. Soc. Med.*, **79**, 289–93.

Shepherd J.H., Praphat H., Ruffulo E. & Cavanagh D. (1982) Diagnostic dilemma of recurrent cervical carcinoma. *In*: Hafez E.S.T. & Smith J.P. (eds), *Carcinoma of the Cervix: Biology and Diagnosis*. Nijhoff (Martinus) Publishers, The Hague, Netherlands.

Shingleton H.M., Gore H., Bradley D.H. *et al.* (1981) Adenocarcinoma of the cervix. I. Clinical evaluation and pathological features. *Am. J. Obstet. Gynecol.*, **139**, 799–814.

Shingleton H.M. & Orr J.W. (1983) *Cancer of the Uterine Cervix Diagnosis and Treatment*. Churchill Livingstone, Edinburgh.

Shingleton H.M. & Palumbo L.J. (1968) Ureteral complications of radical hysterectomy: effects of preoperative radium and ureteral catheters. *Surgery Forum*, **19**, 410–12.

Silva E.G., Kott M.M. & Ordonez N.G. (1984) Endocrine carcinoma intermediate cell type of the uterine cervix. *Cancer*, **54**, 1705–13.

Smales E., Perry C.M., MacDonald J.S. & Baker J.W. (1986) The value of lymphography in the management of carcinoma of the cervix. *Clin. Rad.*, **37**, 19–22.

Soutter W.P., Regorato R.J., Green-Thompson R.W. *et al.* (1983) Nuclear and cytoplasmic oestrogen receptors in squamous carcinoma of the cervix. *In*: Morrow C.P., Bonnar J., O'Brian T.J. & Gibbone W.E. (eds), *Recent Clinical Developments in Gynecologic Oncology*. Raven Press, New York. pp. 23–31.

Stern E. (1969) Epidemiology of dysplasia. *Obstet. Gynecol. Surv.*, **24**, 711–23.

Sudarsanem A., Charyulu K. & Velinson J. (1978) Influence of exploratory celiotomy on the management of carcinoma of the cervix. *Cancer*, **41**, 1049.

Surwit E., Fowler W.C. & Palumbo F.L. (1976) Radical hysterectomy with or without preoperative radiotherapy for stage IB squamous cell carcinoma of the cervix. *Obstet. Gynecol.*, **48**, 130–33.

Talbert L.M., Palumbo L., Shingleton H.M. *et al.* (1965) Urologic complications of radical hysterectomy for carcinoma of the cervix. *South. Med. J.*, **58**, 11–17.

Tamimi H.K. & Figge D.C. (1982) Adenocarcinoma of the uterine cervix. *Gynecol. Oncol.*, **13**, 335–44.

Van Nagell J.R., Donaldson E.S. & Parker J.C. (1977) The prognostic significance of cell type and lesion size in patients with cervical cancer treated by radical surgery. *Gynecol. Oncol.*, **5**, 142–51.

Van Nagell J.R., Rayburn W., Donaldson E.S., Hanson M., Gay E.C., Yoneda J., Marayuma Y. & Powell D.E. (1979) Therapeutic implications of patterns of recurrence in cancer of the uterine cervix. *Cancer*, **44**, 2354–61.

Villard L., Murphy M. & Vessey M.P. (1989) Cervical cancer deaths in young women. *Lancet*, **i**, 377.

Walton R.J. (1982) Cervical screening programmes. Summary of 1982 Canadian Task Force Report. *Can. Med. Asoc. J.*, **127**, 581–89.

Ward B.G., Shepherd J.H. & Monaghan J.M. (1985) Occult advanced cervical cancer. *Br. Med. J.*, **290**, 1301–2.

Webb G.A. (1975) The role of ovarian conservation in the treatment of carcinoma of the cervix with radical surgery. *Am. J. Obstet. Gynecol.*, **122**, 476–84.

Webb M.J. & Symmonds R.E. (1979a) Wertheim hysterectomy: a reappraisal. *Obstet. Gynecol.*, **54**, 140–45.

Webb M.J. & Symmonds R.E. (1979b) Radical hysterectomy: influence of recent conization on morbidity and complications. *Obstet. Gynecol.*, **53**, 290–92.

Welander C.E., Pierce V.K., Nori D., Hilaris B.S., Kostoff C., Clark D.G.C. *et al.* (1981) Pre-treatment laparotomy in carcinoma of the cervix. *Gynecol. Oncol.*, **12**, 336–47.

Wertheim E. (1900) Zur Frage der Radikaloperation beim Uteruskrebs. *Arch. Gynak.*, **61**, 627.

Wertheim E. (1905) Discussion on the diagnosis and treatment of carcinoma of the uterus. *Br. Med. J.*, **2**, 689.

Yamasaki M., Theishi R., Hongo J., Ozaki Y., Inoue M. & Ueda G. (1984) Argyrophil small cell carcinoma of the uterine cervix. *Int. J. Gynecol. Pathol.*, **3**, 146–52.

Zander J., Baltzer J., Lohe K.J. *et al.* (1981) Carcinoma of the cervix: an attempt to individualise treatment: results of a 20 year co-operative study. *Am. J. Obstet. Gynecol.*, **139**, 752–59.

5

The Management of Advanced and Recurrent Cervical Cancer by Pelvic Exenteration

JOHN M. MONAGHAN

Introduction

One-third to one-half of patients with invasive carcinoma of the cervix have residual or recurrent disease after treatment (Disaia & Creasman 1981; Shingleton & Orr 1983), and up to one-quarter of these cases develop a central recurrence which may be amenable to exenterative surgery. Since the first description of pelvic exenteration for advanced and recurrent carcinoma of the pelvis by Brunschwig in 1948, there has developed a slow acceptance of the procedure throughout gynaecology. Initially the high mortality and morbidity of the extensive surgery were considered unjustifiable. However, when it was realized that in those patients for whom no alternative management was available, there was the possibility of good long term survival (20% in early and up to 60% in later series), the procedure became more generally accepted. There has been a steady improvement in preoperative preparation, anaesthesia, postoperative care, the routine use of prophylactic antibiotics, more accurate blood transfusion and better prophylaxis against thromboembolic disease. Consequently there has been a concomitant improvement in survivals, now reaching 40–60% in recently reported large series (Morley & Lindenauer 1976; Rutledge et al. 1977, and in the author's own experience).

The surgery involved is extensive, and the postoperative care complex, so this operation has become part of the repertoire of the gynaecological oncologist, occasionally working alone but frequently combining with the urologist and general surgeon. Unfortunately Britain has tended to lag behind the USA in its appreciation of the role of exenteration and many patients are not considered for this procedure because of low acceptance of the operation and the few centres capable of managing the patients.

Pelvic exenterations are of three types, anterior, posterior and total, the most frequently practised being the anterior and total exenteration (see Fig. 5.1)

Selection of patients for exenteration

Exenterative surgery should be considered for both advanced primary cervical carcinoma and recurrent disease. The majority of operations are now performed

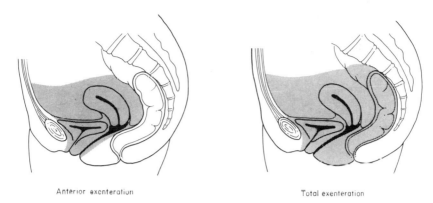

Anterior exenteration   Total exenteration

Fig. 5.1. The shaded portion shows the organs removed during anterior and total exenteration (reproduced by kind permission of W.B. Saunders Co. Ltd).

for carcinoma which has recurred after radical radiotherapy. Further radiotherapy is contraindicated and to date chemotherapy has not shown any consistent long term results. Very occasionally exenterative surgery has been used in the treatment of radiation necrosis without histological evidence of carcinoma (Barber 1969).

The procedures may be extended even further by being combined with hemipelvectomy or removal of some part of the bony pelvis when disease affects these structures (Brunschwig & Barber 1969).

Very few series have advocated using exenterative surgery as a palliative (Deckers *et al.* 1976). However, circumstances may arise when exenteration will offer an improved quality of life in spite of distant metastases or persisting disease. In the author's experience these circumstances are limited to the presence of carcinomatous fistulae in the pelvis associated with cystitis, incontinence, proctitis, severe local pain and pelvic infection. Even in this situation it may be argued that a bypass procedure would achieve a similar result with less trauma (Curry *et al.* 1981; Lyndrup & Sorensen 1983), by using percutaneous nephrostomy (Mann *et al.* 1983) or medical means to relieve symptoms.

Recently Stanhope & Symmonds (1985) have reviewed the survival characteristics of those patients operated upon when there was evidence of distant or nodal metastases. The 2-year survival being 47% and the 5-year 17%, they conclude that as the operative morbidity and mortality are now very small, even exenterative surgery may be used in a palliative manner in selected patients.

Patient assessment

It is relatively easy to be certain of the diagnosis of primary cervical carcinoma, but it is frequently difficult after treatment to be sure that the mass palpable in the pelvis is due to recurrent disease and not to radiotherapy reaction, or to the scarring from infection or the effects of adhesion of bowel to the irradiated area. Every attempt should be made to make an accurate tissue diagnosis including the use of needle biopsy, aspiration cytology or even open biopsy at laparotomy. Some authorities carry out scalene node biopsy under local anaesthetic as it is said that up to 17% of patients with recurrence and para-aortic node metastases will have subclinical spread to the scalene nodes (Shingleton & Orr 1983).

A careful assessment of the patient's physical and mental state is important but age is not a bar to exenterative surgery. Although the average age of patients in most series is in the fifties the range is wide from early childhood to the eighth decade.

Absolute contraindications to exenteration

Distant metastases. If there is evidence of metastases to the extrapelvic lymph nodes, upper abdominal viscera, lungs or bones, there is little value in performing the exenteration. Barber & Jones (1971) made the definitive statement on the value of carrying out exenterative surgery in the presence of nodal metastases, commenting that although in their series 17.4% (29 of 166 patients) with non-involved nodes survived 5 years, only 5.1% (five of 97 patients) with involved nodes lived a similar length of time. Although in more modern series the numbers surviving have increased, the poor survival of those patients with nodal metastases remains.

Relative contraindications

Pelvic side wall spread. If the tumour in the pelvis has extended to the pelvic side wall, either in the form of direct extension of the primary or as nodal metastases, then the prospects for cure are extremely small and the surgeon must decide whether the procedure will materially improve the patient's quality of life.

The triad of (1) unilateral uropathy, renal nonfunction or ureteric obstruction; (2) unilateral leg oedema; and (3) sciatic leg pain is an ominous sign. The prospects for cure are extremely poor.

Mental state. In his earliest writings Brunschwig stated that psychosis was a contraindication to exenteration. Those patients who show signs of being unable to cope with mental or physical stress should be very carefully assessed prior to embarking on surgery.

Obesity. This is always a problem in any surgical procedure, producing intra-operative technical difficulties as well as postoperative respiratory and mobiliz-ation problems. These difficulties are many times magnified during exenterative surgery, up to one-third of obese patients dying in the postoperative period (Barber 1969).

Preoperative preparation

A careful assessment of the patient must be made including full haematological and biochemical testing. Intravenous urography, computerized axial tomography, ultrasound scans of abdomen and pelvis, liver and bone scans and chest X-ray all assist the clinician in his assessment of the patient and the extent of disease.

The patient must be fully informed of her condition and the way in which it is to be managed; she must be seen by a stomatherapist and ideally should meet other patients who have had similar procedures. The patient's abdomen should be examined by the surgeon and the stomatherapist together in order to site any stomata that may need to be made. It is also important to discuss fully with the patient and her husband the full impact of the proposed operation, especially upon sexual function and the alteration to body image. The possibility of producing a neovagina must be considered and the timing of this extra surgery discussed.

The anaesthetist must assess the patient's ability to withstand the operation and determine the feasibility of performing some form of local analgesia such as spinal or epidural. Because of the inevitability of resecting bowel the bowel must be prepared, usually by using a combination of low residue diet and a non-absorbable antibiotic to sterilize the gut flora. These methods have largely replaced the extreme systems of bowel washouts used in years gone by, which all too often left the patient in a poor condition prior to operation.

The final decision to perform the exenteration must await laparotomy.

Evaluation at laparotomy

The author prefers to operate with one team working first abdominally and then at the perineum thereafter returning to the abdomen to make the conduits and stomas. If an anterior exenteration is to be performed the bladder is catheterized and the vagina packed to facilitate dissection of the rectum from the vagina. Having placed the patient in slight Trendelenburg position (Morley & Lindenauer 1976) the abdomen is opened via a high subumbilical muscle cutting transverse incision (Maylard); some authorities recommend a midline incision (Symmonds & Webb 1981). Either of these incisions will give adequate access both to the pelvis and to the para-aortic regions and allow full inspection of the upper abdomen. After the abdomen is opened, the pelvis is assessed to determine if the tumour is mobile. If the surgeon feels that this is so, he should then proceed to inspect the upper abdomen for evidence of metastases, especially in the para-aortic lymph nodes and the upper abdominal viscera. In most centres para-aortic nodes down as far as the common iliac nodes are sampled and sent for frozen section. While this is being carried out, the pelvic side wall is examined in more detail. The round ligaments are divided and the lateral wall of the pelvis exposed, separating the fascia below the external iliac vessels in order to view and palpate the lymph nodes of the external and internal iliac systems and the obturator nodes. The tumour mass can then be assessed down to the pelvic floor. If the para-aortic nodes are negative then the exenteration can proceed.

Operative technique

In the author's department the standard technique for entering the abdomen is to carry out a Maylard transverse muscle cutting incision midway between the umbilicus and the symphisis pubis, incising the peritoneum in the same line. Having assessed that the carcinoma is operable, the peritoneum is separated from the transversalis muscle lateral to the incision by finger dissection. The incision in the peritoneum is then continued in a circular manner around the lateral part of the false pelvis and across the ilio-psoas muscles to reach the midline on the right side over the upper part of the sacral promontory. On the left side this incision of the peritoneum will stop at the inferior mesenteric artery in the mesentery of the sigmoid colon. It is important to preserve as much peritoneum as possible in the lateral parts of the pelvis as this sheet which has been developed anteriorly and posteriorly will form the 'sac' to contain the bowels at the end of the procedure (Way 1974). During the course of this incision, the infundibulo−pelvic ligaments are isolated, clamped and divided. The ureters are also isolated but are not divided at this time.

The final assessment of the pelvis is now made by releasing the bladder anteriorly using a simple finger dissection behind the pubic arch down into the Cave of Retzius. The lateral part of the pelvis can now be finally assessed down to the pelvic floor. This is easily performed by opening up the relatively avascular space in the paravesical and pararectal areas.

If it is decided to carry out the procedure as an anterior exenteration, the peritoneal dissection which has been brought to the sigmoid colon on the left and to the midline on the right is then continued down into the pelvis, crossing the Pouch of Douglas anterior to the rectum and posterior to the cervix. Having incised the peritoneum, the vagina is dissected by finger dissection from the anterior surface of the rectum producing a pillar of tissue between the uterosacral ligaments posteriorly and the paravesical space anterior to the broad ligament.

In a total exenteration the sigmoid colon is divided at or about the level of the pelvic brim. This can be done very swiftly and cleanly using the GIA stapling gun, leaving the rectal stump completely closed and the proximal end stapled to await formation of the colostomy or its use as part of a colonic conduit. After separating the bowel and carefully ligating the lower branches of the inferior mesenteric artery, the rectum is separated from the anterior surface of the sacrum down as far as the pelvic floor by finger dissection. Surprisingly little bleeding is experienced during this manoeuvre.

Now all that remains linking the pelvic side wall to the central tumour mass are the uterine arteries and the lower branches of the internal iliac arteries and ureters. The ureters are divided just below the pelvic brim in a primary procedure, but if following irradiation it is wise to divide the ureters a short distance above the pelvic brim. It is occasionally prudent at this point to isolate and ligate the internal iliac arteries. Long exenteration clamps can now be placed on the lower part of the pedicle that has been developed between the central tumour mass and the pelvic side wall. These clamps (usually two on either side) allow the entire central block of tissue to be isolated down to the pelvic floor. Cutting close to the clamps the central mass is mobilized.

The perineal phase of the operation is now carried out; the patient's legs are raised into stirrups; Morley & Lindenauer (1971) recommend placing the patient in the 'ski position' prior to surgery so as to avoid moving the patient during the operation. The author uses this position when a gracilis myocutaneous neovagina is being formed.

The anterior part of the vulva is preserved, including the clitoris, and the anterior labia minora and majora. The incision will include the urethra and a circumferential cut around the vagina in an anterior exenteration and the anus in a total exenteration. These incisions are then deepened to the pelvic floor musculature. The space behind the pubis is entered by incising the membrane anterior to the urethra, allowing the operator to isolate and grasp the pelvic floor musculature in the lateral parts of the pelvis between finger and thumb. The muscles are then incised under direct vision and the entire tumour mass delivered through the perineal incision. Bleeding usually occurs from the muscle edge of the pelvic floor, and is dealt with by a continuous locked suture, giving isolated vessels individual treatment. Blood loss is small at this stage. The perineum is closed by interrupted sutures with a corrugated plastic drain *in situ*. If a neovagina is to be produced the appropriate surgical team will then continue working at the perineum.

Having completed the perineal phase the surgeon then returns to the abdomen; the pelvis is completely empty except for the two or four exenteration clamps on the pelvic side wall. These pedicles are then stitch ligatured and with haemostasis secure a pelvic lymphadenectomy is performed.

The urinary and bowel bypasses are now made. In total exenterations a colostomy must be produced. This is done in the standard manner bringing the stoma out through the previously marked spot in the left iliac fossa, taking care to check the quality of the blood supply to the stoma and not to stretch the segment as this will jeopardize the venous drainage. This problem may be further exacerbated in the immediate postoperative period as the abdomen distends during the normal period of ileus.

An ileal loop or colonic conduit is now produced in the right side of the abdomen. In some centres the Leadbetter technique of implanting the ureters into the bowel loop is used; the author prefers the Wallace technique (Monaghan 1986). This involves bringing the two ureters together intraperitoneally, splaying out the ends so as to produce a platform and then having canalized the ureters with a T-tube, placing the bowel segment end on onto the platform and suturing the bowel to the ureters, passing the long arm of the T-tube down the bowel segment. The conduit base is anchored to the posterior abdominal peritoneum so that it does not prolapse into the pelvis and also to avoid putting tension onto the ureteric/bowel anastomosis. The distal end of the bowel is then brought out onto the abdomen forming a spout stoma.

Stapling techniques are now being used extensively producing big improvements in speed and cleanliness of operating (Delgado 1980; Orr *et al.* 1982; Monaghan 1987).

Techniques to place the conduit on the right side (i.e. above the mesentery) of the small bowel have been developed to protect the conduit from prolapsing into the pelvis and to reduce the risk of postoperative urinary fistulae (Schoenberg & Mikuta 1973).

All that is now required is to deal with the large empty cavity of the pelvis. The huge raw surface has a massive potential for adhesions, producing postoperative obstruction and fistula formation. Over the years a wide variety of techniques have developed to cope with this problem including the following. Pelvic packing (Brunschwig 1962); omental flaps and pedicles (Valle & Ferraris 1969; Buchsbaum & White 1973; Pearse 1978); peritoneal flaps (Symmonds *et al.* 1968; Morley & Lindenauer 1971; Perticucci 1976); bovine pericardium grafts and collagen film (Green & Patterson 1968); small bowel mesenteric leaf inserts (Alexander *et al.* 1975); amnion−chorion grafts (Massee *et al.* 1962; Trelford-Sauder *et al.* 1977); synthetic pelvic floor sling (Wheeless *et al.* 1971).

The very low obstruction and fistula rates seen in this department are a direct consequence of using the 'sac technique' developed by Stanley Way (1974). This consists of using the flaps of peritoneum developed anteriorly and posteriorly at the beginning of the procedure to form a sac holding the entire bowel contents above the pelvic brim. The large air space in the pelvis can be clearly seen in Fig. 5.2. The integrity of the sac is maintained by the use of slowly absorbable suture materials such as Dexon or Vicryl.

Once the sac is completed the abdominal wall is closed. The average time for the procedure is between 2 and 3 hours and the average blood loss a little over 3 U.

It is now the author's practice to produce a neovagina at the time of the primary surgery by swinging Gracilis myocutaneous flaps into the empty pelvis (Wheeless 1980; Lacey & Stern 1987).

Variations in exenterative technique

There are many variations of exenterative technique, all designed to reduce the extent of the surgery, including the supralevator exenteration where the entire pelvic floor and therefore anal function is preserved. This technique is applicable where the primary or recurrent carcinoma is situated high up in the pelvis; it is really an extended radical hysterectomy.

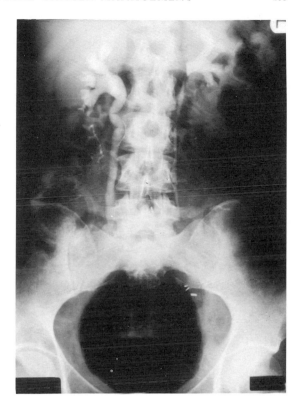

Fig. 5.2. This postoperative IVU radiograph shows the gas filled pelvic cavity, with abdominal contents held above the pelvic brim by the 'sac' of peritoneum (reproduced by kind permission of W.B. Saunders Co. Ltd).

It is occasionally possible to resect the central section of the rectum which has been in the radiation field, and then to perform a primary anastomosis with the mobilized sigmoid colon; this method is facilitated by the use of end-to-end stapling techniques when a very low anastomosis can be achieved outside the radiation field.

A variety of urinary bypass techniques have also been used.

1 Ureterosigmoidostomy.
2 Wet colostomy.
3 Ileal conduit.
4 Colonic conduit, both sigmoid and transverse.

It is now generally accepted that the optimum techniques are the ileal or colonic conduit together with a separate colostomy in total exenteration.

Postoperative care

The postoperative period is the most dangerous period for the exenteration patient. The care must be meticulous and emphasis must be on pre-empting problems rather than treating them when they arise. Unfortunately in most reported series (of American origin) there has developed a remarkable reliance on invasive anaesthetic techniques, including routine postoperative ventilation for up to 48 h, pulmonary artery catheterization and massive fluid replacement programmes. In spite of, or possibly because of, this postoperative 'care', the operative mortality is quoted as 7.8% to 37% (Shingleton & Orr 1983) compared with 4.4% in the author's series.

Prophylactic antibiotics should always be used, usually a combination of a broad spectrum Gram-negative product with one specific for bacteroides infections. The patient must be well hydrated with close attention being paid to fluid balance and urinary output. Renal function can be stimulated for the first few days by the use of diuretics to produce a good flow of urine, of at least 1500 ml per day. A nasogastric tube is put in at operation and is maintained for the first 3 to 4 days. The conduit stents can be removed on the tenth postoperative day; following removal, an intravenous urogram is carried out.

As a prophylaxis against thromboembolic disease subcutaneous heparin 5000 U b.d. is started at the end of the operation after the epidural catheter has been removed. This regimen is maintained for the next ten days during which time the patient is rapidly mobilized.

Long term follow up

It is important that all exenteration patients should be carefully reviewed, paying special attention to renal function, occult sepsis and bowel obstruction. As the risk of infection to the urinary tract is high prophylactic antibiotics should be used. Antibiotics are preferable to antiseptics as adequate levels can be maintained using only one or two tablets per day, whereas antiseptics require many tablets to be taken at regular intervals throughout the day. The patient should have regular visits to the stomatherapy clinic until she is fully confident of handling her stomas.

Results of treatment

Table 5.1 shows the results of a number of large modern series and the earlier series of Brunschwig & Barber.

Complications of exenterative surgery

It is inevitable that there will be a significant number of complications in association with such extensive surgery. The most important factor in the prevention of complications in this series of procedures is the development of an experienced team of doctors and nurses both in the operating theatre and on the wards.

Table 5.1. Five-year survival statistics following pelvic exenteration

	Patients (n)	Survival (%)
Brunschwig (1965)	264	18
Morley & Lindenauer (1976)	70	61.8
Rutledge et al. (1977)	296	42.1
Symmonds & Webb (1981)	198	32
Monaghan (personal series 1988)	72	42

Length of the operative procedure

There is considerable evidence that operations which take longer than 5 hours put patients under considerable stress. Large transfusions of blood and fluid also put a great load on the patient's physiological resources. The author's series of 72 cases recorded an average operation time of two- and three-quarter hours with an average blood replacement of 3 U. This may account for the fact that 43% of patients had no complications.

Operative mortality

In early series up to 40% primary operative mortalities were reported; in modern series the mortality should now be no more than 10%. In the author's own series of 72 patients three patients died in the postoperative period (4.4%).

Anaesthesia

The anaesthesia has to be of the highest order and must be of a type to assist the surgeon by reducing peripheral blood flow and pelvic pooling. This can be achieved by the use of epidural/spinal type analgesia increasing the operability and allowing less invasive anaesthetic techniques to be used. When this type of anaesthesia is combined with heparin prophylaxis for thromboembolic disease there is a theoretical risk of extradural haemorrhage. The value of epidural analgesia in the postoperative period must be weighed against the value of heparin as a prophylactic.

Fluid loss

Intraoperative fluid loss must be steadily replaced by the anaesthetist who should also gauge and project the fluid loss in the immediate postoperative period. The traditional method of continuously assessing fluid replacement needs is to monitor central venous pressure, but in many centres this has been superceded by more invasive techniques such as the use of Swan–Ganz catheters to measure pulmonary artery wedge pressures.

Haemorrhage

There is no doubt that in exenterative surgery the potential for haemorrhage is enormous but with care and an experience of the tissue planes in the pelvis there should not be any excessive loss. When dealing with the irradiated pelvis great care and gentleness should be exercised as any trauma to the tissues will result in bruising and multiple tiny haemorrhages from any damaged surface.

In the irradiated pelvis it is frequently difficult or impossible to define tissue planes so that dissection has to be sharp. Therefore, great skill must be exercised to reduce the risk of bleeding.

Bowel trauma

It is now unusual to perform exenterative surgery for primary disease, most patients having had some form of previous treatment, usually radiotherapy. Consequently any bowel which has been in the radiotherapy field may be compromised and even the most minor trauma will produce a risk of at least petechiae or haemorrhage and at worst perforation and fistula formation. It is therefore important to handle bowel as little as possible and not to use irradiated bowel in any bypass procedure. This particularly applies to the terminal ileum.

Secondary haemorrhage

This distressing complication will occur in 5–10% of cases. It is important to differentiate bleeding from the profuse sero-sanguinous loss which will occur from the drain sites. Vital signs in the postoperative period must be very carefully monitored. The most dangerous sites for secondary haemorrhage are the ligated internal iliac vessels and the incised pelvic floor musculature.

Thromboembolic disease

The exenteration patient is at particularly high risk for the development of this complication; active prophylaxis is mandatory. Previous surgery and radiotherapy will inevitably alter the lymphatic and vascular drainage of the pelvis, as does the presence of recurrent or residual carcinoma. Cachexia and preoperative immobility may also increase the risk but anaemia if present may have a slightly protective effect. Postoperatively the risk is also increased by immobility but even with exenteration the general policy of early mobilization is adhered to.

Postoperative infection of the wound and the empty pelvis

Exenterative surgery presents a greater risk of postoperative infection than most other gynaecological surgery. The extent of surgery is enormous, the bowel must be opened, and large denuded surfaces will be left within the abdomen and pelvis. Approximately 65% of patients will suffer some infectious morbidity, mainly of the urinary tract and the remainder related to the wound or the pelvis.

Prevention

This is best carried out by the use of preoperative bowel preparation and prophylactic antibiotics in the intra- and postoperative period. Meticulous surgical technique with the minimum of tissue handling coupled with scrupulous skin cleansing are the most important preventives. Other precautions that can be taken are to allow adequate drainage of the pelvis and to cover as many denuded surfaces as possible with peritoneum or mobilized omentum. When packing techniques are used to deal with the pelvic space there seems to be an increased risk of infection, which should be dealt with by local cleansing and appropriate antibiotics. In the author's practice the Way 'sac' technique is used to support the abdominal contents above the pelvic brim (Way 1974), leaving the pelvis empty and massively reducing the postoperative obstruction and fistula rate. Unfortunately the empty pelvis is prone to become infected. This 'empty pelvis syndrome' has characteristic symptomatology of malaise, pyrexia with occasional rigors and an increase in discharge from any perineal sinus, which may or may not be purulent.

When patients are given antibiotics, they are singularly unsuccessful in treating the problem. What is required is local therapy to the pelvis which can best be provided by inserting a soft catheter into the space via the perineal drain hole and washing out the cavity with hydrogen peroxide or Eusol until the drain returns are clean. The patient rapidly feels better and recovery is complete.

Biochemical complications

It is inevitable that after such enormous surgery there is a very great stress laid on the liver and its enzyme systems and on the kidneys and their ability to deal with waste and breakdown products. Similarly lung function and their ability to maintain blood pH can be severely stressed. Any previous damage to these organs will further jeopardize the patient. Lung and renal problems may manifest themselves in the form of difficulties in maintaining acid base balance, in achieving acceptable levels of oxygenation and in excreting waste products such as urea and creatinine. In the extreme catabolic phase that follows such surgery the serum potassium may rise to dangerous levels and need to be artificially reduced.

Hepatic stress will show itself as postoperative jaundice, frequently developing between the third and tenth day after operation. This elevation of bilirubin cannot be entirely explained by red cell destruction rates, for there is a significant hepato—cellular component. As well as elevation of the bilirubin, the alkaline phosphatase, the serum transaminase, and the lactic dehydrogenase levels are elevated and the serum protein levels depressed.

Parenteral nutrition must be considered for all patients undergoing exenterative surgery and particularly those who have evidence of being poorly nourished or showing early signs of cachexia preoperatively.

Intestinal obstruction and fistula

Intestinal fistulae following exenteration have been reported to occur in 4—8% of patients. They are almost always intestino—perineal, rarely appearing abdominally except via the operative wound. The interval from surgery to their development is variable ranging from one month to nine years. Postexenteration bowel fistula have a very high mortality and require accurate and early assessment, intensive therapy and treatment if death is to be avoided.

Risk factors include the following:
1 Previous surgery, radiotherapy or chemotherapy.
2 Poor general condition of the patient including diabetes, atherosclerosis, obesity, cachexia, uremia, anaemia and hypoproteinaemia.
3 Poor operative technique, intra- and postoperative sepsis and persistent or recurrent carcinoma also contribute.

Site of bowel fistula

Ileo—perineal fistulae appear most commonly and are usually due to loops of ileum falling into the pelvis and their blood supply being compromised. This risk is much increased if the distal ileum has been subjected to irradiation, or if the small bowel anastomosis comes in contact with a nonperitonized area of pelvis. Where an ileal rather than a colonic conduit has been made the risk of ileo—perineal fistula is also said to be increased, especially close to the resection lines.

Rectoperineal fistula

These tend to develop in one of two circumstances, as follows:
1 Where the rectum has been preserved in an anterior exenteration following a radical level of pelvic irradiation.
2 Where a low rectal anastomosis has been performed in combination with an anterior exenteration, following radical pelvic irradiation. One in four of such procedures may end in fistulae.

Coloperineal fistulae

These are less common, but may be mistaken for the other types. They are however usually successfully managed by resection of the involved segment.

The management is best summarized as *stabilization*; *assessment* and *surgical treatment*.

Stabilization. The patient's general condition, especially fluid and electrolyte pattern, must be normalized. Fistula output must be minimized or eliminated by using total parenteral nutrition (TPN), or prolonged proximal decompression. The fistula must be protected from further irritation and associated sepsis treated by antibiotics and surgical drainage where indicated. Accurately applied stoma appliances will also reduce skin problems. Further catabolism must be reversed by TPN and care taken to allow for fistula loss.

Assessment. Using contrast radiology including IVU, Barium meal and enema, loopograms, sinograms and retrograde endoscopy where appropriate.

Surgical treatment. Rarely is TPN alone curative; however, if the fistula appears to be closing, then the TPN phase should be continued. In most circumstances surgery is necessary, especially when there is evidence of distal obstruction. Four possibilities exist:
1 Closure of the fistula.
2 Resection and removal of the fistula with primary anastomosis.
3 Bypass of the fistula.
4 Isolation of the fistulous loop and production of a mucous fistula (Smith *et al*. 1984).

Psychological and sexual complications

In the immediate postoperative period it is very important to be able to pick up the first signs of psychological stress, manifested as:
1 Heightened pain appreciation;
2 Fatigue;
3 Insomnia;
4 Disorientation, and
5 Paranoia.
The patient should be given considerable psychological support by the whole team, any setbacks should be explained and a clear and confident approach made to their resolution. Care should be used before prescribing anxiolytics and sedatives as these may heighten the problem by increasing the patient's disorientation.

Mental adjustment

Following exenteration this is usually excellent, the patients with the highest risk of the development of postoperative problems being those who have a history of mental and marital disturbances prior to surgery, particularly depression.

Social adjustment

Also of a high order, with many patients returning to work and fully involving themselves in leisure activities, some achieving very high levels of satisfaction both personally and competitively.

Sexual adjustment

By comparison this is much more variable. For all exenteration patients a major alteration in sexual function and activity will occur. For some women with poor to nonexistent sex lives the removal of the vagina will not materially alter function. However, for the majority of women the readjustment will have to be massive. Even for those patients who have had a neovagina made sexual function will not be 'as it was before'. The new vagina is often of the wrong size and shape and intercourse may be accompanied by pain and excessive discharge.

The patient has difficulty in adjusting to her altered body image, and phantomization of the vagina and erotisization of the colostomy have been described. The most important factor in the patient's reconciliation with her altered body image and function after exenteration is the woman's own attitude, but this does not mean that the surgeon and hospital staff can abrogate their responsibilities. Prior to the operation the patient must be encouraged to identify closely with all the ward staff and must be accurately informed of the true nature of the surgery proposed; she must be interviewed alone and with her partner. The couple should then be allowed time to digest the information and to return to the hospital to ask any further questions that have arisen. Some questions are impossible to answer and a frank 'I don't know the answer' is more satisfactory than prevarication.

Urinary tract infection

This may be discovered as an asymptomatic bacteriuria or as symptomatic infection, the former often occurring in spite of the patient being on prophylactic antibiotics. A preoperative UTI or urinary tract pathology increases the risk to the patient. However, the use of urinary antiseptics or antibiotics as a prophylaxis does seem to reduce the risk of progression to pyelonephritis.

Exenterative surgery is an important option to have available for a small highly selected group of patients with recurrent or extensive cancer. Many patients are not given the chance of this option because such procedures are not considered feasible or curative. It is important that all clinicians are aware of this option and are willing to refer to those gynaecological oncologists with the team of skills necessary for the successful performance of exenterative surgery.

References

Alexander J.C., Beazeley R.M. & Chretien P.B. (1975) Mesenteric leaf repair of pelvic defects following exenterative operations. *Ann. Surg.*, **182**, 767–69.

Anderson B.L. & Hacker N.F. (1983) Psychosexual adjustment following pelvic exenteration. *Obstet. Gynecol.*, **61**, 331–38.

Barber H.R.K. (1969) Relative prognostic significance of preoperative and operative findings in pelvic exenteration. *Surg. Clin. North Am.*, **49** (2), 431–47.

Barber H.R.K. & Brunschwig A. (1965) Pelvic exenteration for locally advanced and recurrent ovarian cancer. Review of 22 cases. *Surgery*, **58**, 935–37.

Barber H.R.K. & Jones W. (1971) Lymphadenectomy in pelvic exenteration for recurrent cervix cancer. *JAMA*, **215**, 1945–49.

Brown R.S., Haddox V., Posada A. & Rubio A. (1972) Social and psychological adjustment following pelvic exenteration. *Am. J. Obstet. Gynecol.*, **114**, 162–71.

Brunschwig A. (1948) Complete excision of the pelvic viscera for advanced carcinoma. *Cancer*, **1**, 177.

Brunschwig A. (1962) Reduction of morbidity and mortality in pelvic exenteration. *Surg. Clin. North Am.*, **42**, 1583.

Brunschwig A. (1965) What are the indications and results of pelvic exenteration? *JAMA*, **194**, 160.

Brunschwig A. & Barber H.R.K. (1969) Pelvic exenteration combined with resection of segments of bony pelvis. *Surgery*, **65** (3), 417–20.

Buchsbaum H.J. & White A.J. (1973) Omental sling for management of the pelvic floor following exenteration. *Am. J. Obstet. Gynecol.*, **117**, 407–12.

Curry S.L., Nahhas W.A., Jahshan A.E., Whitney C.W. & Mortel R. (1981) Pelvic exenteration: a 7 year experience. *Gynecol. Oncol.*, **11**, 119–23.

Deckers P.J., Olsson C., Williams L.A. & Mozden P.J. (1976) Pelvic exenteration as palliation of malignant disease. *Am. J. Surg.*, **131**, 509–15.

Delgado G. (1980) Use of the automatic stapler in urinary conduit diversions and pelvic exenterations. *Gynecol. Oncol.*, **10**, 93–97.

Devereux D.F., Sears H.F. & Ketcham A.S. (1980) Intestinal fistula following pelvic exenteration surgery: predisposing causes and treatment. *J. Surg. Oncol.*, **14**, 227–34.

Disaia P.J. & Creasman W.T. (1981) *Clinical Gynaecologic Oncology; Cancer of the Cervix, Pelvic Exenteration*, chapters 2–8. Mosby, New York, pp. 82–88.

Green T.H. & Patterson W.B. (1968) Collagen film pelvic floor reconstruction following total pelvic exenteration. *Surg. Gynecol. Obstet.*, **126**, 309.

Heath P.M., Woods J.E., Podratz K.E., Arnold P.G. & Irons G.B. (1984) Gracilis myocutaneous vaginal reconstruction. *Mayo Clinic Proc.*, **59**, 21–24.

Ketcham A.S., Deckers P.J., Sugarbaker E.V., Hoye R.C., Thomas L.B. & Smith R.R. (1970) Pelvic exenteration for carcinoma of the uterine cervix. *Cancer*, **26**, 513–21.

King T.M. & Frick H.C. (1966) Intestinal fistulas following pelvic exenteration. *Surg. Gynecol. Obstet.*, **123**, 991–94.

Knorr N.J. (1967) A depressive syndrome following pelvic exenteration and ileostomy. *Arch. Surg.*, **94**, 258–60.

Lacey C.G. & Stern J.L. (1987) Gracilis flap vaginal substitution. *In:* Monaghan J.M. (ed) *Operative Surgery: Gynaecology and Obstetrics*. London: Butterworths, 238–43.

Lyndrup J. & Sorensen B.I. (1983) Palliative urinary conduit diversions in cases of intolerable urinary discomfort. *Gynecol. Oncol.*, **16**, 360–64.

Mann W.J., Hatch K.D., Taylor P.T., Partridge E.M., Orr J.W. & Shingleton H.M. (1983) The role of percutaneous nephrostomy in Gynecologic Oncology. *Gynecol. Oncol.*, **16**, 393–99.

Massee J.S., Symmonds R.E., Dockerty M.B. *et al.* (1962) Use of fetal membranes as replacement for pelvic peritoneum after pelvic exenteration in the dog. *Surg. Forum*, **13**, 407.

Monaghan J.M. (1986) Operation for the formation of an ileal conduit. *In:* Monaghan J.M. (ed.), *Bonney's Gynaecological Surgery*, Ninth Edition. Baillière Tindall, London. pp. 253–58.

Monaghan J.M. (1987) Pelvic exenterative surgery. *In:* Monaghan J.M. (ed.), *Rob and Smith's Operative Surgery, Gynaecology and Obstetrics*. Butterworths, London. pp. 206–22.

Morley G.W. & Lindenauer S.M. (1971) Peritoneal graft in total pelvic exenteration. *Am. J. Obstet. Gynecol.*, **110**, 696–701.

Morley G.W. & Lindenauer S.M. (1976) Pelvic exenteration therapy for gynecologic malignancy (an analysis of 70 cases) *Cancer*, **38**, 581–86.

Orr J.W., Shingleton H.M., Hatch K.D., Taylor P.T., Austin J.M., Partridge E.E. & Soong S.J. (1982) Urinary diversion in patients undergoing pelvic exenteration. *Am. J. Obstet. Gynecol.*, **142**, 883–89.

Orr J.W., Shingleton H.M., Hatch K.D., Taylor P.T., Partridge E.E. & Soong S.J. (1983) Gastrointestinal complications associated with pelvic exenteration. *Am. J. Obstet. Gynecol.*, **145**, 325–32.

Partridge E.E., Beasley W.E., Holcomb C., Hatch K.D., Shingleton H.M. & Austin J.M. (1979) The Swan–Ganz catheter and management of patients undergoing pelvic exenteration. *Obstet. Gynecol.*, **53**, 253–55.

Pearse H.D. (1978) Use of omental pedicle graft in exenterative surgery. *J. Urol.*, **119**, 476–77.

Perticucci S. (1976) Pelvic floor reconstruction following gynecologic exenterative surgery. *Obstet. Gynecol.*, **50**, 31–34.

Polk H.C., Butcher H.R. & Bricker E.M. (1966) Perineal fecal fistula following pelvic exenteration. *Surg. Gynecol. Obstet.*, **123**, 308–12.

Rutledge F.N., Smith J.P., Wharton J.T. & O'Quinn A.G. (1977) Pelvic exenteration: analysis of 296 patients. *Am. J. Obstet. Gynecol.*, **129**, 881–92.

Schoenberg H.W. & Mikuta J.J. (1973) Technique for preventing urinary fistulas following pelvic exenteration and ureteroileostomy. *J. Urol.*, **110**, 294–95.

Shingleton H.M. & Orr J.W. (1983) *In:* Singer A. & Jordan J. (eds), *Cancer of the Cervix, Diagnosis and Treatment*. Edinburgh: Churchill Livingstone. p. 170.

Smith D.H., Pierce V.K. & Lewis J.L. (1984) Enteric fistulas encountered on a gynecologic oncology service from 1969 through 1980. *Surg. Gynecol. Obstet.*, **158**, 71–75.

Stanhope C.R. & Symmonds R.E. (1985) Palliative exenteration—what, when and why? *Am. J. Obstet. Gynecol.*, **152**, 12–16.

Symmonds R.E., Pratt J.H. & Welch J.S. (1968) Exenterative operations: experience with 118 patients. *Am. J. Obstet. Gynecol.*, **101**, 66.

Symmonds R.E. & Webb M.J. (1981) *In:* Coppleson M. (ed.), *Pelvic Exenteration. Gynecologic Oncology*. Churchill Livingstone, Edinburgh. Chapter 71, pp. 896–922.

Trelford-Sauder M., Trelford J.D. & Matalo N.M. (1977) Replacement of the peritoneum with amnion following pelvic exenteration. *Surg. Gynecol. Obstet.*, **145**, 699–701.

Valle G. & Ferraris G. (1969) Use of the omentum to contain the intestines in pelvic exenteration. *Obstet. Gynecol.*, **33**, 772–75.

Way S. (1974) The use of the sac technique in pelvic exenteration. *Gynecol. Oncol.*, **2**, 476–81.

Wheeless C.R. (1979) Gracilis myocutaneous flap in reconstruction of the vulva and female perineum. *Obstet. Gynecol.*, **54**, 97.

Wheeless C.R. (1980) *Atlas of Pelvic Surgery*. Lea & Febiger, Philadelphia.

Wheeless C.R., Julian C.G., Burnett L.S. & Dorsey J.H. (1971) Synthetic pelvic floor sling to decrease small bowel complications after total exenteration. *Obstet. Gynecol.*, **38**, 779–83.

6

The Management of Cancer of the Uterine Corpus

DAVID ORAM

Introduction

Endometrial cancer is the commonest female gynaecological cancer in the USA (Casey 1977; Morrow & Schlaerth 1982). It is the second commonest pelvic malignancy in the UK. Although this has evolved through a reduction in the incidence of cervical cancer, evidence exists to support the premise that the incidence of the disease is increasing (Masubuchi *et al*. 1975; Weiss *et al*. 1976). This is probably a true increase associated with increased world-wide development but figures are undoubtedly influenced also by improved diagnosis and reporting, an increasing age of population, a broadening of associated pathological criteria and, arguably, increased oestrogen usage (Greenblatt & Stoddard 1978).

Traditionally, it has been comforting for the gynaecologist to note that the chance of curing this disease is relatively high and some recent evidence suggests that overall mortality figures might be improving slightly. Notwithstanding this, survival rates are poor for all but the most favourable clinical circumstances (Fig. 6.1) and it is sobering to acknowledge that at least 25% of women with endometrial cancer will die of the disease within 5 years of diagnosis (Boronow 1976). Complacency in diagnosis, staging, primary surgery and the individualization of adjuvant therapy has therefore been repeatedly and firmly discouraged.

This chapter attempts to provide a comprehensive account of endometrial cancer but lays emphasis on the need to identify the woman at risk and argues the case for accurate primary surgical assessment and individualization of adjuvant treatment in the belief that the adherence to fixed management criteria will occasion an improvement in associated survival data.

Epidemiological considerations

Age

Endometrial cancer is essentially a disease of postmenopausal women with at least 80% of cases occurring after the cessation of menstruation. The maximum number of cases occur in the sixth decade of life with a median age of presentation of

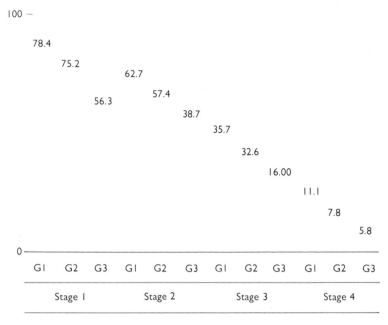

Fig. 6.1. Five-year survival data on 7656 patients treated world-wide between 1973 and 1975 (FIGO 1982).

61 years. Less than 5% of cases occur in women under the age of forty (Mattingly 1977) and there is a decrease in age-specific incidence rates after the age of 65 years.

Obesity

Overweight postmenopausal women have increased conversion of andro-stenedione to oestrone in their peripheral fat. Sex hormone binding globulin levels are decreased causing increased free oestrogens at cellular level. As a result of these changes target organ hyperstimulation might occur. The risk of development of endometrial cancer is proportional to the degree of obesity. Wynder *et al.* (1966) described the risk as being increased 3-fold if the woman was between 21−50 lb overweight and 10-fold if she was greater than 50 lb overweight.

Medical disorders

Diabetes mellitus and hypertension are risk factors associated with endometrial cancer and also occur in conjunction with obesity and increasing age. It would appear that the risk of endometrial cancer is increased 2.8 times in women who are diabetic. Conversely, reports vary regarding the incidence of diabetes mellitus

(5—45%) and hypertension (25—60%) in patients with endometrial cancer (Van Nagell *et al.* 1972).

Immunodeficiency diseases and immunosuppressed states are associated with the development of malignant disease (Husslein *et al.* 1978) and a past history of prior pelvic irradiation might also predispose to the development of gynaecological cancers (Rodriquez & Hart 1982; Gallion *et al.* 1987).

Abnormal hormonal status

Endogenous oestrogen production may occur in patients with hormone secreting tumours and in such conditions as polycystic ovary disease (Kistner 1970). Exogenous oestrogen has been implicated in the aetiology of endometrial cancer in patients with Turner's syndrome (McCarty *et al.* 1978; Oster *et al.* 1978), in women taking sequential oral contraception (WHO 1988) and in women who have inappropriately prescribed or administered hormone replacement therapy (Smith *et al.* 1975). Interestingly, there is some evidence to suggest that the inclusion of a progestogen in opposed hormone replacement therapy reduces endometrial stimulation (Whitehead *et al.* 1982) and results in reduced prevalence of corpus cancer in developed Western populations (Marret *et al.* 1982).

Parity

Between 21 and 34% of patients with endometrial cancer are nulliparous and the risk of endometrial cancer diminishes with increasing number of pregnancies. A nulliparous woman is twice as likely to develop endometrial cancer as the woman who has had one child and is three times more likely to develop the disease than the woman who has had five children (MacMahon 1974; Masubuchi & Nemoto 1972).

Late menopause

The association between the delayed cessation of menstruation and the development of endometrial carcinoma has been long recognized. Women undergoing the menopause after the age of 52 years have a 2—4 times increased risk of developing endometrial cancer over women ceasing menstruation before the age of 49 years.

Family history

Cancer of the uterine corpus occurring in a first degree relative will increase an individual's risk of developing the disease. Positive family histories are present in approximately 15% of cases.

Demography

Endometrial cancer is a disease of North America and northern European countries and is associated with the typical high fat and high protein western diet. Populations from low risk areas that adopt such a diet will assume the higher incidence of the disease.

Pathological considerations

The commonest histological cell type of endometrial cancer is adenocarcinoma, with most series quoting incidence rates between 60 and 80% (Liu 1972). Adenoacanthomas which incorporate adenocarcinomatous changes coexistent with benign squamous metaplasia comprise nearly 20% of tumours and a further 14% are of the adenosquamous variety where both the glandular and squamous elements are considered to be malignant (Silverberg *et al.* 1972; Ng *et al.* 1973). In 1% of cases clear cell carcinomata are identified and mucinous and papillary adenocarcinoma are variants. Primary squamous cell cancer of the endometrium is described but in its true form it is extremely rare and is usually associated with a pyometra (Hopkin *et al.* 1970; White *et al.* 1973; Levine & Sciorsci 1976). The endometrium is a site of secondary spread notably by tumours of the cervix, breast, gastrointestinal tract and kidney. Further, in women with endometrioid ovarian cancer the uterine corpus is involved in one-third of cases either as a function of metastatic spread or as a concomitant primary tumour (Scully 1975).

The histological grade of a particular tumour is important to categorize and the prognostic significance of such accurate analysis will be discussed later. In its most well differentiated form endometrial adenocarcinoma is difficult to distinguish from the more severe grades of atypical hyperplasia. While this is not of great significance in terms of management such lack of pathological agreement will, of course, affect quoted incidence rates and overall survival figures making data difficult to interpret. Bearing this in mind the quoted rates for various grades of adenocarcinoma are as follows (Du Toit 1985):

Grade I   45–55%
Grade II   30–35%
Grade III   15–20%

Mode of spread

Endometrial cancer may disseminate by direct invasion, by lymphatic spread, via the bloodstream or by a combination of these routes.

Direct invasion

The earliest spread of cancer of the corpus is by direct extension into the myometrium and progressively towards the uterine isthmus and cervix. Approximately 50% of all endometrial cancers are confined to the endometrium at the time of diagnosis, a further 26% will exhibit early myometrial invasion and 12% deep myometrial invasion. Extension beyond the uterus at the time of presentation is found in 11% of cases (Reagan & Fu 1981). Adenosquamous tumours tend to be more advanced at the time of detection; in the same series only 35% were limited to the endometrium at initial diagnosis.

Lymphatic spread

Lymphatic spread may involve three groups of nodes; pelvic, para-aortic, and, rarely, the inguinal lymph nodes. The incidence of nodal involvement closely correlates with the size of the central tumour, the histological grade and the depth of myometrial invasion (Berman *et al.* 1980; Disaia & Creasman 1981). An understanding of the pattern of lymphatic spread in this disease is important. In the majority of instances tumour cells will pass into broad ligament lymphatics and from there progress to the external iliac, internal iliac and obturator nodes in the pelvis. The lymphatic flow from the pelvic nodes is in a cephalad direction and para-aortic node involvement can occur on a secondary and progressive basis. Tumours arising from the uterine fundus can, however, spread via lymphatic channels in the infundibulo—pelvic ligament and thereafter follow pathways associated with the primary lymphatic drainage of the ovary leading to metastatic disease in para-aortic lymph nodes at the level of the renal vessels. Once again the prevailing direction of lymph flow is cephalad but retrograde spread is well described and disease may arise in the nodes at the aortic bifurcation by this second pathway. Notwithstanding this, the finding of positive aortic nodes in the absence of pelvic node disease is an uncommon event; conversely, if the pelvic nodes are involved the para-aortic nodes will be positive in approximately 60% of cases (Creasman *et al.* 1976). It is unusual for lymphatic channels in the region of the round ligament to convey tumour to the groin nodes but such lymphatic spread patterns are occasionally encountered.

Spread to the vagina, at the apex of the vaginal vault and also to the lower third of the anterior wall, is a feared complication and occurs in approximately 8% of cases. As will be discussed later this is probably a reflection of retrograde spread in lymphatics rather than cell spillage and implantation.

Blood-borne spread

Spread by the bloodstream tends to occur at a later stage in this disease and most commonly involves the lungs (8.3%), but metastases to liver (5.9%), bone (3.4%), brain and the adrenal glands are also described (Plentl & Friedman 1971).

Clinical features

Cancer of the corpus

Originates in the superficial layers of a thick walled organ. Disruption of the endometrium fortunately will reveal itself at an early stage by inappropriate bleeding. Such bleeding may be preceded by a brownish watery discharge. Therefore, the prime symptom is postmenopausal bleeding. Twenty percent of cases, however, occur in younger women in which case the tumour presents with intermenstrual bleeding or metrorrhagia. Clearly, such symptoms must be taken seriously and acted upon, but it must be noted that the specificity of abnormal bleeding patterns for endometrial cancer is low. Estimates of the incidence of endometrial cancer underlying the symptom of postmenopausal bleeding vary between 1–20%.

Diagnosis and primary assessment

Traditionally the diagnosis of endometrial cancer has been confirmed by histological examination of the specimen obtained at dilatation and curettage. At this procedure examination under anaesthesia will also provide the clinician with an initial assessment of the extent of the pelvic pathology. The size of the uterus can be assessed with a good degree of accuracy and evidence of adnexal pathology can be obtained. Exploration of the uterine cavity and systematic curettage will also provide some impression of the size and extent of tumour burden but gross assessment of curettings is notoriously inaccurate and the precise location and extent of tumour spread cannot be assessed with any great accuracy by this technique. Some authorities advocate the use of fractional curettage in order to obtain evidence of cervical involvement by the tumour. It is the author's feeling that this procedure is also highly imprecise and if treatment modification is to be based on information gained from this technique it is essential that as much care as possible is taken to avoid mixing of specimens obtained from the cervical canal and the uterine cavity. Prior to any manipulative procedure, therefore, the cervical canal must be carefully curetted and any specimen should be obtained prior to sounding or dilatation. In spite of this it is a rare circumstance to find convincing evidence of occult stage II disease at this pretreatment assessment. Because of this, attempts at more accurate methods of assessing the size of the tumour burden and the extent of tumour spread have been made using a variety of visualization techniques. Hysteroscopy is advocated by some as a means of providing such useful information. Both contact and standard hysteroscopy have been employed and those in support of the technique testify to its usefulness in directing biopsy, and in assessing tumour characteristics (Joelsson *et al.* 1971; Sugimoto 1975) such as volume and involvement of the endocervix. A persistent worry associated with hysteroscopy has always been that, theoretically, it could facilitate tumour spread and its detractors are quick to voice this concern (Baggish & Barbot 1983). However, no firm data exist to support this understandable fear. With increased knowledge, hysteroscopy might well prove to be a useful adjuvant investigation in the pretreatment assessment of patients with endometrial cancer. Gas hysteroscopy markedly reduces the risk of tumour dissemination.

Recently there has been increasing interest in the use of imaging techniques in the initial assessment of patients with postmenopausal bleeding (Ross 1988). Ultrasound may demonstrate endometrial thickening, can give an idea of tumour size and will help to identify grossly enlarged regional lymph nodes (Lehtovirta et al. 1987). Whether it is of value as a screening test which may be used to subselect a group of patients with postmenopausal bleeding who do not need a curettage awaits the results of current research trials. Computerized axial tomography (CT) scanning and, more recently, magnetic resonance imaging (MRI) may also be employed to provide information on extended tumour spread. Such techniques in this context, however, are in their infancy, are relatively expensive and in very fat and very thin patients are hampered by size limitation of lesion detected. However, grossly enlarged lymph nodes can be identified and in certain circumstances an idea of the extent and depth of myometrial invasion can be obtained.

Further information regarding tumour spread may be obtained from a chest X-ray, which is essential, but radiological assessment of the urinary and gastrointestinal tract is not performed on a routine basis. Lymphangiography has its advocates but again does not normally constitute part of routine preoperative management, and indeed, with increasing knowledge of the values of magnetic resonance spectroscopy, lymphangiography might assume even less relevance in the future (Galaknoff et al. 1988).

It is, of course, of importance to make as thorough and precise an assessment of each patient and her tumour and to acquire as much knowledge as possible of the disease prior to therapy. Only then can rationalized and planned treatment be directed on an individual basis. Such an assessment would necessarily give credence to acknowledged risk factors which adversely affect survival.

Age

Evidence exists to show that older patients developing endometrial cancer have poorer survival rates. This probably reflects a disproportionately high number of tumours of poor histological differentiation and more advanced stage that occur in women in their 60s and 70s compared with women who develop the disease in their 50s (Frick et al. 1973). The patients' age may also reflect their general health (Oster et al. 1978) and this together with an assessment of obesity may influence their suitability for surgery.

Uterine size

Although this factor has been incorporated into a FIGO clinical substage and while there is some correlation between uterine size and survival (84.5% 5-year survival for normal sized uterus vs. 66.6% 5-year survival if the uterus is enlarged (Jones 1975)), it is well recognized that the uterus may be enlarged by pathology other than corpus cancer. In a review of 100 cases of endometrial cancer Javert & Douglas (1956) report uterine enlargement in half, but cancer was the underlying cause in only eight patients. It must be concluded therefore that uterine size is an unreliable prognostic indicator.

Histological grade

Information regarding the histological grade of the tumour will be obtained at the initial curettage. However, it must be understood that the degree of differentiation in any malignancy may not be homogeneous and that different histological grades may be identified in different areas of the tumour. In these instances the pathologist is obliged to classify the tumour at the lowest histological grade. This can be the reason for discrepancy between tumour differentiation reported at curettage and the grade of tumour which is decided upon in the final hysterectomy specimen. The histopathologist's difficulties may be compounded by the problems implicit in the subjective appraisal of architectural appearance. Grade I and grade III tumours are usually easy to distinguish but grade II lesions are less easy to define and to diagnose with clarity using these standard techniques. Nevertheless, patients with a poorly differentiated or unclassifiable tumour must be recognized as high risk prior to undergoing their definitive surgery (Chambers *et al.* 1987).

Cell type

Cell type is an important prognostic indicator in patients with endometrial carcinoma. Although the majority (85%) are endometrioid adenocarcinomas, the less common histological variants must be recognized as these have a much poorer survival (Table 6.1).

Staging and secondary assessment

At the time of the primary assessment, therefore, patients can be categorized as high risk because of obvious advanced disease, adverse histological features or both. Other risk factors may not be defined with clarity until the time of the initial laparotomy or until the final histological assessment of the hysterectomy specimen is obtained.

It is widely agreed that clinical staging of cancer of the corpus is inaccurate,

Table 6.1. Relative frequency of cell types and associated 5-year survival

	n	Percent of cases	Percent alive	Percent DOD
Adenocarcinoma*	604	61.1	75.2	9.7
Adenoacanthoma	215	21.7	87.0	6.0
Papillary adenocarcinoma	46	4.7	51.1	33.3
Mixed adenosquamous	68	6.9	47.5	42.4
Clear cell carcinoma	56	5.7	35.2	61.1

* Includes secretory and mucinous carcinoma.
DOD = dead of disease (Christopherson 1986).

however, while approximately 75% of these tumours at the time of presentation may be designated stage I as shown in Table 6.2. The majority of patients that die of the cancer have stage I disease. While clinical staging broadly correlates with overall survival it cannot be used as a reliable prognostic indicator on an individual basis. Clinicians have reacted to this state of affairs by frequently publishing data associated with surgicopathological findings rather than clinical stage. While this practice is aesthetically satisfying it has inevitably led to a degree of confusion and it is pleasing therefore that at the most recent FIGO World Congress in Brazil (1988) (Shepherd 1989) the concept of surgical staging in this disease was approved and an official classification was agreed. Table 6.3 outlines the current staging of endometrial cancer together with suggested guidelines from the FIGO Committee on Gynaecological Oncology. Such thorough surgical exploration and accurate clinicopathological assessment will, hopefully, rid us of the dilemmas previously faced when apparent stage I disease was found to have occult ovarian metastases at the time of surgery; when a large uterus with apparent clinical stage Ib disease at laparotomy is found to be a small tumour with a fibroid; when apparent clinical stage III disease is found to be an early endometrial cancer and a benign ovarian cyst; and finally surgical staging will enable the critical factor of lymph node status to be taken into account.

Table 6.2. Endometrial carcinoma: FIGO staging at diagnosis

Series	Stage			
	I	II	III	IV
Morrow et al. (1973)	76.5	8.4	10.4	4.6
Berman et al. (1980)	74.4	12.8	9.4	3.4
Kauppila et al. (1982)	75.9	16.8	10.0	7.3
Du Toit (1983)	70.0	16.0	10.0	4.0

Table 6.3.   Corpus cancer staging (FIGO 1988)

Stage	
IA G123	Tumour limited to endometrium
IB G123	Invasion to < 1/2 myometrium
IC G123	Invasion to > 1/2 myometrium
IIA G123	Endocervical glandular involvement only
IIB G123	Cervical stromal invasion
IIIA G123	Tumour invades serosa and/or positive peritoneal cytology
IIIB G123	Vaginal metastases
IIIC G123	Metastases to pelvic and/or para-aortic lymph nodes
IVA G123	Tumour invasion bladder and/or bowel mucosa
IVB	Distant metastases including intraabdominal and/or inguinal lymph node

Histopathology: degree of differentiation

Cases of carcinoma of the corpus should be grouped with regard to the degree of differentiation of the adenocarcinoma as follows.

G1 = 5% or less of a nonsquamous or nonmorular solid growth pattern
G2 = 6–50% of a nonsquamous or nonmorular solid growth pattern
G3 = more than 50% of a nonsquamous or nonmorular solid growth pattern

Notes on pathological grading

1 Notable nuclear atypia, inappropriate for the architectural grade, raises the grade of a grade I or grade II tumour by 1
2 In serous adenocarcinomas, clear cell adenocarcinomas, and squamous cell carcinomas, nuclear grading takes precedent
3 Adenocarcinomas with squamous differentiation are graded according to the nuclear grade of the glandular component

Rules related to staging

1 Since corpus cancer is now surgically staged, procedures previously used for differentiation of stages are no longer applicable, such as the finding of D & C to differentiate between stage I and stage II
   (a) It is appreciated that there may be a small number of patients with corpus cancer who will be treated primarily with radiation therapy. If that is the case, the clinical staging adopted by FIGO in 1971 would still apply but designation of that staging system would be noted
2 Ideally, width of the myometrium should be measured along with the width of tumour invasion

Cytological washings

On opening the peritoneal cavity the Pouch of Douglas and pelvic peritoneum should be washed with saline and the aspirate sent for cytological examination. In the absence of a randomized study, the significance of positive cytological washings at the present time is uncertain. A positive result is obtained in up to

15% of endometrial cancers and Creasman and Rutledge have reported impaired survival in such cases (Creasman & Rutledge 1971; Lewis 1980). The finding is more frequently associated with high grade lesions and those tumours invading the outer third of the myometrium. In these selected cases a positive result may be obtained in 50% of washings taken, and can only be assumed to constitute an extra adverse feature of this disease process. However, Konski et al. (1988) deny that positive cytology is an independent prognostic factor. A retrospective study of 163 patients by Kennedy et al. (1987) failed to demonstrate a significant association between positive washings and other risk factors, and as only two patients underwent treatment modification as a result of the cytology result they conclude that pelvic washings have a limited role in the management of early stage endometrial cancer.

Myometrial invasion

On removing the uterus the specimen should be opened carefully in a longitudinal fashion until the endometrial cavity is displayed. Macroscopic assessment enables the clinician to assess the bulk of tumour present and in the majority, but not all, an idea can be gleaned as to the depth of involvement of the underlying myometrium. Impaired survival with increasing depth of myometrial invasion is a feature reported by most series. Patients with superficial myometrial invasion would appear to have no worse a prognosis in terms of 5-year survival than patients with tumour confined to the endometrium; however, if there is deep myometrial involvement the survival rates fall from 80 to 60% in stage 1 disease (Jones 1975). The proximity of tumour invasion to the serosal surface is of prognostic significance (Lutz et al. 1978).

Adnexal spread

At the time of primary surgical assessment spread to the adnexae may be identified in 7–8% of cases. Frequently this is a microscopic detection which is reported at the time of the final histological report. If it is representative of solitary disease then it need not signify poorer survival. Once again, however, this finding most frequently occurs in conjunction with other risk factors such as poor histological differentiation, myometrial invasion and cervical involvement.

Lymph node status

Clearly, the risk factors of histological grade and myometrial invasion are inter-linked. Only 12% of well differentiated lesions exhibit deep myometrial invasion compared with a 46% incidence in grade III lesions (Cheon 1977). If at the time of primary or secondary assessment a patient is deemed to be of high risk due to any of the above risk factors then lymph node sampling may be considered.

Tables 6.4 and 6.5 demonstrate the incidence of pelvic lymph node involvement with worsening degrees of myometrial invasion and increasing histological grade.

The woman at risk

Assimilation of all of the preceding information allows the clinician to identify the woman who is destined to fail treatment. This selection process allows individualized management that is crucial if survivals in endometrial cancer are to be improved (Creasman *et al.* 1987). It has been proposed that using the above risk criteria patients may be divided into four clinicopathological groups, as illustrated in Table 6.6.

Management

Screening and prevention

In purely theoretical terms endometrial cancer is a disease that should lend itself to the screening process, but in practice no studies of large scale screening of an asymptomatic female population have been reported. In all probability this reflects the failure of any single test to emerge with adequate fulfillment of basic screening

Table 6.4. Stage I endometrial cancer: incidence of lymph node metastases associated with varying degrees of myometrial invasion

	Myometrial invasion		
Authors	Superficial (%)	Intermediate (%)	Deep (%)
Lewis *et al.* (1970)	0	14.3	36.2
Creasman *et al.* (1976)	7.5	10.0	43.0
Berman *et al.* (1980)	3.0	14.0	41.0
Disaia & Creasman (1981)	5.5	13.3	46.4

Table 6.5. Stage I endometrial cancer: incidence of lymph node metastases against histological grade

	Histological grade		
Authors	1 (%)	2 (%)	3 (%)
Lewis *et al.* (1970)	5.5	10.0	26.0
Creasman *et al.* (1976)	3.1	10.9	36.0
Berman *et al.* (1980)	3.0	11.0	26.0

Table 6.6. Surgicopathological prognostic groups and management

Prognostic group	Disease criteria
1 Excellent prognosis	EAC in stage I with G1 or G2 *and* My– or My0
2 Very good prognosis	EAC in stage I with G1 or G2 *and* My1
3 High risk group	PC, ASC, CCC and UCC in stages I, II, or III with spread only to ovaries, tubes or pelvic nodes, with any G and any My EAC in stage I with G3, *or* with My2, My3 or My4 (a) any stage II, histologically confirmed (b) any stage III if spread is only to ovaries, tubes or pelvic nodes, histologically confirmed All cell types of tumour in (a) any stage III with spread to pelvic tissues other than ovaries, tubes, nodes and/or with incomplete tumour excision (b) any stage IVa or IVb, any recurrence

Staging quoted is FIGO staging. Tumour terminology is that of International Academy of Pathology (Appendix D).

Abbreviations:

EAC	Endometrioid adenocarcinoma	My–	No residual tumour	G	Histological grade (1, 2 or 3)
PC	Papillary carcinoma	My0	No muscle invasion	TAH	Total abdominal hysterectomy
ASC	Adenosquamous carcinoma	My1	1/3 muscle invasion	BSO	Bilateral salpingo-oophorectomy
CCC	Clear cell carcinoma	My2, My3	2/3, 3/3 muscle invasion	IVR	Intravaginal radiotherapy
				MVT	Megavoltage radiotherapy
UCC	Unclassifiable carcinoma	My4	Serosal invasion		

requirements. A variety of techniques exist which permit sampling of endometrial cells by both cytological and histological means. The standard Papanicolaou cervical smear has inadequate specificity for use as a screening test for endometrial cancer, being positive, probably, in no more than 50% of cases (Jones *et al.* 1972; Frick *et al.* 1975). Some authorities suggest that concomitant sampling of the vaginal pool will increase the diagnostic yield, but even so sufficient accuracy is still not achieved. Endometrial samples are generally obtained by a variety of techniques which include some form of scraping, aspirating or suction of the uterine cavity. Cytological assessment of endometrial cells which are obtained by brushing or washing the endometrial cavity has a limited diagnostic accuracy for endometrial cancer and the ability to detect precursor lesions is even less satisfactory (Pacifico *et al.* 1982). Histological analysis of specimens obtained by suction aspiration techniques provides greater accuracy and has a higher ability to identify precursor lesions and accuracy rates in excess of 96% have been reported for instruments such as the Kevorkian curette and the Vabra aspirator. Specimens obtained by these techniques are adequate for laboratory assessment by both cytological and histological means. Cytology requires special skills in interpretation. A negative result will not necessarily exclude endometrial pathology but false positive results are uncommon. The main limitation of these techniques, however, is the discomfort caused by the passage of the cannula through the cervical canal, particularly in postmenopausal patients with a degree of atrophic change and cervical stenosis.

The incidence of hyperplasia of the endometrium in asymptomatic women is unknown but the problem is greatest in the perimenopausal age group and in postmenopausal women taking oestrogen with inadequate progestogenic balance. Consideration may be given to the application of some of these screening techniques alone or in combination for use in selected instances in what might be defined as a high risk population for endometrial cancer (Ewertz *et al.* 1988). In practice, a form of screening in a selected population already exists as diagnostic curettage is performed on all women with abnormal bleeding patterns in their 40s and 50s. It is in this group of symptomatic women that screening using ultrasound, hysteroscopy or magnetic resonance imaging might be most beneficial.

The purpose of the implementation of a screening programme would be to diagnose early asymptomatic endometrial cancers in the hope, albeit unsubstantiated, that the detection of the disease at an asymptomatic screened stage would result in improved survival figures over disease diagnosed at symptomatic presentation. Secondly, an opportunity would be provided for the identification of endometrial cancer precursors such as adenomatous hyperplasia.

The identification of atypical hyperplasia in these groups provides an opportunity for counselling the patient towards hysterectomy and the consequent prevention of endometrial cancer (Fox & Buckley 1982; Scully 1982).

Management of established disease

Endometrial cancer has a less predictable behaviour pattern than other gynaecological malignancies and its management in terms of curative treatment remains a source of controversy amongst gynaecologists. Agreement can be reached on the basic premise that the cornerstone of treatment is surgery; however it is to be hoped that there is a growing acknowledgement of the benefit and advisability of individualization of therapeutic options. The concept of a single treatment regimen for endometrial cancer is simplistic and unacceptable in modern oncological practice. The woman with a small, well differentiated lesion has a greatly different prognosis and necessarily requires different treatment to the patient with a poorly differentiated lesion demonstrating cervical involvement or deep myometrial invasion. The prevailing opinion therefore is to proceed from the diagnostic curettage to a laparotomy which permits a very thorough and accurate assessment of the tumour burden and the extent of disease spread (Creasman et al. 1987). Treatment modifications based on surgicopathological findings may then be logically made.

The fact that confusion persists, however, is understandable and arises from the failure to identify a clearly superior treatment plan. This in turn is due to a paucity of well controlled prospective randomized trials and a continuing inability to draw comparisons between studies because of inconsistency in staging and design. The dilemma of selecting optimum therapy is added to by the number and variation of biological patterns of tumour behaviour that can influence prognosis. In the absence of convincing data from well planned clinical trials, efforts to rationalize treatment regimens have evolved which are based on these biological methods of tumour spread. Considering these in detail will, it is hoped, ease the frustration for the student and clinician alike and help to identify a reasoned and defensible approach to therapy.

Stage I disease

Seventy-five percent of cases of endometrial cancer present at this early stage. The majority of management decisions and dilemmas exist within this group of patients. The major issues that influence attitudes and fire prejudices concern the use and timing of radiotherapy in relation to surgery, and the degree of radicality that is required of the operative procedure itself. It must be clear that answering these questions honestly and scientifically is often difficult. For instance, in well differentiated stage I tumours 5-year survival rates in excess of 90% are described. In order to show survival advantages of statistically significant difference between therapies, long term studies of large numbers of patients would be required. Understandably, such data are lacking. Nevertheless certain issues are clear:
1 Endometrial cancer is radiosensitive.

2 Survival is better when surgery is used alone than when radiotherapy is used alone.

3 The survival benefit of combining surgery and radiotherapy is unproven.

In spite of this radiotherapy continues to be an integral part of current management schemata and debate persists as to the optimum dosage, method and timing of administration.

Preoperative vs. postoperative radiotherapy

Much of clinical practice has been influenced by the underlying concern regarding the risk of recurrent disease at the vaginal vault. Comfort has been gained from the belief that irradiating the vagina decreases the incidence of this complication even if assurance of ultimate survival benefit is lacking. The incidence of vault recurrence is affected by the histological grade of the primary tumour and the depth to which it invades the myometrium. Poorly differentiated lesions which are confined to the endometrium rarely metastasize to the nodes but the risk of vault recurrence is appreciable. As previously mentioned disease in the vault arises as a result of retrograde spread in paravaginal lymphatics and not by tumour cell dissemination and implantation at the time of surgery (Truskett & Constable 1968). The incidence of vault recurrence is extremely low (1%) if the tumour is only superficial and does not penetrate the myometrium (Brown *et al.* 1986) and occurs in only 2.5% of cases if the tumour is well differentiated (Price *et al.* 1965). In the same series the incidence of this complication in patients treated by surgery alone having anaplastic tumours or with deep myometrial invasion rises to 13.6 and 15.1%, respectively. This can be reduced by the addition of adjuvant radiotherapy but whether this is given pre- or postoperatively appears immaterial.

Proponents of preoperative radiotherapy stress the following advantages.

1 By giving intrauterine and vaginal applications paravaginal and paracervical lymphatics are treated, not just vaginal epithelium, thus reducing the incidence of vault recurrence.

2 Tissue oxygenation is maximum prior to surgery.

3 Preoperative irradiation obviates the need to remove a vaginal cuff.

4 If surgery follows rapidly the specimen is not necessarily affected.

5 The morbidity of local radiotherapy applications is low.

6 Decreased viability of tumour cells reduces any theoretical chance of intra-operative dissemination.

Arguments against preoperative irradiation include:

1 Because of the low incidence of endometrial cancer vault metastases a high percentage of patients would have unnecessary irradiation.

2 No data exist to support the view that vault recurrence is less following preoperative than postoperative radiotherapy.

3 Tumour characteristics are obscured even if operation follows reasonably soon after therapy.

4 It is rational to assess the extent of disease before embarking on treatment.

5 Some tumours are radio-resistant and preoperative radiotherapy would occasion an unnecessary delay in surgery.

The majority of endometrial cancers are stage I grade I lesions with an associated 5-year survival rate in excess of 90%. Vault recurrence associated with such lesions following surgery alone is rare (less than 3%). Whether it is justified to give radiotherapy to all patients with stage I endometrial cancer, acknowledging that it is over treatment for the majority but beneficial to the few women who would be missed by postoperative selection, is the issue that underpins this whole debate.

Radical vs. nonradical surgery

Current surgical trends dictate that endometrial cancer should be treated by extrafascial hysterectomy with bilateral salpingo-oophorectomy. The inclusion of a cuff of upper vagina with the specimen is favoured by some in the belief that upper vaginal vault recurrence will be prevented. This is not borne out in practice, however (Price *et al.* 1965) and it is argued that for favourable tumours this procedure is unnecessary and for more aggressive tumours it is inadequate.

Poorly differentiated lesions and tumours invading the myometrium more than one-third have a propensity for lymphatic spread. In such high risk cases surgical removal of regional lymph nodes should be considered.

Lymphadenectomy

Selective lymphadenectomy may be of value. Information gained may be used as a prognostic indicator and also as a treatment modifier. Balanced against the beneficial individualization of patient care is the possibility of increasing morbidity by extending surgery in women who often have a poor general medical status. The technique of lymphadenectomy, whether pelvic or para-aortic, is not a difficult one (Oram & Bridges 1987) but is considerably hampered by obesity in such patients. Access is restricted, small vessel bleeding from fatty tissue is a nuisance and landmark anatomy is obscured. The use of occlusive clips to secure haemostasis and lymphostasis is recommended.

Pelvic lymphadenectomy

Pelvic nodes are involved by tumour in approximately 10% of clinical stage I disease overall (Boronow *et al.* 1984). This percentage is higher in poorly differentiated tumours, unfavourable cell type and those exhibiting myometrial invasion. It might reasonably be argued that the performance of complete pelvic lymphadenectomy in these cases is justifiable. These patients fall into a high risk category and should be considered for postoperative pelvic irradiation. Knowledge gained from the status of the regional lymph nodes will affect this therapeutic decision. In particular, if following complete pelvic lymphadenectomy no evidence of metastatic nodal spread is evident the patient will be spared unnecessary adjuvant radiotherapy following her surgery. If positive pelvic nodes are found the situation is less clear. It is debatable whether lymphadenectomy is curative in its own right and equally it is not clear if the addition of pelvic irradiation in these cases will improve survival. In such instances it is also worthy of note that 60% of pelvic node positive cases will have involved para-aortic nodes.

Para-aortic lymphadenectomy

As previously described, the para-aortic nodes may be involved as a result of direct spread from fundal endometrial tumours, but more commonly disease arises in this area as a result of progressive lymphatic spread from pelvic nodes. Para-aortic lymphadenectomy is indicated in high risk endometrial cancers when the patient's general medical condition permits. The status of the para-aortic nodes in these cases will have therapeutic implications. It is widely described that clinical assessment of these nodes is notoriously inaccurate. Palpably enlarged nodes can be due to reactive hyperplasia and normal sized non-palpable nodes are capable of containing micrometastatic deposits. The only means of accurately assessing the nodal status therefore is by removing the lymphoid tissue and subjecting it to histological examination. Should tumour be found in the para-aortic lymph nodes then this is of prognostic significance and therapeutic import-ance. These nodes lie outside conventional treatment fields. The attack on gynaecological tumours, be it surgical or radiotherapeutic, is primarily directed at the pelvis. Disease in the para-aortic nodes is therefore not treated by these traditional regimens. The identification of para-aortic nodal disease will modify treatment either by extending the irradiation field to include this nodal group or adding systemic chemotherapy to the treatment plan. Conversely, if the para-aortic nodes are proven to be free of disease then the clinician has the assurance that treatment of the pelvis will encompass the extent of the disease spread.

This approach is well thought out and rational. It is defensible on the basis that it is fundamentally important for the clinician to know the precise nature of the tumour and the exact extent of disease spread, and to this extent is laudable in that it permits logical and reasoned therapy which is tailored to the individual patient and her tumour. It is a theory that requires the support of the modern gynaecological oncologist. In the course of providing practical patient care how-ever, theoretical neatness should be tempered by clinical judgement and two points should be firmly noted. First, in elderly women who are overweight and often medically unfit for radical surgery, it has been estimated (Kneale 1977) that lymphadenectomy is feasible in no more than 30−40% of cases. Secondly, whether treatment modification based on the knowledge gained from nodal status leads to improved overall survival rates remains to be proven.

In summary, extensive nodal sampling will identify a proportion of high risk patients who do not require radiotherapy, and a small number of patients who might benefit from extended field irradiation and systemic chemotherapy. A treatment schema for stage I disease is shown in Table 6.7. Because of the variables inherent in this disease process and the marked differences in survival figures within these various groups it is necessarily complex.

Grade I lesions rarely invade the myometrium to any significant degree and may be regarded as minimal risk. In poorly differentiated lesions myometrial invasion and lymphatic spread are encountered with increasing frequency. Lymphadenectomy is recommended in such instances and it is in this minority (20%) of patients with endometrial cancer that tertiary referral to a gynaecological oncology centre might be considered.

Stage II disease

Notwithstanding the doubtful benefits of fractional curettage and the increasingly accepted advantages of hysteroscopy, the identification of cervical involvement by tumour in endometrial cancer is frequently undiagnosed pre-operatively. Extension to the cervix is found most commonly when the uterus is opened following its removal at surgery, or in the absence of such macroscopic change, disease spread is identified for the first time in the histological report. Treatment guidelines may be affected by the timing of this knowledge. Traditionally those patients with stage II disease diagnosed preoperatively were treated by radical hysterectomy and pelvic lymphadenectomy. However, as previously discussed, radical surgery in these women is often difficult and has no survival benefit over irradiation and simple hysterectomy. This is borne out when the pattern of recurrent disease in stage II is considered. Studies have shown that the majority who fail treatment present with distant metastases rather than recurrent pelvic disease. In such circumstances in spite of the propensity for stage II disease to metastasize to pelvic lymph nodes, radical surgery makes little sense. At the present time it must be concluded that stage II corpus cancer should be treated by a combination of simple hysterectomy and bilateral salpingo-oophorectomy, combined with pelvic irradiation.

If stage II disease is diagnosed prior to laparotomy arguments can be made in favour of preoperative intracavity and vaginal vault caesium applications, whole pelvic external beam irradiation, followed by surgery. If, as is more commonly the case, cervical extension is noted following staging laparotomy then external beam irradiation to the whole pelvis supported by vaginal vault application is the treatment of choice.

Table 6.7.   Treatment schema for stage Ia disease

	Myo 0/I	Myo II	Myo III
G I	TAH + BSO	TAH + BSO + LNS	
G II	TAH + BSO + LNS		
	+ve = MVT + IVR	+ve or not performed = MVT + IVR	
G III	−ve/not performed	−ve = IVR	
	= IVR		

TAH: total abdominal hysterectomy; BSO: bilateral salpingo-oophorectomy;
LNS: lymph node sampling; MVT: megavoltage radiotherapy; IVR:
intravaginal radiotherapy; Myo O/I: no muscle or 1/3 muscle invasion; Myo
II: 2/3 muscle invasion; Myo III: 3/3 muscle invasion.

Advanced stage disease

Fortunately, advanced stage disease at the time of presentation is relatively uncommon. Attention is drawn to the possibility of tumour spread beyond the
uterus at the time of the initial clinical appraisal.

   The management of patients with stage III disease is dictated by the time at
which it is identified. If the overall clinical assessment provides conclusive
evidence of adnexal spread, then preoperative whole pelvic irradiation followed
by total abdominal hysterectomy and bilateral salpingo-oophorectomy is acceptable. More often, adnexal spread is identified intraoperatively or postoperatively on histological review of the surgical specimen. If disease spread of
this nature is identified during primary laparotomy then a thorough metastatic
survey should be performed including selective para-aortic and pelvic node
sampling. Postoperative irradiation and/or chemotherapy should be given on an
adjuvant basis depending on the extent of the tumour dissemination. Unsuspected
adnexal spread diagnosed at histological examination would be treated in a
similar but possibly less precise fashion. Stage IV disease identified either preoperatively or at the initial surgical assessment should be treated initially by
radiotherapy if confined to the pelvis, with or without adjuvant chemotherapy.
Radical surgery in these cases has little place because of the potential for distant
spread in such circumstances.

Recurrent disease

Tumour recurrences are more likely in the defined high risk groups and in
approximately 80% of cases will occur within two years of primary therapy.
Treatment is directly related to the site of recurrence and whether it is solitary or
multifocal. Vaginal recurrences classically occur in two sites, at the apex of the
vaginal vault and in the lower third of the vagina in a retrourethral position on
the anterior wall. These can usually be treated by surgery, radiotherapy or a
combination of both. Patients frequently do well and long term survivors are
described. In such circumstances, however, it is important to ascertain that this

apparent solitary recurrence is exactly that, and not a local manifestation of more widespread disease. Recurrent disease occurring in more distant sites, e.g. lungs, should be treated by hormonal or chemotherapy. The place of radical or exenterative surgery is extremely limited and should only be considered if recurrent disease is confined to the centre of the pelvis with no evidence of further spread. This is an uncommon clinical occurrence.

Hormonal and chemotherapy

Hormonal therapy

The use of anti-oestrogens (Tamoxifen) and progestogens in the treatment of endometrial cancer is widespread. Studies reporting objective response rates of up to 60% in advanced or recurrent disease have been described (Batteli *et al.* 1982). However, the use of adjuvant hormonal therapy in the treatment of primary disease is less clear. The oestrogen/progesterone receptor status of the tumour appears to correlate well both with the response to progesterone therapy and also to 5-year survival (Chambers *et al.* 1988). A decrease in receptor concentration appears to occur with the worsening histological grade and advancement of the disease. In the same series it was also suggested that oestrogen receptor status was a better predictor of survival than tumour grade. Nevertheless, treatment modification based on receptor status must be viewed with caution. Lack of receptor homogeneity within any individual tumour can be found when multiple blocks of tissue are examined. Further, the expression of receptors by single tumour cells may be varied or cyclical in nature rather than a constant phenomenon. The use of progestogens in early stage disease in those tumours with a high receptor content is still to be evaluated; this is difficult because of the excellent survival in this group of patients. Results from a prospective randomized trial of progestogen therapy in high risk patients is awaited and is currently being performed by the COSA – UK collaborative group. Recent data however (MacDonald *et al.* 1988) suggest that progestogens are of no value in this group of patients. Moreover these studies report a worryingly high incidence of thromboembolic disorders occurring in the treatment arm. At present, therefore, the blanket use of progestogen therapy in patients with endometrial carcinoma cannot be justified. The selective use of progestogens as primary adjuvant therapy must be weighed against the possible risks of intercurrent disease associated with the drug and its relatively high cost.

Tamoxifen has been demonstrated to invoke tumour response in advanced and recurrent disease (Swenerton *et al.* 1979). Quinn & Campbell (1989) have recently described a 20% overall response rate in such cases. These authors speculate that as Tamoxifen not only has anti-oestrogen activity but is also capable of enhancing progestogen response, the use of the hormones in combination may be an attractive proposition. The results of randomized trials are awaited.

Chemotherapy

Few large randomized controlled trials exist to support the use of cytotoxic agents in the treatment of endometrial carcinoma. However, adriamycin and cisplatinum appear to be the most effective single agents with response rates of up to 45% reported. Although overall response rates of up to 85% with combined agent chemotherapy are described, these data are small, and as yet the benefit of these regimens is inconclusive.

Results and treatment

Table 6.8 illustrates a selection of reported survival data according to broad clinical stage of disease at presentation. The overall 5-year survival for all stages of this disease has not improved substantially in recent years and is reported as 63% between the years 1962−68 and 67.7% between the years 1976−78 (FIGO Annual Report, Stockholm). Risk factors within clinical stages affect survival and Tables 6.9 and 6.10 illustrate the effect of histological grade and myometrial invasion on overall 5-year survival as reported by collected series.

Table 6.8.   Stage vs. survival in endometrial cancer

| | Survival | | | |
Series	Stage I (%)	Stage II (%)	Stage III (%)	Stage IV (%)
Kottmeier (48)	72	50	31	9
Morrow (67)	76	51	26	9
Salt (81)	90	50	24	9

Table 6.9.   Stage I endometrial carcinoma: histological grade vs. 5-year survival

Series	Grade 1 (%)	Grade 2 (%)	Grade 3 (%)
Frick *et al.* (1973)	86.1	63.4	54.5
Jones (1975)	81.0	74.0	50.0
Connelly *et al.* (1982)	84.1	73.9	51.1

Table 6.10.   Stage I endometrial carcinoma: myometrial invasion vs. 5-year survival

| | Myometrial invasion | | |
Series	> 1/3 (%)	Middle 1/3 (%)	Outer 1/3 (%)
Frick *et al.* (1973)	81.7	73.3	45.2
Connelly *et al.* (1982)	94.3	71.4	47.8

Acknowledgements

I am indebted to Miss Jane Bridges, Gynaecological Oncology Research Fellow and Miss Adrienne Westmoreland, Gynaecological Cancer Unit Co-ordinator, for their help in the preparation of the manuscript.

References

Baggish M.S. & Barbot J. (1983) Contact hysteroscopy. *Clin. Obstet. Gynaecol.*, **26** (2), 219.

Battelli J., Saccani F., Saccani Jotti G. *et al.* (1982) Hormonal therapy associated with combination chemotherapy in the treatment of advanced endometrial cancer. In: Cavalli F., McGuire W.L., Pannuti F., Pellegrini A. & Robustelli Della Cuna G. (eds), *Proceedings of the International Symposium on Medroxyprogesterone Acetate.* Excerpta Medica, Amsterdam. pp. 397−406.

Berman M.L., Barlow S.C., Lagasse L.D. *et al.* (1980) Prognosis and treatment of endometrial cancer. *Am. J. Obstet. Gynecol.*, **136**, 679.

Boronow R.C. (1976) Endometrial cancer − not a benign disease. *Obstet. Gynecol.*, **47**, 630.

Boronow R.C., Morrow C.P., Creasman W.T. *et al.* (1984) Surgical staging in endometrial cancer: clinical pathological findings of a prospective study. *Obstet. Gynecol.*, **63**, 825.

Brown J.M. *et al.* (1986) Vaginal recurrence of endometrial carcinoma. *Am. J. Obstet. Gynecol.*, **100**, 544−49.

Casey M.J. (1977) Age specific incidence rates of endometrial cancer. *JAMA*, **238**, 213.

Chambers J.T., MacLusky N., Eisenfield A., Kohorn E.I., Lawrence R. & Schwartz P.E. (1988) Estrogen and progestin receptor levels as prognosticators for survival in endometrial cancer. *Gynecol. Oncol.*, **31**, 65−77.

Chambers S.K., Kapp D.S., Peschel R.E. *et al.* (1987) Prognostic factors and sites of failure in FIGO stage I, grade 3 endometrial carcinoma. *Gynecol. Oncol.*, **27**, 180−88.

Cheon H.K. (1977) Prognosis of endometrial carcinoma. *Obstet. Gynecol.*, **34**, 680.

Christopherson W.M. (1986) Significance of pathologic findings. In: Creasman W.T. (ed), *Endometrial Cancer. Clinics in Obstetrics and Gynaecology.* W.P. Saunders, London.

Connelly P.J., Alberhashy R.C. & Christopherson W.M. (1982) Carcinoma of the endometrium III. Analysis of 865 cases of adenocarcinoma and adeno-acanthoma. *Obstet. Gynecol.*, **59**, 569.

Creasman W.T., Boronow R.C., Morrow C.P. *et al.* (1976) Adenocarcinoma of the endometrium: its metastatic lymph node potential. *Gynecol. Oncol.*, **4**, 239−43.

Creasman W.T., Morrow C.P., Bundy B.N., Homesley H.D., Graham J.E. & Heller P.B. (1987) *Cancer*, **60**, 2035−41.

Creasman W.T. & Rutledge F.N. (1971) The prognostic value of peritoneal cytology in gynecologic malignant disease. *Am. J. Obstet. Gynecol.*, **110**, 773.

Disaia P.J. & Creasman W.T. (1981) Adenocarcinoma of the uterus. In: Disaia P.J. & Creasman W.T. (eds), *Clinical Gynecologic Oncology.* Mosby, St. Louis. p. 139.

Ewertz M., Schou G. & Boice J.D. Jnr. (1988) The joint effect of risk factors on endometrial cancer. *Eur. J. Cancer Clin. Oncol.*, **24** (2), 189−94.

Fairweather D.V.I. (1989) Corpus cancer staging. FIGO news. *Int. J. Gynecol. Obstet.*, **28**, 190.

Fox H. & Buckley C.H. (1982) The endometrial hyperplasias and their relationship to endometrial neoplasia. *Histopathology*, **6** (5), 493.

Frick H.C. II, Munnel E.W. & Richart R.M. (1973) Carcinoma of the endometrium. *Am. J. Obstet. Gynecol.*, **115**, 663.

Galaknoff C., Masselot J., Dau N., Pejovic M.H., Prade P. & Duvillard P. (1988) Lymphography in the initial evaluation of endometrial carcinoma. *Gynecol. Oncol.*, **31** (2), 276.

Gallion H., Van Nagell J.R. Jnr., Donaldson E. & Powell D. (1987) Endometrial cancer following radiation therapy for cervical cancer. *Gynecol. Oncol.*, **27** (1), 76.

Greenblatt R.B. & Stoddard L.B. (1978) The estrogen/cancer controversy. *JAM Geriat. Soc.*, **26**, 1.

Homesley H.D. *et al.* (1976) Treatment of adenocarcinoma of the endometrium. *Obstet. Gynecol.*, **47**, 100.

Hopkin I.D., Harlow R.A. & Stevens P.J. (1970) Squamous carcinoma of the body of the uterus. *Br. J. Cancer*, **24**, 71.

Husslein H., Breitenecker G. & Tatra G. (1978) Pre-malignant and malignant uterine changes in immuno-suppressed renal transplant recipients. *Acta Obstet. Gynecol. Scand.*, **57**, 73.

Javert C. & Douglas R. (1956) Treatment of endometrial carcinoma. *Am. J. Roentgenol.*, **75**, 580.

Joelsson I., Levine R.U. & Moberger G. (1971) Hysteroscopy as an adjunct in determining the extent of carcinoma of the endometrium. *Am. J. Obstet. Gynecol.*, **64**, 780.

Jones H.W. (1975) Treatment of adenocarcinoma of the endometrium. *Obstet. Gynecol. Survey*, **30**, 147.

Jones W.E., Kanner H.M., Kanner H.H. *et al.* (1972) Adenocarcinoma of the endometrium. Twenty-five years experience in private practice. *Am. J. Obstet. Gynecol.*, **113**, 549.

Kauppila A., Gronroos M. & Niemineu U. (1982) Clinical outcome of endometrial cancer. *Obstet. Gynecol.*, **60**, 473.

Kennedy A.W., Peterson G.L., Becker S.N., Nunez C. & Webster K. (1987) Experience with pelvic washings in stage I and II endometrial carcinoma. *Gynecol. Oncol.*, **28**, 50—60.

Kistner R.W. (1970) The effects of progesteronal agents on hyperplasia and carcinoma *in situ* of the endometrium. *Int. J. Gynecol. Obstet.*, **8**, 561.

Kneale B.L.G. (1977) Studies in the behaviour of cancer of the endometrium. *Thesis*, University of Melbourne.

Konski A., Poulter C., Keys H., Rubin P., Beecham J. & Doane K. (1988) Absence of prognostic significance, peritoneal dissemination and treatment advantage in endometrial cancer patients with positive peritoneal cytology. *Int. J. Radiation Oncol. Biol. Phys.*, **4**, 49—55.

Lehtovirta P., Cacciatore B., Wahlstrom T. & Ylostlo P. (1987) Ultrasonic assessment of endometrial cancer invasion. *J. Clin. Ultrasound*, **15**, 519—24.

Levine S. & Sciorsci E.F. (1976) Squamous cell carcinoma of the uterine corpus and its relation to pyometra. *Cancer*, **19**, 485.

Lewis B., Stallworthy J.A. & Cowdell R. (1970) Adenocarcinoma of the body of the uterus. *J. Obstet. Gynaecol. Br. Commonwealth*, **77**, 343.

Lewis G.C. (1980) Endometrial cancer—surgical treatment. *Am. Soc. Natl. Conf., Gynecol. Cancer*, 1980.

Liu C.T. (1972) A study of endometrial adenocarcinoma with emphasis on morphologically variant types. *Am. J. Clin. Pathol.*, **57**, 562.

Lutz M.H., Underwood P.B. Jr & Kreutner A.J. *et al.* (1978) Endometrial carcinoma: a new method of classification of therapeutic and prognostic significance. *Gynecol. Obstet.*, **6**, 83.

McCarty K.S. Jnr., Barton T.K., Peete C.H. Jnr. & Creasman W.T. (1978) Gonadal dysgenesis with adenocarcinoma of the endometrium. An electron microscopic and steroid receptor analysis with a review of the literature. *Cancer*, **42**, 512.

MacDonald R.R., Thorogood J. & Mason M.K. (1988) A randomised trial of progestogens in the primary treatment of endometrial carcinoma. *Br. J. Obstet. Gynaecol.*, **95** (2), 166.

MacMahon B. (1974) Risk factors for endometrial cancer. *Gynecol. Oncol.*, **2**, 122.

Marret L.D., Meigs J.W. & Flannery J.T. (1982) Trends in the incidence of cancer of the corpus uteri in Connecticut in relation to consumption of exogenous estrogens. *Am. J. Epidemiol.*, **116**, 57.

Masubuchi K. & Nemoto H. (1972) Epidemiologic studies on uterine cancer at Cancer Institute Hospital, Tokyo, Japan. *Cancer*, **30**, 268.

Masubuchi K., Nemoto H. & Masubuchi S. Jnr. (1975) Increasing incidence of endometrial carcinoma in Japan. *Gynecol. Oncol.*, **3**, 335.

Mattingly R.F. (1977) Malignant tumours of the uterus. *In: Te Lindes Operative Gynecology*. J.B. Lippincott, Philadelphia.

Morrow C.P., DiSaia P.J. & Townsend D.E. (1973) Current management of endometrial cancer. *Obstet. Gynecol.*, **60**, 339.

Morrow C.P. & Schlaerth J.B. (1982) Surgical management of endometrial carcinoma. *Clin. Obstet. Gynaecol.*, **25** (1), 81.

Ng A.B.P., Reagan J.W., Storaasli J.P. & Wentz W.B. (1973) Mixed adenosquamous carcinoma of the endometrium. *Am. J. Clin. Pathol.*, **59**, 765.

Oram D.H. & Bridges J.E. (1987) Para-aortic lymphadenectomy. *Clin. Obstet. Gynaecol.*, **1** (2), 369—81.

Oster A.G., Fortune D.W., Evans J.H. & Kneale B.L. (1978) Endometrial carcinoma in gonadal dysgenesis with and without oestrogen therapy. *Gynecol. Oncol.*, **6**, 316.

Pacifico E., Miraglia M. & Miraglia F. (1982) Diagnosis of endometrial carcinoma and its precursors by means of cytologic examination of jet-washing material. *Acta Cytol.*, **26**, 630.

Plentl A.A. & Friedman A.E. (1971) *Lymphatic System of the Female Genitalia*. W.B. Saunders, Philadelphia.

Price J.J., Hahn G.A. & Rominger C.J. (1965) Vaginal involvement in endometrial carcinoma. *Am. J. Obstet. Gynecol.*, **91**, 1060–65.

Quinn M.A. & Campbell J.J. (1989) Tamoxifen therapy in advanced/recurrent endometrial carcinoma. *Gynecol. Oncol.*, **32**, 1–3.

Reagan J.W. & Fu Y.S. (1981) Pathology of endometrial carcinoma. *In*: Coppleson M. (ed), *Gynaecologic Oncology*. Churchill Livingstone, Edinburgh.

Rodriquez J. & Hart W.R. (1982) Endometrial carcinoma occurring in ten or more years after pelvic irradiation for pelvic carcinoma. *Int. J. Gynecol. Pathol.*, **1**, 135.

Ross L.D. (1988) Pelvic ultrasound—should it be used routinely in the diagnosis and screening of postmenopausal bleeding? Discussion paper. *J. Roy. Soc. Med.*, **81**, 723.

Scully R. (1982) Definition of endometrial carcinoma precursors. *Clin. Obstet. Gynaecol.*, **25** (1), 39.

Scully R.E. (1975) Recent progress in ovarian cancer. *Hum. Pathol.*, **1**, 73.

Shepherd J.H. (1989) Revised FIGO staging for gynaecological cancer. *Br. J. Obstet. Gynaecol.*, **96**, 889

Silverberg S.G., Bolin M.G. & DeGeorgio L.S. (1972) Adenoacanthoma and mixed adenosquamous carcinoma of the endometrium; a clinico pathologic study. *Cancer*, **30**, 1307.

Smith D.C., Prentice R. & Thompson D.J. (1975) Association of exogenous estrogen and endometrial carcinoma. *New Engl. J. Med.*, **293**, 1164.

Sugimoto A. (1975) Hysteroscopic diagnosis of endometrial carcinoma. *Am. J. Obstet. Gynecol.*, **121**, 105.

Swenerton K.D., Shaw D., White G.W. & Boyes D.A. (1979) Treatment of advanced endometrial carcinoma with tamoxifen. *N. Engl. J. Med.*, **301**, 105.

Du Toit J.P. (1985) Carcinoma of the uterine body. *In*: Shepherd J.H. & Monaghan J.M. (eds), *Clinical Gynaecologic Oncology*. Blackwell Scientific Publications, Oxford.

Truskett I.D. & Constable W.C. (1968) Management of carcinoma of the corpus uteri. *Am. J. Obstet. Gynecol.*, **101**, 689–94.

Van Nagell J.R. Jnr., Roddick J.W. & Wallace J.O. (1972) Clinical correlates of endometrial carcinoma. *Am. J. Obstet. Gynecol.*, **112**, 936.

Weiss N.S., Szekely D.R. & Austin D.F. (1976) Increasing incidence of endometrial cancer in the United States. *New Engl. J. Med.*, **294**, 1259

White A.J., Buchsbaum H.J. & Macasaet M.A. (1973) Primary squamous cell carcinoma of the endometrium. *Obstet. Gynecol.*, **41**, 912.

Whitehead M.I., Townsend P.T., Pryse-Davies J. *et al.* (1982) Effects of various types and dosages of progestogens on the post menopausal endometrium. *J. Reprod. Med.*, **27**, 539.

Wynder E.L., Escher G.C. & Mantell N. (1966) An epidemiological investigation of cancer of the endometrium. *Cancer*, **19**, 489.

7

The Management of Carcinoma of the Vulva

JOHN M. MONAGHAN

Introduction

Vulvar carcinoma is rare, representing only 3–5% of genital cancers; however, this proportion may be changing. Green (1978) noted an increase in incidence to approximately 8%. It is said that each gynaecologist in Britain will on average see only one case per annum. Consequently very few individuals or even referral centres can build up an adequate experience of handling this disease. The cancer is a problem mainly of the aged, the average age at presentation being in the late seventh decade, although the range of age of presentation is wide, occasionally being reported in girls in their teens and not infrequently in women in their 20s and 30s.

Aetiology

No clear aetiological agent has been incriminated in the development of carcinoma of the vulva. In older women there is almost invariably a long history of vulval irritation and pruritus, often associated with a vulval skin dystrophy. These skin changes appear to have a malignant potential only if there is evidence of atypia (Jeffcoate & Woodcock 1969). It has also been observed that these changes are not solely confined to vulval skin. The same changes can occur in perianal skin and transposed or transplanted skin to the vulval site. This has led to suggestions that there may be a vaginal factor promoting these changes. At the present time a viral factor, possibly the herpes or papilloma viruses are the most popular aetiological agents proposed. Human papilloma virus is the most likely factor supported by the frequent association of vulval condylomata and carcinoma. In condylomatous carcinoma of the vulva Downey et al. (1988) have shown the presence of human papillomavirus in 55% of cases with equal distribution of types 6 and 16. In VIN and vulvar dystrophies atypia has been associated closely with evidence of infection with type 16 human papilloma virus.

In younger women carcinoma of the vulva and vulvar intraepithelial neoplasia are seen in association with other cancers and precancers of the genital tract (Hammond & Monaghan 1983). This association has also been confirmed by

Sherman *et al.* (1988) in a case controlled study. They demonstrated an increased association of between 3.5 and 29.8 times for the development of prior or concurrent anogenital cancer, but no association with prior or concurrent non-anogenital cancers. The younger patient also shows a marked tendency to develop multifocal disease on the vulva and perianal region (Figs 7.1, 7.2). In common with the generally increased incidence of cancer and precancer in immunosuppressed patients, vulval cancer has been found to develop more frequently in renal transplant recipients (Penn 1986). He reported a 100-fold increase in the incidence of cancer of the vulva and anus in transplanted patients when compared with the normal population.

Histopathology and differentiation

Most carcinomas of the vulva are squamous in type (85%). Approximately 5% are melanomas and the remaining 10% are made up of carcinomas of the Bartholin's gland (1–3%), sarcomas and other rarer cancers.

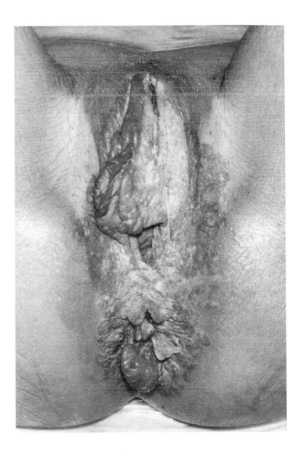

Fig. 7.1. Wide area of multifocal VIN 3 and early invasive carcinoma in a young woman.

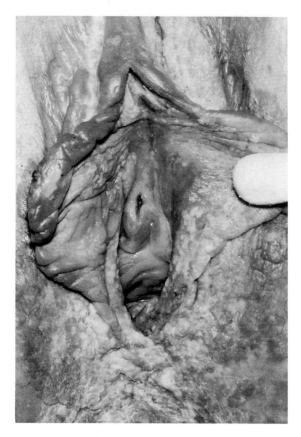

Fig. 7.2. Intraepithelial carcinoma of the vagina (VAIN 3) in association with multifocal VIN 3.

Squamous carcinoma

Among the squamous carcinomas are included basal cell carcinomas and verrucous carcinomas, both of which are relatively benign.

Thus it is important that an adequate biopsy is taken prior to any decision about the extent of surgery. Both basal cell and verrucous carcinomas have a very low propensity for lymphatic metastases (Japaze *et al.* 1981); therefore a vulvectomy or a wide local excision is usually sufficient. The verrucous carcinoma is similar to the giant condyloma of Buschke–Lowenstein. It should not be treated by radiotherapy as transformation of the tumour into a poorly differentiated and highly malignant carcinoma can occur.

In those patients affected by squamous cell carcinomas the degree of differentiation is closely related to the metastatic potential. In 1960 Way showed almost a 2-fold increase in metastases when anaplastic squamous carcinomas were compared with well differentiated tumours. Iversen *et al.* (1981) found no difference in the two groups. Andreasson *et al.* (1982) found a lower metastatic rate in better differentiated tumours only in those cases less than 4 cm in diameter, but the author has found a statistically significant difference when squamous carcinoma differentiation is related to nodal metastases (Table 7.1).

Melanoma

Malignant melanoma is the second most common carcinoma of the vulva. It may be melanotic or amelanotic, examples of both cell lines being seen both in the primary tumour and in the metastases (Edington & Monaghan 1980). It is an extremely variable cancer, sometimes being very aggressive with widespread metastases developing even when the primary is small. At other times the cancer responds to very conservative care and disappears completely. This variability has resulted in considerable disagreement over treatment methods with fluctuating vogues of radical and conservative therapy. An improvement in assessment has been advocated by Clark et al. (1969) (Clark's levels), and by Breslow (1970) by assessing and measuring the depth of penetration of the tumour into the dermal layers. A progressive decrease in survival is seen as the melanoma reaches the lower levels of the epithelium (level II−V), so that when the disease reaches the subcutaneous levels (level V) then the survival drops rapidly and the recurrence rate reaches 78% (Podratz et al. 1983). It also appears that only those patients with disease in levels IV and V exhibit nodal metastases. There has been considerable acceptance that an *en bloc* dissection of the inguinal and/or pelvic lymph nodes with radical vulvectomy is the optimum management for lesions reaching these deeper levels. In recent times Davison et al. (1987) have questioned the need for radicality comparing the disease when it affects the vulva with that of the anorectal region. They found in a retrospective review of 32 patients no advantage in using more radical approaches and advocated dealing with nodal metastases as and when they arose. In the author's series groin node metastases occurred in 50% of patients whereas none had involvement of the pelvic nodes.

Carcinoma of the Bartholin's gland

Primary carcinoma of the Bartholin's gland is rare, representing approximately 1−3% of all vulval tumours. This disease is characterized by a high groin node

Table 7.1. Vulvar carcinoma histology and nodal metastases (September 1984)

Tumour		Groin nodes		Pelvic nodes	
		n	+ve	n	+ve
Squamous cell	Well differentiated	108	20(18.5%)	55	2(3.6%)
	Moderately differentiated	30	16(53%)	17	1(6%)
	Poorly differentiated	40	18(45%)	18	3(16.6%)
			$x^2 = 15.51$	$P < 0.001$	
Melanoma		7	3(43%)	2	0
Total		185		92	

metastasis rate (37.3%, Leuchter *et al.* 1982; 47%, Copeland *et al.* 1986); in the former series there was also an 18% pelvic node involvement rate. Even those patients with negative groin nodes have a poor 5-year survival of 52% (Leuchter *et al.* 1982). This compares very badly with squamous carcinoma of the vulva where similar node negative patients can expect to have a 94% chance of surviving 5 years (Monaghan & Hammond 1984). However, Copeland *et al.* (1986) demonstrated a high 5-year survival of 84% in their series where management was individualized and consisted of surgery with or without radiotherapy. It has been frequently written that carcinoma of the Bartholin's gland has a capacity for direct spread to the pelvic lymph nodes; however, the only case reported is that of Barclay *et al.* (1964). Pelvic node dissection as part of the basic management is not necessary unless more than four groin nodes are involved (Curry *et al.* 1980), or the tumour is larger than 4 cm in diameter (Monaghan & Hammond 1984).

Adenoid cystic cancer of the vulva

This tumour is a rare variant of adenocarcinoma of the Bartholin's gland, representing 10% of such cases. Forty-two cases have been reported in the literature and the author has managed a further two. The tumour is characterized clinically by an infiltrating pattern of growth frequently extending subdermally for a considerable distance beyond the apparent margins of the lesion. Lymph node metastases are said to be uncommon but in the author's two cases both had groin node involvement. Lung metastases also occurred in one of the cases, as has been reported elsewhere. Currently management should consist of radical vulvectomy and groin node dissection with careful assessment of the margins of resection and the possible use of adjuvant radiotherapy (Amichetti & Aldovini 1988).

Sarcoma of the vulva

These rare carcinomas can present difficult diagnostic and management problems. The histological appearance may not be that of a malignant tumour, but any lesion with more than 10 mitoses per high power field must be regarded as such. They tend to grow rapidly and frequently give the appearance of arising from the Bartholin's gland; the centre of the tumour becomes necrotic and can be scooped out at surgery. Radical surgery is the basis of management, but radiotherapy and chemotherapy may be necessary as adjuvant treatment.

Secondary cancers of the vulva

The vulva is the site of secondary cancers from a variety of primary sites, including cervix and vagina, the ovary, the gastrointestinal tract, the renal tract and distant sites such as the breast and thyroid.

Symptoms and mode of presentation

Over two-thirds of patients with cancer of the vulva present with irritation and pruritus of the vulval region, usually of long duration, varying from a few months to many years. A mass or ulcer is also commonly seen but it is relatively uncommon for patients to complain of bleeding or discharge (Table 7.2). There is frequently a delay in diagnosis partially due to the patient's reluctance to attend and partially due to the referring doctor's failure to properly examine. In the author's series of 335 cases 32 patients presented after a delay of more than 24 months, whereas only 35 patients attended within 3 months of first symptoms. Similar delays were noted over forty years ago by Taussig (1940). Hacker *et al.* (1981) reported a mean delay of 10 months with a range of 1 to 36 months in a Californian practice.

Medical condition of the patient

Carcinoma of the vulva is most commonly seen in women in the seventh decade of life; consequently these patients often have significant medical problems including hypertension, obesity, diabetes and heart and lung disease. It is important that these complicating factors are assessed prior to any decision about the type of operative procedure to be performed. This assessment must be made by the surgeon and his anaesthetist. The judgement must be made in the light of their experience; if they work closely together in a department dealing with a large number of such cases then the operability rate will inevitably be high, increasing further with the use of spinal and epidural anaesthesia. Reports from major centres commonly quote operability rates of the order of 96% (Podratz *et al.* 1982; Monaghan & Hammond 1984).

Choice of operation

For approximately 40 years it has been accepted that carcinoma of the vulva should be treated by radical vulvectomy together with groin and possibly pelvic node dissection. This belief is founded on the work of Stoeckel (1930), Taussig (1940) and Way (1954), each of whom demonstrated the very much improved survival statistics when patients were treated radically. In spite of these im-

Table 7.2. Symptoms as percent of total number

IRRITATION	71
LUMP	57
PAIN	35
BLEEDING	28
DISCHARGE	23

335 patients: no recorded symptoms in two

provements, critics have been unhappy about the extent of these radical procedures. When carried out on old women they may result in death or prolonged
stay in hospital awaiting the healing of large groin wounds. Little, if any,
evidence was available to show that this standard approach could be modified or
tailored to the individual patient until the early 1970s. At this time it was
suggested (Rutledge *et al.* 1970) that those patients with small tumours, less than
2 cm in diameter (T1, N0, M0) with a depth of invasion of less than 5 mm, may
not require a groin node dissection, there being little evidence of nodal metastases
in this group of patients. Wharton *et al.* (1974) subsequently reported on a series
of 25 patients who met these criteria, 15 of whom were treated with radical
vulvectomy alone and 10 of whom had additional groin node dissection. They
reported a 100% 5-year survival rate.

These reports stimulated a considerable amount of study and interest; unfortunately it rapidly became clear that the parallel with microinvasive carcinoma of
the cervix could not be drawn. Many authorities subsequently reported cases and
series showing nodal metastases and deaths in patients with T1, N0, M0 tumours
with less than 5 mm of invasion (Nakao *et al.* 1974; Diapola *et al.* 1975; Parker *et
al.* 1975; Jafari & Cartnick 1976; Yasigi *et al.* 1978).

A number of factors must be considered before accurate individualization of
treatment can become a reality for carcinoma of the vulva.

Stage of tumour

Staging of carcinoma of the vulva continues to be unsatisfactory; it clearly requires an operative staging system (Friedrich & Diapola 1977) but over the years
has been hampered by using the TNM non-operative method of staging (Table
7.3). This system was adopted by FIGO in 1988.

Errors in clinical staging of vulval squamous carcinoma can be unacceptably
high, reaching 25% (Podratz *et al.* 1980), and in a series of malignant melanomas
from the same institution 31% inaccurate assessments were noted (Podratz *et al.*
1983). The TNM system has more serious staging limitations in malignant
melanoma in that many tumours are less than 2 cm in diameter but conversely
are extremely aggressive and tend to have widespread metastatic patterns (Podratz
et al. 1983; Monaghan & Hammond 1984).

Size of tumour

Podratz *et al.* (1982) showed that the larger the tumour the greater the chance of
metastases. In the author's published series of over 150 groin and/or groin and
pelvic node dissections it has been observed that there is a clear cut-off point at
4 cm diameter between those with pelvic node metastases (>4 cm) and those
without (<4 cm) (Monaghan & Hammond 1984). A similar observation was
noted by Andreasson *et al.* (1980). Thus by reserving pelvic node dissection only

Table 7.3. Definitions of the clinical stages in carcinoma of the vulva (correlation of the FIGO, UICC and AJCC nomenclatures)

Stage 0	
Tis	Carcinoma *in situ*, intraepithelial carcinoma
Stage I	
T1 N0 M0	Tumour confined to the vulva *and/or perineum* — 2 cm or less in greatest dimension. Nodes are not palpable
Stage II	
T2 N0 M0	Tumour confined to the vulva *and/or perineum* — more than 2 cm in greatest dimension. Nodes are not palpable
Stage III	
T3 N0 M0	Tumour of any size with
T3 N1 M0	(1) Adjacent spread to the lower urethra and/or the vagina, or the anus, and/or
T1 N1 M0	(2) *unilateral regional lymph node metastasis*
T2 N1 M0	
Stage IVA	
T1 N2 M0	Tumour invades any of the following:
T2 N2 M0	*Upper urethra, bladder mucosa, rectal mucosa, pelvic bone and/or bilateral regional node metastasis*
T3 N2 M0	
T4 Any N M0	
Stage IVB	
Any T Any N M1	Any distant metastasis including pelvic lymph nodes

for those patients with tumours greater than 4 cm a small but significant salvage would be achieved without subjecting all patients to the procedure.

Conversely, the smallest carcinoma in the author's series of 300 patients to develop groin node metastases was 3×3 mm, affecting the clitoris.

Site of tumour and lymphatic drainage

Most carcinomas of the vulva affect the labia, the left slightly more often than the right; the second commonest site is the clitoris. It has been thought that carcinomas affecting the clitoris require more aggressive management. The lymphatics of the clitoris were said to communicate directly with the pelvic lymphatics (Parry-Jones 1963). This direct communication has never been satisfactorily demonstrated. Recent work by Iversen & Aas (1983) did not find any evidence of such a communication. They also demonstrated the frequent bilateral flow of the clitoral lymphatics and evidence of contralateral flow alone from laterally placed injection of a radionuclide (technetium) in the labia (28/42, 67%). They did not demonstrate higher lymph flow rates from any particular part of the vulva. However, care must be used in interpreting this study as they used patients with *carcinoma of the cervix* and no allowance was made or could be made for any disturbance of lymphatic drainage in the presence of *vulvar carcinoma*.

There is no evidence that the pelvic nodes should be routinely dissected simply because the clitoris is involved unless the groin nodes are heavily infiltrated, and in these circumstances the salvage is low.

In the author's series the clitoris was involved in 54 out of 200 cases, 47 of which had nodal dissections. Twenty-five (53%) had metastases to the groin nodes but only two (4.2%) had metastases to the pelvic nodes, thus giving little support for the routine dissection of pelvic nodes. Piver & Xynos (1977) in a similar sized series came to the same conclusion.

Laterality

It has been proposed that when a vulvar carcinoma affects the labia alone and does not impinge on the clitoris, urethra, vagina, fourchette or perianal region, it may be reasonable to carry out a local excision or vulvectomy plus an ipsilateral groin node dissection, the contralateral nodes being preserved. This proposal is based on the belief that contralateral spread alone and bilateral spread from a laterally placed tumour are extremely rare. Hacker *et al.* (1984a) stated that they had never seen positive contralateral nodes with negative ipsilateral nodes; they developed their argument further by stating that if ipsilateral nodes are found to be negative then a contralateral dissection is unnecessary. In general this has not been the author's experience (Table 7.4); a small but significant number of patients with very small tumours have contralateral alone or bilateral spread. However, in an analysis when the author's series had reached 244 patients, it was found that of 50 stage I carcinomas where the groin nodes had been dissected, although eight (16%) were involved, in those patients where the tumour was laterally placed only three patients had nodes involved. All these involved nodes were on the same side as the carcinoma. Thus this particular group may well benefit from a more limited approach. It is of interest that contralateral and bilateral spread did occur in those carcinomas which affected midline structures.

In a more recent analysis of 71 FIGO stage I tumours, nine (12.5%) had positive groin nodes and five of these had laterally placed tumours. All three

Table 7.4. Site of tumour: 200 cases, 199 had site recorded (from Studd J. (1985) *Progress in Obstetrics and Gynaecology*. Churchill Livingstone, Edinburgh, with permission)

Left side tumours *n* = 44				Right side tumours *n* = 41		
			NODE METASTASES			
Ipsilateral	Contralateral	Bilateral		Ipsilateral	Contralateral	Bilateral
7	2	0		6	1	1

n: node dissections

cases on the left side had ipsilateral nodes whereas one of two on the right side had a contralateral groin node involved. Thus although the risk of bilateral and contralateral node metastases is very low it is not nil and care should be taken before dispensing with the contralateral node dissections.

Groin node status

Palpation of groin nodes has always been notoriously inaccurate. Benedet *et al.* (1979) quoted error rates of between 13 and 39%. In the author's experience (Table 7.5), similar inaccuracies have been found.

Lymphography has also been disappointing in spite of the relative accessibility of the groin nodes, giving false positive results for fatty nodes and false negative for nodes totally replaced by tumour. This technique demands great skill and interest of the radiologists.

Fine needle aspiration may be able to assist in confirming significant metastases, but is of lower accuracy where there are small metastases and peripheral sinus emboli.

Intraoperative sampling has been used to determine whether to proceed to removal of deep inguinal nodes, or to carry out pelvic node dissection. Curry *et al.* (1980) stated that where four or more nodes were involved in the groin then pelvic node dissection should be carried out. Disaia *et al.* (1979) have recommended that a 'sentinel' node lying above the femoral fascia may be removed and if not involved no further treatment is necessary. If involved, a dissection of the groin should proceed. Similarly, Patsner & Mann (1988) have suggested a 'sneak' superficial inguinal lymphadenectomy may be used on the same basis.

Monoclonal radionuclide labelling may have a role to play in the assessment of involvement of nodes by metastatic disease.

Table 7.5. Palpation of groin nodes vs. metastases

	Number cases *n*	Groin nodes	
		−ve	+ve
Not palpable	157	128 (81.5%)	29 (18.5%)
Palpable — mobile	50	28 (56%)	22 (44%)
Palpable — fixed	5	1 (20%)	4 (80%)

'Microinvasion'

After the initial enthusiasm of Rutledge *et al.* (1970) and Wharton *et al.* (1974) it was shown in some studies that lymph node metastases could occur with depths of invasion below 3 mm (Yasigi *et al.* 1978; Andreasson *et al.* 1982; Hacker *et al.* 1983). It is not uncommon to see node metastasis rates of from 8−20% quoted for tumours invading less than 5 mm. Clearly it is not only depth of invasion which determines the carcinoma's capacity for metastasis. These other factors include vascular space involvement, plasma cell/lymphocyte infiltration, confluence of tumour and perineural invasion.

Vascular space involvement

Parker *et al.* (1975) and Iversen *et al.* (1981) both commented that vascular space involvement by tumour was the most important prognostic factor in determining metastases in tumours invading less than 5 mm.

Plasma cell/lymphocytic infiltration

Andreasson *et al.* (1982) found improved survivals with severe or moderate local immune cellular reaction. In recent work from the author's own department Price *et al.* (1988) have shown the reduced metastatic potential of tumours which generate a profuse lymphocytic response and also an increase in Ig-A containing cellular infiltrate. Conversely, Rowley *et al.* (1988) in a much smaller series did not find a significant relationship.

Confluence

Depth of invasion and confluence and nodal metastases were found to be strongly related by Hoffman *et al.* (1983). Their series showed that 17 of 47 cases (36%) exhibiting confluence had nodal metastases, whereas none of 31 cases without confluence had any nodal spread.

Perineural invasion. In a recent review of prognostic parameters Rowley *et al.* (1988) found that perineural invasion was strongly associated with metastatic lymph node disease in a group of stage I cancers of the vulva.

Conclusion. It is now clear that it is not justifiable to dispense with groin node dissection unless the depth of invasion is less than 1 mm (Hacker *et al.* 1984a). In the author's view the groin node dissection must include all nodes. No attempt should be made to distinguish between the superficial and the deep inguinal node systems.

Modifications to the original butterfly incision

It is generally agreed that for almost all patients a dissection of the groin nodes is an essential part of the surgical treatment. Unfortunately this groin node dissection frequently results in breakdown and infection of the wounds resulting in a markedly increased morbidity and prolongation of hospitalization.

Although the classic butterfly incision has been the mainstay of management for many years there have been frequent and ingenious attempts to modify this incision in order to reduce the risk of sloughing.

1 The use of rotational skin flaps (Trelford *et al.* 1984) and myocutaneous flaps; gracilis (Wheeless *et al.* 1979) tensor fascia lata (Chafe *et al.* 1983) and gluteal thigh flap (Achauer *et al.* 1984).

2 The use of a lower midline abdominal incision with wide undercutting to reach the groin (Goldberg *et al.* 1979).

3 The use of minor modifications of the original butterfly incision so as to preserve the mons (Abitol 1973).

4 The technique of leaving the groin wounds open and allowing them to heal by secondary intention (Daly & Pomerance 1979).

5 Dissection of the superficial inguinal nodes as sentinel nodes in the groin and then skin grafting (Disaia *et al.* 1979).

6 Separate groin incisions (Taussig 1940; Byron *et al.* 1962; Ballon & Lamb 1975; Hacker *et al.* 1981).

7 'Sneak' superficial inguinal lymphadenectomy via a single elliptical vulvar incision (Patsner & Mann 1988).

Each of these variations has been developed by enthusiasts prompted by dissatisfaction with the significant wound breakdown rates of the more traditional incisions. All clinicians handling large numbers of patients work very hard to reduce the morbidity from this radical procedure.

It is intriguing for the student of the history of surgery to see that most of the variations in operative technique so painstakingly described during the twentieth century were summarized by W. Stoeckel writing in the 1930s based on his experiences in the early part of this century (Stoeckel 1930).

Spread of vulvar carcinoma — embolization or permeation?

When surgery for carcinoma of the vulva is limited to vulvectomy alone the results are very poor. The extremely high survival rates in patients with negative nodes (Table 7.6) frequently tempts less experienced operators to adopt a more conservative technique, dispensing with the groin node dissection. The usual end result is a disastrous recurrence. It is clear that the groin node dissection not only deals with gross metastases in the nodes, but also effectively removes micrometastases which are not detectable. These are usually dealt with when the

Table 7.6. Results of radical surgical treatment of cancer of the vulva

Authors	Year	n	Rad.V.GND Node stat	5-year survival (%)	Rad. V.GND+PND Node Stat	5-year survival (%)
Monaghan, personal series	1988	330	Negative Positive	95 62	Negative Positive	89 26.5
Benedet et al.	1979	204	Negative Positive	86 55.6	Negative Positive	81.8 50
Morley	1976	229	Negative Positive	93 28.7	Negative Positive	57 16.7
Way	1978	354	Negative Positive	Not reported 52.2	Negative Positive	83.7 21.2

Rad.V.GND: radical vulvectomy and groin node dissection.
Rad.V.GND+PND radical vulvectomy and groin node dissection + pelvic node dissection.

groin nodes are removed in direct continuity with the vulvar dissection. There are no large series comparing the results of dissection in continuity with those of separate incisions. The success of procedures using separate groin incisions will depend on the hypothesis that squamous carcinoma of the vulva spreads primarily by embolization and not by permeation (Willis 1973).

The author believes that small tumours spread by embolization primarily and then later will partially obstruct or fill the lymphatic channels and thereafter spread by permeation. It is frequently seen that in large tumours the groin lymphatics become obstructed and then retrograde lymphatic permeation occurs especially down the lymph channels running alongside the saphenous vein.

It is important that the relative merits of separate groin incisions versus the traditional dissection in continuity with the vulva should be fully evaluated. In the meantime separate incisions should be reserved for small tumours (FIGO stage I). The author has now carried out 71 procedures where separate groin node incisions have been performed since 1985. Nine patients had positive groin nodes and so far no recurrences in the skin bridge have occurred. Christopherson et al. (1985) have reported a case of recurrence in the skin bridge between the groin and vulvar incisions following excision of a stage I carcinoma. At the present time it is important that any deviation from an *en bloc* dissection to separate incisions be critically assessed and not routinely practised.

Is it safe to consider that separate incisions are adequate treatment for patients who have positive groin nodes?

Hacker *et al.* considered in 1984 that for patients with fewer than two microscopically involved nodes the risk of metastases in the skin bridge is nil. Christopherson *et al.* (1985) are clearly sceptical.

Plan of management

From the information now available it is clear that a high degree of individualization of management can be achieved for patients with carcinoma of the vulva.

The author proposes the following role for the use of separate groin incisions:
1 For patients with stage I laterally placed tumours a radical vulvectomy with an ipsilateral groin node dissection may be performed through separate incisions.
2 For stage I disease encroaching on midline structures a radical vulvectomy with bilateral groin node dissection may be performed through separate incisions or using a 'butterfly incision'.

Metastatic vulvar carcinoma

Vulvar carcinoma is a disease characterized by delay; consequently, the patient frequently presents with widespread disease (Fig. 7.4). It is important to realize

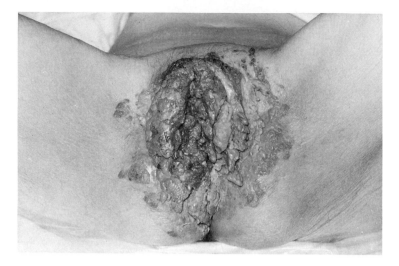

Fig. 7.3. Extensive carcinoma of the vulva affecting the vulva thigh and anus. The groin nodes were clear of metastases.

that, even with diseases involving the pelvic organs or fungating groin nodes, it may still be possible to cure the patient or at worst improve her state to such an extent that she can live (and die) with a degree of dignity.

Distant metastases are not a contraindication to carrying out a radical vulvectomy and groin node dissection. It is often possible to completely remove all local disease and leave the patient with a clean vulva and groin; thus although the patient will die from the distant metastases, the mode of death will be much improved.

Fungating groin nodes (Fig. 7.4) should be removed in continuity with the vulva, and ideally combined with a pelvic node dissection. Occasionally it is found that the pelvic nodes are clear of tumour and the prospects for the patient are very much improved. More interest has developed in the use of preoperative radiotherapy as a tumour reductive agent for this group of patients.

Pelvic organ involvement including the bladder, anus, rectum and vagina demands a more aggressive approach. If the patient is fit she should be considered for an exenterative procedure using the techniques of total, anterior or posterior exenteration to achieve clearance of all tumour. Lesions which extend into the anus but do not invade further than the pectinate line may be treated by radical anovulvectomy after colostomy, rather than by posterior exenteration.

Occasionally it may be possible to reduce the tumour mass by using radiotherapy, thus rendering the patient operable and allowing a less invasive procedure to be performed (Hacker *et al*. 1984b).

If the tumour invades bone, the bones of the pubic arch being most commonly affected, then the tumour may be removed by resecting a segment of bone with the specimen. A patient so treated is able to walk without difficulty in spite of the loss of a segment of her bony pelvis.

Recurrent disease

Up to 26% of treated cases will develop recurrences (Podratz *et al.* 1982). Following radical vulvectomy and groin node dissection most recurrences occur on the vulva with very few in the groin. This may be due to new lesions developing in areas that have undergone precancerous modification, but also due to residual disease being left at primary surgery, because although most surgeons will produce adequate lateral margins for the resection it is very common to see structures such as the terminal urethra being preserved at all costs; by removing the end 1–1.5 cm the risk of recurrence can be markedly reduced. Most recurrences should be managed by surgery using the standard principles of adequate margins and wide local excision. Occasionally surgery may be combined with radiotherapy or chemotherapy to deal with a recurrence in a difficult position.

Groin recurrences are very difficult to deal with and unless they are small and can be removed by surgery, local radiotherapy is probably the only prospect.

As with all cancers *the first chance of treatment is the best chance*.

Operative technique

After Bassett (1912) described the combined vulvectomy and groin node dissection for vulvar carcinoma, the procedure did not progress until the work of Stoeckel (1930), Taussig (1935) and Way (1948). Since that time there has been a general acceptance that a combination of radical vulvectomy and *en bloc* groin node dissection is the minimum procedure for the treatment of vulvar carcinoma.

The traditional incision has been the 'butterfly incision'; unfortunately if used as described by Way (1978) it involved removal of wide areas of skin in the groins and over the symphisis pubis, resulting in either failure to achieve primary closure or at best the wounds being brought together under enormous tension. Frequently patients had to be nursed for some days postoperatively with the knees and hips flexed and even bandaged together. This immobilization and restriction increased the risk of thromboembolic disease, and all too often the wounds broke down resulting in long stays in hospital (Fig. 7.5).

Many surgeons have attempted to minimize these risks and problems in a variety of ways, including the use of extended plastic surgery incisions to mobilize flaps of skin, primary skin grafting, secondary skin grafting having left the wound open, grafting with porcine skin to cover the defect and a bewildering variety of separate vulvar and groin incisions. The author considers that a simple modification of the original 'butterfly incision' (Fig. 7.6) will allow virtually all

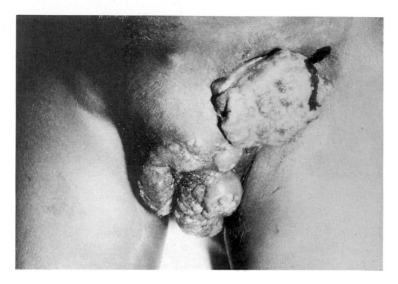

Fig. 7.4. Fungating groin nodes in a young negro woman. Complete surgical removal gave an improved quality of life.

tumours to be removed and at the same time achieve primary closure without tension, the patient being nursed prone with full movement in the postoperative period (Monaghan & Mathias 1982).

It is now becoming accepted that a considerable degree of individualization of treatment can be applied to cancer of the vulva particularly in relationship to the extent of surgery performed. Figure 7.7 shows the pattern of incisions used

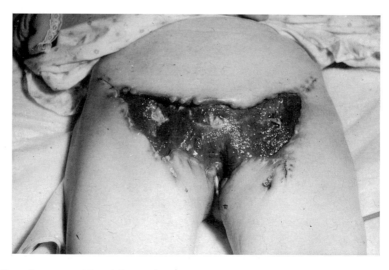

Fig. 7.5. Complete wound breakdown after radical vulvectomy and groin node dissection. Clean granulation tissue is present and re-epithelialization is beginning to occur.

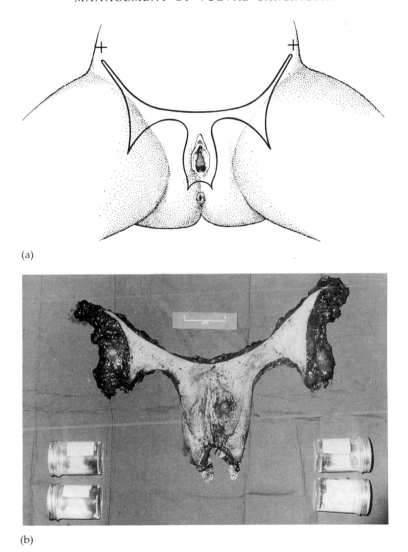

(a)

(b)

Fig. 7.6.   (a) Modified 'butterfly incision'. (b) Vulval specimen showing the modified 'butterfly incision'.

by the author in a series of 72 patients. These modifications have resulted in a marked increase in wound healing rates without jeopardizing the results of surgery. There has not been a groin or skin bridge metastasis in this series to date.

Suction drainage of the groin wounds should always be used as 250–300 ml of serosanguinous fluid can drain on either side each day in the postoperative period. Antibiotics are now routinely used prophylactically as a 'one shot' intra-operative bolus. This technique makes a significant difference to postoperative pyrexia and wound breakdown rates. As many of the patients undergoing this radical surgery are old with many medical problems it is important that the procedure is carried out in departments where all the staff are of the highest standard; this is best achieved by treating the patient in major oncological centres where such experience can be developed.

Complications

Wound disruption and infection

It is the author's experience that more than half of patients will achieve primary wound healing (Fig. 7.8), the remainder having some degree of wound breakdown varying from minor to total. This breakdown is most commonly associated with infection, usually of the skin edges only, but occasionally of extreme degree. This extensive infection may progress to necrotizing fasciitis, a rare, rapidly progressing and often fatal infection of the superficial fascia and the subcutaneous tissues. The patients at highest risk of developing wound infection are the obese and the diabetics. After the infection has been dealt with by local cleansing with antiseptic solutions such as Eusol and irrigated with hydrogen peroxide, it has been shown that liquid honey will promote healthy granulation tissue growth. In recent times hyperosmolar techniques have been applied to the wound with some success in promoting rapid healing. Wide areas of separation in the wounds may be treated by skin grafting.

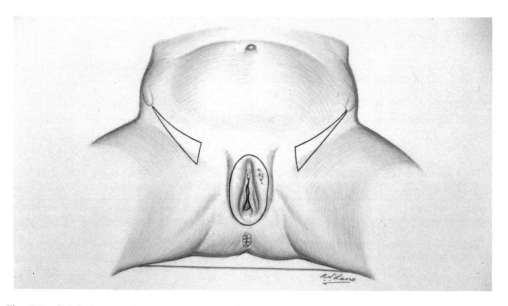

Fig. 7.7.   Triple incision for stage I lesions.

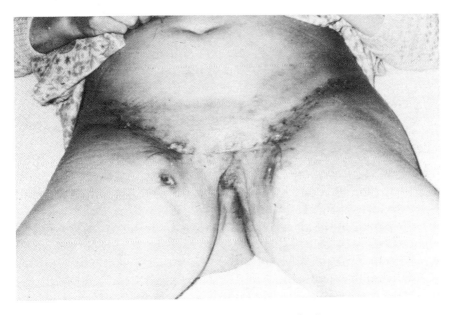

Fig. 7.8. Ten days postoperative photograph showing primary healing.

Thromboembolic disease

Patients with carcinoma of the vulva are at high risk of developing thrombo-embolic disease because of their age, obesity and both pre- and postoperative immobility. It is therefore vital that the surgeon considers using some method of prophylaxis, such as calf muscle pumps, subcutaneous heparin or antiembolism stockings. Since 1976 the author has used subcutaneous heparin (5000 U b.d. for 10 days postoperatively). During this time 300 patients have been so treated and although a number of patients have had leg thromboses and two had pulmonary emboli, only one patient weighing over 100 kg has succumbed. Because of the risk of extradural haemorrhage care must be taken when using heparin in association with epidural anaesthesia; therefore it is now the author's policy to begin heparin at the end of the surgical procedure after removal of the epidural catheter. In 1983 Piver et al. reported a significant relationship between the use of prophylactic heparin and the development of femoro–inguinal lymphocysts (eight of 19 patients (42%) developed lymphocysts). The author could not substantiate these findings. It is the author's opinion that the benefits of heparin prophylaxis far outweigh the disadvantages.

Secondary haemorrhage

Meticulous haemostasis is important as the raw area beneath the skin flaps is very extensive. In the author's view the risk of disruption of the femoral vessels

has been exaggerated and therefore techniques such as sartorious muscle transplant can be dispensed with. In a recent review Cavanagh *et al*. (1986) found that
only four patients in a series of 346 had had femoral artery or vein rupture in a
period covering 38 years. In the author's series of 335 patients one patient has
disrupted the femoral vein and one the femoral artery; both were saved by the
prompt action of the nursing staff.

Leg oedema

Leg oedema is one of the most important and most distressing complications
for the patient and is reported to occur in between 8% and 65% of patients
(Calame 1980; Monaghan & Hammond 1984; Cavanagh *et al*. 1986). There is
enormous variation in the development of oedema from patient to patient; as a
prophylaxis support stockings should be worn for at least 3 months following the
operation. Patient compliance, however, is poor. It is important to treat any
tendency to lymphangitis because if not actively managed this will leave long
term damage to the lymphatics leading to chronic lymphoedema (Fig. 7.9). The
infection is commonly caused by streptococcal infection and responds rapidly to
the use of penicillins. If acute lymphangitis is allowed to develop the patients
may become very toxic requiring fluid replacement and intensive antibiotic
therapy.

TREATMENT OF LYMPHOEDEMA

The broad principles of treatment involve the following.
1   Elevation of the limb whenever the patient is sitting or resting during the day

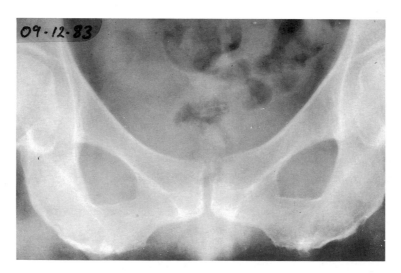

Fig. 7.9.   Preoperative X-ray of pubic bones.

with the addition of slight elevation of the foot of the bed during sleeping, although frequently some resolution of the oedema occurs at night due to improved renal function.

2 Progressive exercise should be encouraged even though the group of patients to be managed rarely if ever take exercise and indeed find great problems in mobilizing.

3 Compression stockings and bandaging should be worn during waking hours but may need to be applied by professionals with special training in oedema care.

4 Massage either performed by the patient or by physiotherapist can be of long standing help in reducing existing oedema. Following massage compression pumps may be of value but are generally only available in specialist centres. Diuretics are of little long term value but are commonly prescribed.

Femoral nerve resection

The small branches of the femoral nerve are frequently damaged or cut during groin node dissections, resulting in parasthesia over the anterior surface of the thigh. This can be distressing and at times painful. The patient should be reassured, as with time some recovery does occur.

Osteitis pubis

This can be a severely debilitating and sometimes fatal complication. The author has seen only three cases in a series of 335 patients, one of which was fatal and the others requiring many months of antibiotic therapy. The problem is characterized by extreme pubic pain especially noticed once the patient begins to mobilize. The diagnosis is usually confirmed by X-ray and should be carefully followed using serial X-rays (Figs 7.9, 7.10 and 7.11). Antibiotics specific for the bacteria and bone infections should be employed, often having to be given for many months.

Herniae

Following dissection of the pelvic nodes herniae will occur occasionally. It is a rare problem, the author finding only two herniae among 96 patients undergoing pelvic node dissection, and one hernia in a patient who did not have a pelvic node dissection.

Urinary tract complications

Troublesome urinary tract infection accompanied by stasis is commonly seen postoperatively (56% of patients). This is probably related to the presence of the

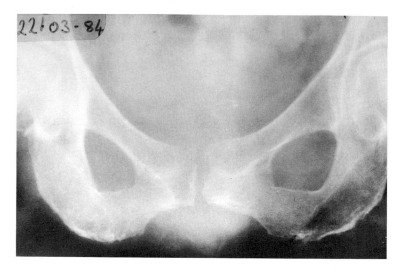

Fig. 7.10. X-ray photograph of early osteitis pubis developing in patient shown in Fig. 7.9.

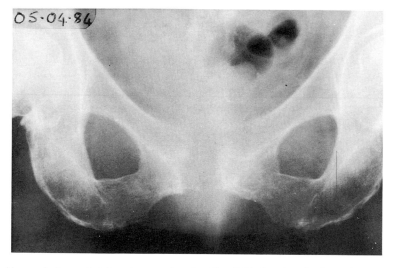

Fig. 7.11. X-ray photograph taken two weeks after Fig. 7.10 showing further advancement of the osteitis pubis.

urethral catheter which is maintained *in situ* for 10 days in order to keep the vulva as dry as possible. It may be that suprapubic catheterization would reduce this complication.

Long term urinary problems including misdirection of the stream due to hooding and scarring of the urethral orifice and varying degrees of incontinence may also occur; appropriate surgery should be used.

Introital scarring and vaginal prolapse

These two problems will be seen from time to time, and may require surgical correction.

Sexual function and body image

There is enormous variation in patients' reactions to radical surgery; each patient must be treated individually and counselled about the alteration to her genitalia and the inevitable scarring that will occur. In the author's experience all his patients have accepted the need for the surgery and have accepted the scarring involved, indeed the youngest patient in the series, aged 25, has recently delivered of her second child since her radical vulvectomy and groin node dissection. Every effort must be made to reduce the amount of disfigurement without reducing the effectiveness of the treatment.

Radiotherapy

From time to time there is a resurgence of interest in the use of radiotherapy in the treatment of vulvar carcinoma. The results have generally been poor; 3-year survivals as low as 10% have been quoted (Lifshitz *et al*. 1982). These poor results are probably due to a combination of the relative insensitivity of the carcinoma, with the extreme radiosensitivity of the vulvar skin. Radiation necrosis of the skin often occurs producing exquisitely painful ulceration which takes a very long time to heal.

There may now be a role for radiotherapy as a preoperative cancer reductive agent in those departments where surgery is not the primary skill available, and also in those few patients who are not fit for operation.

A small number of reports have shown the value of preoperative radiotherapy in those patients who have tumours affecting the fourchette, perineum and anus. It has been noted that apparently inoperable cases can be rendered operable and the required procedure reduced in magnitude using this combined technique (Fairey *et al*. 1985).

Homesley *et al*. (1986), reporting a gynecological oncology group multicentre study, have shown a statistically significant improvement in 3-year survival when patients with positive groin nodes were treated with radiotherapy to the groins and over the pelvic nodes as compared to a group who had pelvic node dissection performed. The morbidity was similar in the two groups which showed two major poor prognostic factors, clinically suspicious or fixed and ulcerated nodes and two or more involved nodes on histological examination. Radiotherapy should also be considered for patients with recurrent disease and as a palliative for inoperable nodal masses.

Chemotherapy

There is at present no single agent or combination treatment available to effectively treat carcinoma of the vulva. Deppe (1979) found that only regimens containing bleomycin and methotrexate produced significant tumour responses.

Results of surgical treatment

Table 7.6 summarizes some of the larger reported series, the excellent results when groin nodes are negative, but the poor prospects for those women with involved pelvic nodes. This suggests that pelvic node dissection should no longer be part of the routine management, but should be reserved for those patients with tumours 4 cm in diameter and possibly for the poorly differentiated squamous lesion. It is debatable whether pelvic node dissection should be carried out for malignant melanoma as the poor survival may not justify the increased morbidity.

The results shown in Table 7.6 are a reflection of the combined skills and experience of members of those departments. There is no place in modern gynaecology for the occasional radical surgeon.

References

Abitol M.M. (1973) Carcinoma of the vulva: improvements in the surgical approach. *Am. J. Obstet. Gynecol.*, **117**, 483–89.

Achauer B.M., Braly P., Berman M.L. & Disaia P.J. (1984) Immediate vaginal reconstruction following resection for malignancy using the gluteal flap. *Gynecol. Oncol.*, **19**, 79–89.

Amichetti M. & Aldovini D. (1988) Primary adenoid cystic carcinoma of the Bartholin's gland: a clinical, histological and immunocytochemical study of a case. *Eur. J. Surg. Oncol.*, **14**, 335–39.

Andreasson B., Bock J.E. & Visfeldt J. (1982) Prognostic role of histology in squamous cell carcinoma in the vulvar region. *Gynecol. Oncol.*, **14**, 373–81.

Andreasson B., Bock J.E. & Weberg E. (1980) Invasive cancer in the vulva region. *Ugeskr. Laeg.*, **1942**, 1067–71.

Ballon S.C. & Lamb E.J. (1975) Separate inguinal incisions in the treatment of carcinoma of the vulva. *Surg. Gynecol. Obstet.*, **140**, 81–84.

Barclay D.L., Collins C.R. & Macey A.B. (1964) Cancer of the Bartholin gland: a review and report of 8 cases. *Obstet. Gynecol.*, **24**, 329.

Bassett A. (1912) Traitement chirurgical operatoire de l'epithelioma primitif du clitoris. *Rev. Chir. Paris*, **46**, 546.

Benedet J.L., Turko M., Fairey R.N. & Boyes D.A. (1979) Squamous carcinoma of the vulva: results of treatment, 1938 to 1976. *Am. J. Obstet. Gynecol.*, **134**, 201–7.

Breslow A. (1970) Thickness, cross sectional areas and depth of invasion in the prognosis of cutaneous melanoma. *Ann. Surg.*, **172**, 902–8.

Byron R.L., Lamb E.J., Yonemoto R.H. & Kase S. (1962) Radical inguinal node dissection in the treatment of cancer. *Surg. Gynaecol. Obstet.*, April, 401–8.

Calame R.J. (1980) Pelvic relaxation as a complication of radical vulvectomy. *Obstet. Gynecol.*, **55**, 716.

Cavanagh D., Roberts W.S., Bryson S.C.P., Marsden D., Ingram J.M. & Anderson W.R. (1986) Changing trends in the surgical treatment of invasive carcinoma of the vulva. *Surg. Gynecol. Obstet.*, **162**, 164–68.

Chafe W., Fowler W.C., Walton L.A. & Currie J.L. (1983) Radical vulvectomy with use of tensor fascia lata flap. *Am. J. Obstet. Gynecol.*, **145**, 207−13.

Christopherson W., Buchsbaum H.J., Voet R. & Lifschitz S. (1985) Radical vulvectomy and bilateral groin lymphadenectomy utilising separate groin incisions: report of a case with recurrence in the intervening skin bridge. *Gynecol. Oncol.*, **21**, 247−51.

Clark W.H., From L., Bernadino E.A. & Mihm M.C. (1969) The histogenesis and biologic behavior of primary human malignant melanomas of the skin. *Cancer Res.*, **29**, 705−26.

Copeland L.J., Nour Sneige, Gershenson D.M., McGuffie V.B., Abdul-Karim F. & Rutledge F.N. (1986) Bartholin gland carcinoma. *Obstet. Gynecol.*, **67**, 794−801.

Curry S.L., Wharton J.T. & Rutledge F.N. (1980) Positive lymph nodes in vulvar squamous carcinoma. *Gynecol. Oncol.*, **9**, 63−67.

Daly J.W. & Pomerance A.J. (1979) Groin dissection with prevention of tissue loss and postoperative infection. *Obstet. Gynecol.*, **53**, 395−99.

Davison T., Kissin M. & Westbury C. (1987) Vulvo-vaginal melanoma−should radical surgery be abandoned? *Br. J. Obstet. Gynaecol.*, **94**, 473−76.

Deppe G. (1979) Chemotherapy of squamous cell carcinoma of the vulva: a review. *Gynecol. Oncol.*, **7**, 345−48.

Diapola G.R., Gomez-Rueda N. & Arrighi L. (1975) Relevance of microinvasion in carcinoma of the vulva. *Obstet. Gynecol.*, **45** (6), 647−49.

Disaia P.J., Creasman W.T. & Rich W.M. (1979) An alternate approach to early cancer of the vulva. *Am. J. Obstet. Gynecol.*, **133**, 825−30.

Downey G.O., Okagaki T., Ostrow R.S., Clark B.A., Twiggs L.B. & Faras A.J. (1988) Condylomatous carcinoma of the vulva with special reference to human papillomavirus DNA. *Obstet. Gynecol.*, **72**, 68−73.

Edington P.T. & Monaghan J.M. (1980) Malignant melanoma of the vulva and vagina. *Br. J. Obstet. Gynaecol.*, **87**, 422−24.

Fairey R.N., Mackay P.A., Benedet J.L., Boyes D.A. & Turko M. (1985) Radiation treatment of carcinoma of the vulva, 1950 1980. *Am. J. Obstet. Gynecol.*, **151**, 591−97.

Friedrich E.G. & Diapola G.R. (1977) Postoperative staging of vulvar carcinoma: a retrospective study. *Int. J. Gynecol. Obstet.*, **15**, 270−74.

Goldberg M.I., Belinson J.I., Ford J.H. & Averette H.E. (1979) Surgical management of invasive carcinoma of the vulva utilizing a lower midline incision. *Gynecol. Oncol.*, **7**, 296−308.

Green T.H. (1978) Carcinoma of the vulva; reassessment. *Obstet. Gynecol.*, **52**, 462−68.

Hacker N.F., Berek J.S., Juillard G.J.F. & Lagasse L.D. (1984) Preoperative radiation therapy for locally advanced vulvar cancer. *Cancer*, **54**, 2056−61.

Hacker N.F., Berek J.S., Lagasse L.D. & Nieberg R.K. (1983) Microinvasive carcinoma of the vulva. *Obstet. Gynecol.*, **62**, 134−35.

Hacker N.F., Berek J.S., Lagasse L.D., Nieberg R.K. & Leuchter R.S. (1984) Individualisation of treatment for stage I squamous cell vulvar carcinoma. *Obstet. Gynecol.*, **63**, 155 62.

Hacker N.F., Leuchter R.S., Berek J.S., Castaldo T.W. & Lagasse L.D. (1981) Radical vulvectomy and bilateral inguinal lymphadenectomy through separate groin incisions. *Obstet. Gynecol.*, **58**, 574−79.

Hammond I.G. & Monaghan J.M. (1983) Multicentric carcinoma of the female genital tract. *Br. J. Obstet. Gynaecol.*, **90**, 557−61.

Hoffman J.S., Kumar N.B. & Morley G.W. (1983) Microinvasive squamous carcinoma of the vulva: search for a definition. *Obstet. Gynecol.*, **61**, 615−18.

Homesley H.D., Bundy B.N., Sedlis A. & Adcock L. (1986) Radiation therapy versus pelvic node resection for carcinoma of the vulva with positive groin nodes. *Obstet. Gynecol.*, **68**, 733−40.

Iversen T. & Aas M. (1983) Lymph drainage of the vulva. *Gynecol. Oncol.*, **16**, 179−89.

Iversen T., Abeler V. & Aalders J. (1981) Individualized treatment of stage I carcinoma of the vulva. *Obstet. Gynecol.*, **57**, 85−89.

Jafari K. & Cartnick E.N. (1976) Microinvasive squamous cell carcinoma of the vulva. *Gynecol. Oncol.*, **4**, 158−66.

Japaze H., Van Dinh T. & Woodruff J.D. (1981) Verrucous carcinoma of the vulva: study of 24 cases. *Obstet. Gynecol.*, **60**, 462−66.

Jeffcoate T.N.A. & Woodcock A.S. (1969) Premalignant conditions of the vulva with particular reference to chronic epithelial dystrophies. *Br. Med. J.*, **2**, 127—32.

Leuchter R.S., Hacker N.F., Voet R.L., Berek J.S., Townsend D.E. & Lagasse L.D. (1982) Primary carcinoma of the Bartholin gland: a report of 14 cases and review of the literature. *Obstet. Gynecol.*, **60**, 361—68.

Lifshitz F., Savage J.E., Yates S.J. & Buchsbaum H.J. (1982) Primary epidermoid carcinoma of the vulva. *Surg. Gynecol. Obstet.*, **155**, 59—61.

Monaghan J.M. & Hammond I.G. (1984) Pelvic node dissection in the treatment of vulval carcinoma — is it necessary? *Br. J. Obstet. Gynaecol.*, **91**, 270—74.

Monaghan J.M. & Mathias I. (1982) (Video tape) *Radical Vulvectomy with Deep Pelvic Node Dissection*. TS81/222/P(M) Audiovisual Centre, The University, Newcastle-Upon-Tyne.

Morley G.W. (1976) Infiltrative carcinoma of the vulva, results of surgical treatment. *Am. J. Obstet. Gynecol.*, **124**, 874—88.

Nakao C.Y., Nolan J.F., Disaia P.J. & Futoran R. (1974) 'Microinvasive' epidermoid carcinoma of the vulva with an unexpected natural history. *Am. J. Obstet. Gynecol.*, **120**, 1122—23.

Parker R.T., Duncan I., Rampone J. & Creasman W. (1975) Operative management of early invasive epidermoid carcinoma of the vulva. *Am. J. Obstet. Gynecol.*, **123**, 349—55.

Parry-Jones E. (1963) Lymphatics of the vulva. *Br. J. Obstet. Gynaecol.*, **70**, 751—65.

Patsner B. & Mann W.J. (1988) Radical vulvectomy and 'sneak' superficial inguinal lymphadenectomy with a single elliptical incision. *Am. J. Obstet. Gynecol.*, **158**, 464—69.

Penn I. (1986) Cancers of the anogenital region in renal transplant recipients. Analysis of 65 cases. *Cancer*, **58**, 611—16.

Piver M.S., Malfetano J.H., Lele S.B. & Moore R.H. (1983) Prophylactic anticoagulation as a possible cause of inguinal lymphocyst after radical vulvectomy and inguinal lymphadenectomy. *Obstet. Gynecol.*, **62**, 17—21.

Piver M.S. & Xynos F.P. (1977) Pelvic lymphadenectomy in women with carcinoma of the clitoris. *Obstet. Gynecol.*, **49**, 592—95.

Podratz K.C., Gaffey T.A., Symmonds R.E., Johansen K.L. & O'Brien P.C. (1983) Melanoma of the vulva: an update. *Gynecol. Oncol.*, **16**, 153—68.

Podratz K.C., Symmonds R.E. & Taylor W.F. (1982) Carcinoma of the vulva: analysis of treatment failures. *Am. J. Obstet. Gynecol.*, **143**, 340—51.

Podratz K.C., Symmonds R.E., Taylor W.F. & Williams T.J. (1980) Treatment of invasive squamous cell carcinoma of the vulva at the Mayo clinic 1955—1975 (Abstract). *Gynecol. Oncol.*, **10**, 362.

Price J.H., Heath A.R., Sunter J.P., Sinha D.P. & Monaghan J.M. (1988) Inflammatory cell infiltration and survival in squamous-cell carcinoma of the vulva. *Br. J. Obstet. Gynaecol.*, **95**, 714—19.

Rowley K.C., Gallion H.H., Donaldson E.S., van Nagell J.R., Higgins R.V., Powell D.E., Kryscio R.J. & Pavlik E.J. (1988) Prognostic factors in early vulvar cancer. *Gynecol. Oncol.*, **31**, 43—49.

Rutledge F.N., Smith J.P. & Franklin E.W. (1970) Carcinoma of the vulva. *Am. J. Obstet. Gynecol.*, **106**, 1117—30.

Sherman K.J., Daling J.R., Chu J., McKnight B. & Weiss N.S. (1988) Multiple primary tumours in women with vulvar neoplasms: a case-control study. *Br. J. Cancer*, **57**, 423—27.

Stoeckel W. (1930) Zur Therapie des Vulvakarzinoms. *Zentralblatt fur Gynakologie*, **1**, 47—71.

Taussig F.J. (1935) Primary cancer of the vulva, vagina and female urethra: five year results. *Surg. Gynecol. Obstet.*, **60**, 477.

Taussig F.J. (1940) Cancer of the vulva: an analysis of 155 cases (1911—1940). *Am. J. Obstet. Gynecol.*, **40**, 764—79.

Trelford J.D., Deer D.A., Ordorica E., Franti C.E. & Trelford-Sauder M. (1984) Ten year prospective study in a management change of vulvar carcinoma. *Am. J. Obstet. Gynecol.*, **150**, 288—96.

Way S. (1948) The anatomy of the lymphatic drainage of the vulva, and its influence on the radical operation for carcinoma. *Annals of the Royal College of Surgeons of England*, **3**, 187.

Way S. (1954) Results of a planned attack on carcinoma of the vulva. *Br. Med. J.*, **2**, 780.

Way S. (1960) Carcinoma of the vulva. *Am. J. Obstet. Gynecol.*, **79**, 692—98.

Way S. (1978) Surgery of vulval carcinoma: an appraisal. *In*: Lees D. & Singer A.S. (eds), *Clinics in Obstetrics and Gynaecology*. W.B. Saunders, London. **5**, 623—28.

Wharton J.T., Gallagher S. & Rutledge F.N. (1974) Microinvasive carcinoma of the vulva. *Am. J. Obstet. Gynecol.*, **118**, 159—62.

Wheeless C.R., McGibbon B., Dorsey J.H. & Maxwell C.P. (1979) Gracilis myocutaneous flap in the reconstruction of the vulva and female perineum. *Obstet. Gynecol.*, **54**, 97–102.

Willis R.A. (1973) *The Spread of Tumours in the Human Body*. 3rd edn. Butterworth, London. pp. 19–30.

Yasigi R., Piver S.M. & Tsukada Y. (1978) Microinvasive carcinoma of the vulva. *Obstet. Gynecol.*, **51**, 368–70.

8

The Presentation and Management of Cancer of the Vagina

JOHN M. MONAGHAN

Carcinoma of the vagina has been commonly held to have a very poor prognosis. Taussig (1935) stated that 'Primary cancer of the vagina is rare and almost always universally fatal'. Recently a number of series have shown a much improved prospect (Brown et al. 1971; Prempree et al. 1977; Al Kurdi & Monaghan 1981; Perez & Camel 1982; Benedet et al. 1983). This chapter is based on a review of 130 cases managed in the author's department over a 40-year period.

Most cancers occurring in the vagina arise by direct spread or metastases from the cervix, body of uterus, vulva, bladder, rectum or sigmoid colon. Primary carcinoma of the vagina is rare and represents only 1–2% of all genital malignancies. It is consequently difficult for individual practitioners to build up a large series; hence most reports are the accumulated experience of large institutions over a long period of time (Al Kurdi & Monaghan 1981; Wharton et al. 1981; Ball & Berman 1982; Benedet et al. 1983; Kucera et al. 1985; Peters et al. 1985; Dancuart et al. 1988). This frequently leads to difficulties in adopting standard treatment methods and results are often not readily comparable.

Considerable skill is required to determine the best method of management. Vaginal cancer demands individualization of treatment as the site and size of tumour vary enormously; the treatment may involve a combination of modalities to provide the best possible prospect for patients.

The age range of presentation for vaginal cancer is very wide although the majority occur in women in their sixth and seventh decades.

Histopathology

Most cancers are squamous in type (93%). Primary adenocarcinoma of the vagina is rare and will occur in only 4–5% of cases. In recent years considerable interest has been shown in clear cell adenocarcinomas of the genital tract particularly those of the vagina, developing in young women with a history of maternal ingestion of diethylstilboestrol during pregnancy. There also appears to have been an overall background increase in prevalance of clear cell adenocarcinomas of the genital tract, both related and unrelated to stilboestrol ingestion. This increase has been observed in patients of all age groups (Wharton et al. 1981).

Rare cancers

Other tumours include malignant melanomas which represent 1% of all vaginal carcinomas, verrucous squamous cell carcinoma and rare childhood cancers including sarcoma botryoides and endodermal sinus tumours (Monaghan 1988). Some of these rarer tumours are described in detail later.

Aetiology

No single aetiological agent has been identified in the development of squamous vaginal carcinoma. In previous series venereal disease, chronic infection and the chronic irritation associated with procidentia and prolapse and the wearing of vaginal pessaries were commonly impuned (Table 8.1). There is no doubt that carcinoma of the vagina does occur in these circumstances (Fig. 8.1), but they are rare as aetiological factors. In more recent times greater significance has been

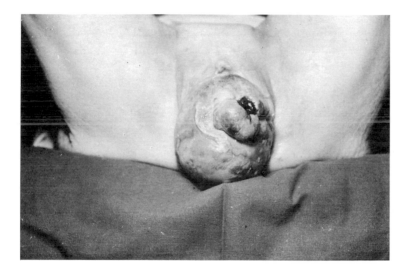

Fig. 8.1. Carcinoma of the vagina developing on a procidentia in an 82-year-old patient.

Table 8.1. Aetiological agents suggested for carcinoma of the vagina (from Williams & Whitehouse 1985. Reproduced by kind permission of John Wiley & Sons Limited)

Author	Cases n	Prolapse	Pessary
Johnston *et al.* (1983)	45	1	1
Al-Kurdi & Monaghan (1981)	99	6	3
Underwood & Smith (1971)	35	2	0
Benedet *et al.* (1983)	97	5	

placed on the role of previous radiotherapy (Pride *et al.* 1979; Peters *et al.* 1985) although this aetiological factor has been discounted by Perez & Camel (1982). Wharton *et al.* (1981), in their series, noted that 48% of patients had had a preceding total abdominal hysterectomy for unrelated disease; 16.7% had had previous CIN or clinical carcinoma of the cervix. Ireland & Monaghan (1988) showed the high risk of invasive cancer developing in patients who had either persistent or recurring abnormal vaginal cytology following hysterectomy. They emphasized the high risk of cancers developing above the vault suture line. Peters *et al.* (1985) noted that in 35 of their reported series of 68 patients there had been 37 previous malignancies, 32 of which had been invasive or preinvasive carcinomas of the cervix. Other authorities have noted a similar association with previous cervical disease (Benedet *et al.* 1983) and endometriosis (Kapp *et al.* 1982; Granai *et al.* 1984).

The possibility of a multicentric origin for vaginal carcinoma has been discussed, but is not as clear as the relationship between vulval neoplasia (both intraepithelial and invasive) and carcinoma of the cervix (Hammond & Monaghan 1983) (Figs 8.2, 8.3, 8.4). Recent interest in viral aetiological factors for genital cancers has focused attention on the Herpes simplex type II and the Papova virus family, particularly types 16 and 18. These may be involved in the development of multifocal disease including the vagina (Weed *et al.* 1983).

Symptomatology

Almost all patients present with some form of abnormal vaginal bleeding, particularly postmenopausal bleeding. Discharge is also frequently seen and may be related to infection of the necrotic surface of the tumour or stimulation of vaginal secretions. Pain can be a feature and is related to the size of the cancer and surrounding tissue reaction. Other symptomatology is related to the position of the carcinoma which may induce urinary or bowel symptoms (Table 8.2). However, it is not unusual for the lesion to be found incidentally at routine pelvic examination, usually during the taking of a cervical smear. If a careless approach is used and the vagina and vulva are not meticulously inspected, it is possible for the cancer to be missed. There is frequently a long delay prior to presentation and diagnosis (Brady 1978).

Mode of spread

Cancer of the vagina spreads primarily by local invasion and lymphatic permeation with embolization as do carcinoma of the cervix and vulva. The vagina has a fine capillary network throughout the mucosa and the muscularis both of which anastomose freely; however in spite of these anastomoses, regular defined channels of drainage do occur (Plentl & Friedman 1971). The lymphatics of the vault drain to the lateral and posterior pelvic nodes, the central portion of the vagina to

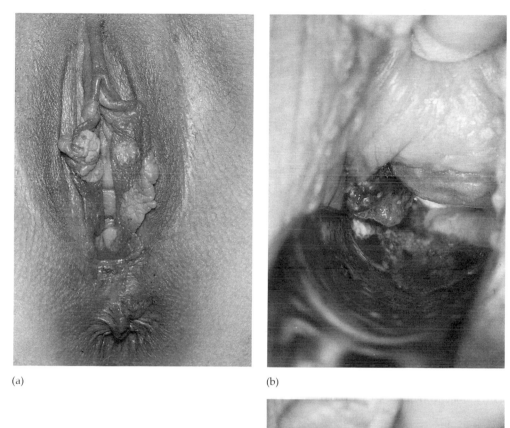

(a)

(b)

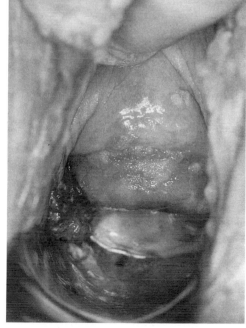

Fig. 8.2. Multicentric carcinoma of the female genitalia: (a) shows vulvar intraepithelial neoplasia III, (b) shows an invasive squamous carcinoma of the right vaginal wall and (c) shows cervical intraepithelial neoplasia III.

(c)

the lateral nodes, from the anterior part into the paravesical lymphatics and from the posterior wall to the deep pelvic nodes. The distal vagina drains, as does the vestibule, vulva and anus, to the nodes in the inguinal region. Many variations of this system have been reported which may in part account for the poor results of local treatment of the carcinoma.

Site of carcinoma

More than half of carcinomas of the vagina occur in the posterior wall of the upper one-third of the vagina. The second commonest site is the anterior wall of the lower one-third of the vagina. Attempts have been made to implicate various aetiological agents to account for this site specificity. It is, however, impossible to isolate one agent to produce tumours in such diverse sites.

The prospect for cure is said to be greater in those patients where the tumour occurs in the upper third of the vagina (Disaia *et al.* 1975), probably because it spreads in a similar manner to carcinoma of the cervix. This better prognosis may also be due to the fact that the upper vagina is more elastic and distensible than the lower so that infiltration of subjacent tissues is a later event. The difference may also be related to the fact that lower vaginal tumours have a tendency to spread to both the pelvic and inguinal lymphatics, making management more complicated (Table 8.3). Thus site of carcinoma as well as staging must be taken into account when treatment is considered reinforcing the need for individualization of management.

Staging

Primary carcinoma of the vagina is a diagnosis of exclusion. If there is evidence of a primary tumour in an adjacent organ, then primary carcinoma of the vagina cannot be presumed. It is important that a complete examination of the patient should be made to eliminate the possibility that the tumour present in the vagina is not a secondary from another site.

FIGO staging is shown in Table 8.4. The close proximity of the bladder and rectum to the vaginal wall can produce difficulties and there may be fine distinction between stage I and stage IV carcinomas. Equally with large tumour masses it is not easy to differentiate between stages I and II.

Variations of this simplistic and rigid staging system have been proposed including subdivisions of stages I, II and IV (Perez & Camel 1982; Pride *et al.* 1979; Prempree *et al.* 1977).

Inevitably, some later stages of cancer of the vagina have to be categorized as arising from cervix or vulva. It is often impossible to be certain of the 'centre of gravity' of the cancer. This problem, coupled with the rigidity of the staging definitions, can cause marked underestimations of the extent and number of cases of cancer of the vagina.

Table 8.2. Frequency of presenting symptoms in carcinoma of the vagina (from Williams & Whitehouse 1985. Reproduced by kind permission of John Wiley & Sons Limited)

Author	Cases n	Bleeding %	Discharge %	Pain %	Mass %	Incidental finding %	Mean delay (weeks)
Underwood & Smith (1971)		51	23	6	6	14	n.k.
Pride et al. (1979)	43	53	16	4.6		21	n.k.
Al-Kurdi & Monaghan (1981)	65	97	63	30	11		45
Ball & Berman (1982)	58	59	7		3.4	19	20
Johnston et al. (1983)	45	36	11			13	5
Benedet et al. (1983)	97	69	69	5	2	13.4	n.k.

n.k. = not known.

Table 8.3. Lymph node involvement related to site of vaginal carcinoma (from Williams & Whitehouse 1985. Reproduced by kind permission of John Wiley & Sons Limited)

Site of tumour	Lymph node dissections	Patients with positive nodes			
		Pelvic cases	Nodes %	Inguinal cases	Nodes %
Upper vagina	13	3	23	0	
Middle vagina	3	0		0	
Lower vagina	13	3	23	5	38
Whole vagina	6	4	67	1	17

Table 8.4. FIGO staging system for primary carcinoma of the vagina

Stage	Degree of involvement
I	Carcinoma limited to the vaginal wall
II	Carcinoma has involved subvaginal tissues, but not extended to the pelvic wall
III	Carcinoma has extended to the pelvic wall
IV	Carcinoma has extended beyond the true pelvis or has involved mucosa of bladder or rectum: bullous oedema as such does not permit a case to be allotted to stage IV

	Proposed modifications to FIGO
IIA	Subvaginal infiltration not into parametrium or paracolpos
IIB	Parametrial infiltration not extending to pelvic wall

Preoperative assessment

Having established that the vaginal cancer is primary rather than secondary, careful pelvic examination, ideally under general anaesthesia, with cystoscopy and proctosigmoidoscopy should be carried out. This is combined with the preoperative use of imaging techniques including ultrasound, computerized axial tomography, magnetic resonance imaging and contrast radiology, particularly of the bowel and urinary tract. In order to fully assess the extent of the disease an adequate representative biopsy or biopsies of the tumour are essential to produce an accurate histopathological assessment. This assessment should include the use of staining and/or immunocytochemistry techniques to differentiate in particular bowel and genital adenocarcinomas, in order to confirm the primary nature of the carcinoma.

Treatment

Radiotherapy

In the majority of centres radiotherapy is the preferred method of treatment. Wharton *et al.* (1981), Perez & Camel (1982) and Kucera *et al.* (1985) have advocated radiotherapy as the treatment of choice because of 'the excellent control (of tumour) and the good functional results'. They were also critical of the use of surgery because of the total or partial loss of vaginal function unless the patient was willing to go through the long process of the production of a neovagina. In their series surgery was only used for the treatment of recurrent disease after failed radiotherapy usually in the form of exenterative operations.

These three large centres have each developed their own techniques of radiotherapy, thereby further individualizing treatment. Wharton *et al.* use the Fletcher Shrinking Field technique, utilizing the external beam in all tumours with a greater diameter than 2 cm to shrink down the tumour, at the same time reducing the field size so that the tumour receives an increasing dose of radiation. The treatment is completed by applying interstitial sources to the tumour. Carcinomas of the upper one-third of the vagina are treated as though they were carcinomas of the cervix, but if the cervix has been previously removed a transvaginal cone source is used. Some anterior wall tumours were treated by interstitial implants, a suprapubic cystotomy being performed to improve the accuracy of the placement of the sources. Most later stage disease is treated by external beam irradiation alone.

Perez & Camel combined external beam irradiation with intracavitary and interstitial methods. The vagina and pelvic nodes were treated by anterior and posterior portals, the groins being included in the field or irradiated separately when the lower vagina was involved. They used a variety of intracavitary applicators and preferred caesium 137 for the interstitial sources.

Kucera *et al.*, reporting on a large series of 362 cases, confirmed the individual approach to therapy. They separately assessed a subgroup of 99 patients treated between 1971 and 1977, commenting on the benefit of teletherapy for more advanced lesions, whereas intrauterine devices improved the prospects for stages I and II.

In an earlier series Underwood & Smith (1971) stated that external irradiation must be added to internal systems in order to improve survival, but Perez & Camel qualified this when they found that external beam irradiation was essential in stages II, III and IV, but did not make any improvement in stage I.

As most large series have been built up over many years and considerable individualization has occurred it is not unusual to see up to 13 different treatment methods being used (Perez & Camel 1982).

Surgery

Very few series have treated their patients with surgery alone. The author found improved 5-year survivals in stage I and stage IV disease. Johnston *et al.* (1983) stated that surgery was equal to radiotherapy in the treatment of stage I disease, but Ball & Berman (1982) went further and stated that surgery was superior to radiotherapy when strictly comparing survivals in stage I disease (84% 5-year survival compared with 55% for radiotherapy). The author has gained considerable experience in the use of radical vaginectomy or hysterovaginectomy for early stage cancers of the vagina (Monaghan 1987). When combined with plastic surgical procedures to replace the vagina long term results have been excellent. Table 8.5 shows the range of possible treatments by stage.

Results

Table 8.6 shows the 5-year survival statistics for the various FIGO staging and modified staging categories (Monaghan 1985). Stage IV disease is only successfully treated in a radiotherapeutic series by Wharton *et al.* (1981). Al-Kurdi & Monaghan (1981) reported on a mainly surgical series quoting a 22% 5-year survival in stage IV, seven of these patients being treated by exenteration with two surviving (29%).

Complications of treatment

Following surgery and radiotherapy for small tumours the complications are very few, involving mainly scarring and shortening of the vagina. When larger lesions

Table 8.5. Range of treatments used for different FIGO stages

FIGO staging	Treatment modality
I	Local excision — total or partial vaginectomy Radical hysterectomy + total or partial vaginectomy +/− pelvic or inguinal lymphadenectomy Pelvic exenteration External beam irradiation Interstitial radiotherapy Vaginal moulds (Colpostats)
II	External beam irradiation +/− interstitial or intracavitary irradiation
III	As for stage II
IV	Anterior, posterior or total exenteration External beam irradiation +/− interstitial or intracavitary irradiation

Table 8.6. 5-year survival rates, all treatment methods

	Cases (n)	I (%)	II (%)	III (%)	IV (%)
			FIGO staging		
Prempree *et al.* (1977)	64	83	65 (IIa) 64 (IIb)	40	0
Pride *et al.* (1979)	43	66	66 (IIa) 31 (IIb)	23	0
Al-Kurdi & Monaghan (1981)	65	71	29	25	22
Wharton *et al.* (1981)	112	64	59	36	40
Ball & Berman (1982)	58	76	37	17	0
Perez & Camel (1982)	134	90	58 (IIa) 32 (IIb)	40	0
Johnston *et al.* (1983)	45	78	55	0	0
Kucera *et al.* (1985)	362	75	45.3	30	40
Manetta *et al.* (1988)	29	71	47	33	33

are treated by radiotherapy a moderate degree of vaginal stenosis and scarring is inevitable, as are proctitis and cystitis. Major complications such as necrosis of rectum, bladder and urethra are reported in 8–11% of cases (Pride *et al.* 1979; Chu & Beechinor 1984; Kucera *et al.* 1985). These complications are both stage and dose related, the highest complication rates occurring in late stage and recurrent disease that has been treated with greater than 5–6000 rad.

When surgery is used complications rise markedly in later stage disease, including intraoperative, intestinal conduit and stoma problems.

Thus it appears that although radiotherapy is the treatment of choice for carcinoma of the vagina, surgery probably has a place in some selected cases of stage I disease; and has a significant place in stage IV disease and that recurring after radiotherapeutic treatment. In a recent review Peters *et al.* (1985) have shown that surgery has given very good results in the management of primary sarcoma of the adult vagina, exenteration being the treatment of choice. The main difference between the two modalities is that with surgery there is usually a total or significant loss of vaginal function. It is possible for those patients with a small vagina or pliable perineum to achieve lengthening and dilatation to the point at which the vagina can be functional. This is more difficult following radiotherapy but patients must be encouraged to use vaginal dilators and creams to lubricate and facilitate lengthening.

Verrucous squamous cell carcinoma

This extremely rare variation of carcinoma of the vagina has been reported less than 20 times (Jones *et al.* 1981). It was said to be first described by Martens & Tilesius in 1804 (Ramzy *et al.* 1976). There does not appear to be a clear aetiological agent although the tumour probably develops due to stimulation by the Papova virus and may be similar to the large condyloma acuminatum found in the male, the giant condyloma of Buschke—Loewenstein. The disease is characterized by a relatively benign 'pushing' pattern of growth almost never metastasizing and involving other organs in the pelvis only very late in its life cycle. The gross appearance is of a fungating, verrucous, brown, trabeculated tissue. Microscopically the tumour is markedly acanthotic with prominent rounded rete ridges, pushing into surrounding tissues but rarely showing clear invasive appearances. The cellular pattern is characterized by abundant oesinophilic cytoplasm. The nuclei are generally round with prominent nucleoli. Mitotic figures are few. There is often a marked tissue reaction to be found along the margins of the tumour, including giant cells exhibiting a foreign body response to the keratotic material in the carcinoma.

Clinical features

Bleeding does not commonly occur as a primary symptom, the tumour being most frequently diagnosed following routine examination when a massive fungating mass in the vagina is noted. Procidentia and a mass appearing at the vulva are frequent presentations.

The most important and valuable investigation is to perform an adequate biopsy. This should be carried out as a formal procedure under anaesthetic when a large piece of tissue to include the growing edge of the tumour should be taken.

Management and prognosis

Surgery. The optimal management appears to be to perform a wide local excision. Unfortunately because of the large size of these tumours at presentation the margin is frequently found to be inadequate and recurrence occurs. In the author's experience the patient may have had a large series of small procedures before presenting to an oncologist. Extensive surgery may then be necessary to effect a cure. It seems that lymphadenectomy is a debatable part of the primary management (Powell *et al.* 1978).

Radiotherapy is not advised as there is a poor cure rate (Goethals *et al.* 1963) and a significant risk of malignant transformation of the tumour into an anaplastic carcinoma (Kraus & Perez-Mesa 1966).

Chemotherapy. There is currently no effective chemotherapeutic agent available. It is often found that the tumour has been treated ineffectually in the past with podophylline.

Basal cell carcinoma

This tumour is extraordinarily rare in the vagina; Blaustein records only one case of 'basal cell-like carcinoma', reported by Naves *et al.* in 1980. They discussed the possibility that the tumour which they had described may have arisen from a group of cell rests and may have had features of the 'cylindromas or basal adenoid carcinomas' of the cervix reviewed by Rosen & Dolan (1975).

Management and prognosis

Surgery. Wide local excision is all that is required to cure the cancer. Widespread metastases do not occur.

Radiotherapy. This modality is of value when the vagina has to be preserved.

Carcinoma arising in a neovagina

This extremely rare event has been reported on a number of occasions, the first squamous carcinoma in a grafted vaginal epithelium occurred in 1959 (Jackson 1959). Over the years a number of other reports have been made, and recently even a verrucous carcinoma has been reported to arise in a split thickness skin grafted vagina (Abrenio *et al.* 1977).

Malignant melanoma of the vagina

Primary malignant melanoma of the vagina is extremely rare. Pomante (1975) had collected 39 cases and in 1980 the author added two more (Edington & Monaghan 1980). Lee *et al.* (1984), in a major review, have updated the world's collected series to 106.

Vaginal bleeding and discharge are the commonest presenting symptoms. It is important to make an adequate biopsy of the lesion as occasionally the abnormality may still be confined to the epithelium (melanomatous intraepithelial neoplasia) (Fig. 8.3) and an excision biopsy is all that is required. Unfortunately when the lesion is invasive the prospects for cure are very poor, both radical surgery and radiotherapy have been used with little success. If the lesion is of the lower one-third of the vagina, radical excision combined with radical vulvectomy is the treatment of choice (Edington & Monaghan 1980). Recent evidence suggests that it is important to consider the disease as a systemic problem, therefore adjuvant therapy should be used (Lee *et al.* 1984). Chemotherapy has been used but with relatively little success. Of the drugs used dacarbazine (DTIC) and hydroxyea probably are the most effective. Immunotherapy may improve the effectiveness of drug treatments.

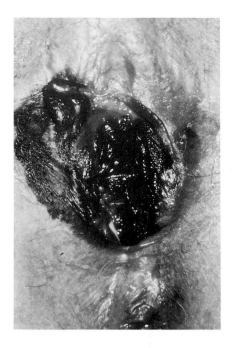

Fig. 8.3. Vulvo–vaginal melanoma *in situ*.

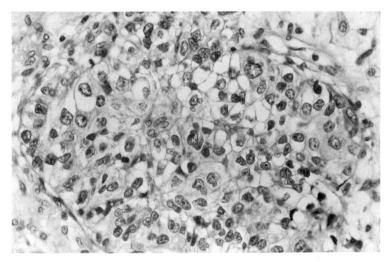

Fig. 8.4. Clear cell adenocarcinoma of the vagina (× 40).

The propensity for melanomas to metastasize widely by both the lymphatic and haematological routes makes them a lethal and unpredictable cancer. They also appear to have a capacity to lie dormant for a number of years and then to reappear after minor stress especially surgical procedures.

Clear cell carcinoma of the vagina

Although clear cell carcinomas of the vagina occur rarely, in 1970 Herbst & Scully reported an unusually high frequency in a short space of time in Boston, USA. They reported on seven young women who had developed the tumour, and in six they were able to show that their mothers had taken diethylstilboestrol (DES) during the course of their pregnancies (Herbst *et al.* 1971). Many more reports followed from the USA where DES had been used extensively to maintain high risk pregnancies, especially those with a past history of abortion, diabetes and twin pregnancies.

The tumour has a very characteristic appearance (Fig. 8.4) with vacuolated or clear areas in the cells and 'hob nail' nuclei.

It was not until 1977 that the first case was seen in Britain (Monaghan & Sirisena 1978) and since that time four more cases have been seen. Herbst and Scully have maintained a registry of cases; to date more than 500 cases of clear cell carcinoma of the vagina and cervix have been recorded worldwide.

Stilboestrol is known to be teratogenic, the characteristic stigmata in the female being vaginal and cervical adenosis, coxcombing and hooding of the cervix and the development of a transverse ridge in the vagina. This teratogenic effect will only occur if the stilboestrol is given prior to 18 weeks gestation. There is no solid evidence that the drug is carcinogenic, but the tumour probably develops because the ectopic columnar epithelium in the vagina is of a endometrioid type and is susceptible to carcinogens present within the vaginal environment. The cancer risk to those females with the stigmata appears to be very low of the order of 1:1000 to 1400 (Herbst & Scully 1983).

Many different modalities of treatment have been used but it appears that local excision is inferior to more radical methods. Lymph node metastases are of the same order as with carcinoma of the cervix, 18% for stage I and 30% for stage II. Five-year actuarial survivals of 90% stage I, 80% stage II and 37% stage III have been reported (Herbst & Scully 1983). Recurrences occur more commonly after local treatments and are best treated by surgery or radiotherapy. To date no effective chemotherapeutic agent has been reported.

For a number of years there has been confusion and disagreement over the risk of cervical and vaginal dysplasia developing in DES-exposed young women. Mattingley and Stafl predicted in 1974 that exposed women would be at increased risk of the development of dysplasia. Since that time a variety of comments have been made. Robboy *et al.* in 1984, reviewing the experience of the National Collaborative DES Project, stated that the incidence of dysplasia and carcinoma *in situ* was significantly higher in the exposed group than in a matched cohort. These higher rates only occurred if the squamous metaplasia extended to the outer half of the cervix or onto the vagina. The possibility of a precancerous atypical vaginal adenosis has been mooted by Davis *et al.* (1981) and more recently by Robboy *et al.* (1983). This appears to be characterized by tuboendo-metrial glandular epithelium consisting of mucin free, often ciliated, cells.

Vaginal sarcomas

Sarcomas of the vagina may occur in both young and old patients. Leiomyosar-comas, spindle cell sarcomas, alveolar soft part sarcomas, angiosarcomas, fibro-sarcomas, neurofibrosarcomas and mixed mesodermal tumours of the vagina occur predominantly in older patients but are extremely rare (2% of all malignant vaginal tumours).

Embryonal rhabdomyosarcomas (sarcoma botryoides) develop in young girls between 6 months and 16 years of age.

Sarcomas of the elderly

Leiomyosarcomas are the most common of the adult sarcomas. They often grow slowly and the tumour may occasionally be responsive to wide local excision.

Epidemiology and aetiology

There are no clear aetiological agents but Peters *et al.* (1985) report that one-third of 17 patients had previous pelvic irradiation for carcinoma of the cervix.

The tumour generally develops alongside the vaginal epithelium presenting as a lump which may cause problems with micturition, defecation or intercourse. Because they are subdermal, bleeding and discharge are late features.

Management and prognosis

Surgery. Extremely wide local excision is essential. The tumour mass often has a false compression capsule consisting of cancer tissue. This 'capsule' must be widely excised with a good margin of normal tissue. As the vagina is so close to other vital organs this wide excision will often dictate that an exenterative procedure is performed; in the Peters *et al.* series this form of treatment produced the only long term survivals.

Radiotherapy has only rarely been used, mainly by Rutledge from the MD Anderson Hospital with mixed results.

Chemotherapy. Unfortunately treatment of adult sarcomas with chemotherapy does not produce the excellent results found in paediatric sarcomas. Chemotherapy may possibly be useful as a tumour reductive agent prior to extensive surgery.

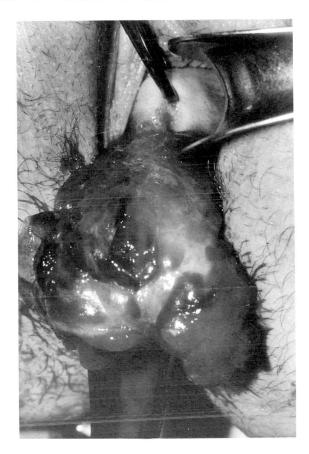

Fig. 8.5. Sarcoma botryoides in a 15-year-old girl.

Sarcomas of the young

Embryonal rhabdomyosarcomas (sarcoma botryoides) and endodermal sinus tumours

These rare tumours develop in young infants with a mean age of 2 years (Hilgers *et al.* 1970). Both tumours present with bleeding or bloody discharge and occasionally with a mass presenting at the introitus. The sarcoma botryoides is characteristically described as a mass of grape-like structures (Fig. 8.5), and the endodermal sinus tumour as a polypoid lesion. Delay in seeking advice is a common feature.

The treatment of sarcoma botryoides has traditionally been by radical surgery including exenteration, but survival figures are poor. Huffman (1968) found that only 12 of 150 cases survived 5 years. More recently it has been shown that chemotherapy is of great value (Hilgers *et al.* 1973). Ortega (1979) showed that preliminary or complete treatment with chemotherapy was at least equal to radical

Edington P.T. & Monaghan J.M. (1980) Malignant melanoma of the vulva and vagina. *Br. J. Obstet. Gynaecol.*, **87**, 422—24.

Goethals P.L., Harrison E.G. Jr & Devine K.D. (1963) Verrucous squamous carcinoma of the oral cavity. *Am. J. Surg.*, **106**, 845—51.

Granai C.O., Walters M.D., Safaii H., Jelen I., Madoc-Jones H. & Moukhtar M. (1984) Malignant transformation of vaginal endometriosis. *Obstet. Gynecol.*, **64**, 592—95.

Hammond I.G. & Monaghan J.M. (1983) Multicentric carcinoma of the female lower genital tract. *Br. J. Obstet. Gynaecol.*, **90**, 557—61.

Harris N.L. & Scully R.E. (1984) Malignant lymphoma and granulocytic tumours of the vagina in adolescence; a report of seven cases including six clear cell carcinomas (so called mesonephromas). *Cancer*, (Philad.) **25**, 745—47.

Herbst A.L. & Scully R.E. (1983) Newsletter—Registry for Research on Hormonal Transplacental Carcinogenesis.

Herbst A.L., Ulfelder H. & Poskanzer D.C. (1971) Adenocarcinoma of the vagina: association of maternal stilboestrol therapy with tumour appearance in young women. *N. Engl. J. Med.*, **284**, 878.

Hilgers R.D. (1977) Prenatal oncogenesis and the development of malignant tumours in the infant and adolescent vagina—a review and hypothesis. *Gynecol. Oncol.*, **5**, 262—72.

Hilgers R.D., Ghavimi F., D'Angio G.J., *et al.* (1973) Memorial Hospital experience with pelvic exenteration and embryonal rhabdomyosarcoma of the vagina. *Gynecol. Oncol.*, **1**, 262—70.

Hilgers R.D., Malkasian G.D. & Soule E.H. (1970) Embryonal rhabdomyosarcoma (botryoid type) of the vagina. *Am. J. Obstet. Gynecol.*, **107**, 484—502.

Huffman J.W. (1968) *The Gynecology of Childhood and Adolescence.* W.B. Saunders Company, Philadelphia.

Ireland D. & Monaghan J.M. (1988) The management of the patient with abnormal vaginal cytology following hysterectomy. *Br. J. Obstet. Gynaecol.*, **95**, 973—75.

Jackson G.W. (1959) Primary carcinoma of an artificial vagina. *Obstet. Gynecol.*, **14**, 534.

Johnston G.A. Jr., Klotz J. & Boutselis J.G. (1983) Primary invasive carcinoma of the vagina. *Surg. Gynecol. Obstet.*, **156**, 34—40.

Jones M.J., Levin H.S. & Ballard L.A. (1981) Verrucous squamous cell carcinoma of the vagina. Case report. *Cleve. Clin. Q.*, **48**, 305—13.

Kapp D.S., Merino M. & Livolsi V. (1982) Adenocarcinoma of the vagina arising in endometriosis: long-term survival following radiation therapy. *Gynecol. Oncol.*, **14**, 271—78.

Kraus F.T. & Perez-Mesa C. (1966) Verrucous carcinoma; clinical and pathological study of 105 cases involving oral cavity, larynx and genitalia. *Cancer*, **19**, 26—38.

Kucera H., Langer M., Smekal G. & Weghaupt K. (1985) Radiotherapy of primary carcinoma of the vagina: management and results of different therapy schemes. *Gynecol. Oncol.*, **21**, 87—91.

Lee R.B., Buttoni L., Dhru R. & Tamini H. (1984) Malignant melanoma of the vagina: a case report of progression from preexisting melanosis. *Gynecol. Oncol.*, **19**, 238—45.

Manetta A., Pinto J.L., Larson J.E., Stevens C.W., Pinto J.S. & Podczaski E.S. (1988) Primary invasive carcinoma of the vagina. *Obstet. Gynecol.*, **72**, 77—81.

Mattingly R. & Stafl A. (1976) Cancer risk in diethylstilbestrol-exposed offspring. *Am. J. Obstet. Gynecol.*, **126**, 543—48.

Monaghan J.M. (1985) The management of carcinoma of the vagina. *In*: Shepherd J.S. & Monaghan J.M. (eds), *Clinical Gynaecological Oncology.* 1st Edition. Blackwell Scientific Publications, Oxford. p. 155.

Monaghan J.M. (1987) Radical vaginectomy. *In*: Monaghan J.M. (ed), *Operative Surgery: Gynaecology and Obstetrics.* Butterworths, London. pp. 200—5.

Monaghan J.M. (1988) Uncommon vaginal cancers. *In*: Williams C. *et al.* (eds), *Textbook of Uncommon Cancer.* Wiley, Chichester. pp. 121—32.

Monaghan J.M. & Sirisena L.A.W. (1978) Stilboestrol and vaginal clear cell adenocarcinoma syndrome. *Br. Med. J.*, **1**, 1588—90.

Naves A.E., Monti J.A. & Chichoni E. (1980) Basal cell-like carcinoma in the upper third of the vagina. *Am. J. Obstet. Gynecol.*, **137**, 136.

Ortega J.A. (1979) A therapeutic approach to childhood pelvic rhabdomyosarcoma without pelvic exenteration. *J. Paediatr.*, **94**, 205—9.

Perez C.A. & Camel H.M. (1982) Long term follow-up in radiation therapy of carcinoma of the vagina. *Cancer*, **49**, 1308—15.

Peters W.A., Kumar N.B., Anderson W.A. & Morley G.W. (1985) Primary sarcoma of the adult vagina. *Presented at the 16th meeting of the Society of Gynecologic Oncologists, Miami, Florida, February 1985*.

Peters W.A., Kumar N.B. & Morley G.W. (1985) Carcinoma of the vagina. Factors influencing treatment outcome. *Cancer*, **55**, 892—97.

Plentl A.A. & Friedman E.A. (1971) *Lymphatic System of the Female Genitalia*. W.B. Saunders Co., Philadelphia. p. 55.

Pomante R.G. (1975) Malignant melanoma — primary in the vagina. *Gynecol. Oncol.*, **3**, 15—20.

Powell J.L., Franklin B.W., Nickerson J.F. & Burrell M.O. (1978) Verrucous carcinoma of the female genital tract. *Gynecol. Oncol.*, **6**, 565—73.

Prempree T., Tang C., Halef A. & Forster S. (1983) Angiosarcoma of the vagina: a clinicopathological report. *Cancer*, **51**, 618—22.

Prempree T., Viravanthana T., Slawson R.G., Wizenberg M.J. & Cuccia C.A. (1977) Radiation management of primary carcinoma of the vagina. *Cancer*, **40**, 109—18.

Pride G.L., Schultz A.E., Chuprevich T.W. & Buchler D.A. (1979) Primary invasive squamous carcinoma of the vagina. *Obstet. Gynecol.*, **53** (2), 218—25.

Ramzy I., Smout M.S. & Collins J.A. (1976) Verrucous carcinoma of the vagina. *Am. J. Clin. Pathol.*, **65**, 644—53.

Robboy S.J., Noller K.L., O'Brien P., *et al.* (1984) Increased incidence of cervical and vaginal dysplasia in 3980 diethylstilbestrol-exposed young women. *JAMA*, **252**, 2979—83.

Robboy S.J., Young R.H., Welch W.R., Truslow G.Y., Prat J., Herbst A.L. & Scully R.E. (1983) Atypical vaginal adenosis and cervical ectropion. *Cancer*, **54**, 869—75.

Rosen Y. & Dolan T.E. (1975) Carcinoma of the cervix with cylindromatous features believed to arise in mesonephric duct. *Cancer*, **36**, 1739.

Rutledge F. (1967) Cancer of the vagina. *Am. J. Obstet. Gynecol.*, **97**, 635.

Taussig F.J. (1935) Primary cancer of the vulva, vagina and female urethra: five-year results. *Surg. Gynecol. Obstet.*, **60**, 477.

Underwood P.B. & Smith R.T. (1971) Carcinoma of the vagina. *JAMA*, **217** (1), 46—52.

Weed J.C., Lozier C. & Daniel S.J. (1983) Human papilloma virus in multifocal, invasive female genital tract malignancy. *Obstet. Gynecol.*, **62**, 83s—87s.

Wharton J.T., Fletcher G.H. & Delclos L. (1981) Invasive tumors of vagina: clinical features and management. *Gynecol. Oncol.*, **27**, 345—49. Churchill Livingstone, Edinburgh.

9

Pathology of Ovarian Cancer

HAROLD FOX

The term 'ovarian cancer' is used here to include not only the malignant epithelial tumours of the ovary but also the various malignant germ cell and sex cord stromal neoplasms.

Epithelial neoplasms

The epithelial tumours of the ovary are so called because they are usually, though not invariably, derived from the surface epithelium (i.e. the serosal covering) of the ovary. Within this broad grouping a number of specific histological types can be defined, these being:

1 serous tumours
2 mucinous tumours
3 endometrioid tumours
4 Brenner tumours
5 clear cell tumours.

Each of these neoplasms can exist in a benign form, may show a histological pattern classed as being of borderline malignancy or can be frankly malignant. The malignant forms are collectively classed as 'ovarian adenocarcinoma'.

It is, of course, recognized that not all epithelial neoplasms fit neatly into this classification. Some malignant tumours are so poorly differentiated that no diagnosis more specific than 'undifferentiated adenocarcinoma' can be made, while others, though better differentiated, do not show features which allow them to be identified in specific terms, these being categorized as 'adenocarcinomata of unclassified type'. Furthermore, a significant proportion of epithelial neoplasms contain more than one type of epithelium, it being not uncommon, for instance, to encounter a mixture of serous and mucinous epithelium within a single neoplasm. Such tumours are classified in terms of the predominant type of epithelium present and are only diagnosed as 'mixed' if the second epithelial component is a prominent feature of the neoplasm.

Histogenesis of epithelial tumours

There is considerable evidence that most epithelial tumours of the ovary arise from the surface epithelium of the organ (Langley & Fox 1987). The ovarian serosal covering is derived from, and is the adult equivalent of, the coelomic epithelium which, during embryogenesis, overlies the nephrogenital ridge. This gives rise, by a process of invagination, to the Müllerian ducts from which the tubal epithelium, endometrium and endocervical epithelium are derived. It is a basic histogenetic concept in ovarian neoplasia that tumours are derived from indifferent cells in adult tissues which have the same potentiality for differentiation as do the embryonic cells from which the adult tissue was derived. Hence it is thought that indifferent cells in the ovarian surface epithelium can undergo a neoplastic change while retaining their embryonic potentiality to differentiate along various Müllerian pathways. Thus differentiation of neoplastic epithelial cells along a tubal pathway produces the serous group of tumours, differentiation along an endocervical route results in mucinous neoplasms and differentiation along endometrial lines yields the endometrioid tumours. In all these three groups of neoplasms the mimicry by their epithelia of normal or neoplastic tubal, endocervical and endometrial epithelium has been fully confirmed at both light and electron microscopic levels (Fenoglio 1980) while the ability of the surface epithelium to undergo various forms of Müllerian metaplasia, either in its normal surface site or when included in a germinal inclusion cyst, is well documented (Blaustein 1981). It is, in fact, thought that many of these neoplasms originate from invaginations of the surface epithelium into the underlying stroma (a process resembling the embryonic derivation of the Müllerian ducts), the neck of the invagination subsequently being pinched off so that an inclusion cyst is formed from which the neoplasm arises.

The origin of the Brenner tumour from the surface epithelium is less obvious in so far as it appears to consist of epithelial islands set in a fibrous stroma. Reconstruction studies have, however, shown that the apparent islands are in reality branches of a richly arborizing tree-like structure cut in cross section and continuity of these branches with the surface epithelium can often be traced (Arey 1961). The nature of the epithelial component of the Brenner tumour has long been a matter of dispute but electron microscopic studies have clearly shown it to be identical with uroepithelium (Fox & Langley 1976). It is thought, therefore, that these neoplasms arise from the surface epithelium by a process of Wolffian, rather than Müllerian, differentiation. A residual capacity of the cells in the serosa to differentiate along a Wolffian pathway is not surprising in view of the close embryological relationship between the coelomic epithelium of the developing gonad and that of the nephric ridge.

The clear cell tumours are not, as was previously thought, of mesonephric (i.e. Woffian) nature. Neoplasms of similar type occur in the endometrium and vagina and electron microscopic studies have indicated that the vast majority are of Müllerian origin (Scully 1979). Further evidence of their Müllerian nature is derived from the observation that they commonly are associated with ovarian endometriosis, some clearly arising in endometriotic foci. This latter observation should not detract, however, from the fact that most clear cell tumours arise from the surface epithelium and thus fall clearly into the epithelial category.

This unitary concept of the epithelial tumours having a common origin but showing differing patterns of differentiation is almost certainly true but is too · all-embracing, for some neoplasms within this broad group are of different histogenesis. Thus, not all mucinous tumours are formed of endocervical-type epithelium for in a significant proportion the epithelium is of gastrointestinal type, often containing not only goblet cells but also argentaffin, argyrophil or Paneth cells. These enteric-type mucinous neoplasms could be derived from the surface epithelium by a process of gastrointestinal metaplasia (Fenoglio 1980) but it is likely that some are monophyletic teratomata, a view supported by the observation that mucinous tumours associated with mature cytic teratomata (a common combination) are invariably of enteric type (Fox & Langley 1976).

Furthermore, not all endometrioid tumours have their origin in the surface epithelium for some develop in, and from, a focus of pre-existing ovarian endo-metriosis. It is difficult to assess the proportion of endometrioid tumours which arise in this manner for a neoplasm may, as it develops, effectively obliterate any residual evidence of a preceding endometriotic lesion, but it would be a reason-able estimate that between 10 and 15% of endometrioid adenocarcinomata orig-inate in this fashion (Scully 1979).

It is also clear that some Brenner tumours, those which are localized to the hilar region, are not derived from the surface epithelium. These could have their origin from hilar mesothelium but it is more probable that they originate from structures of Wolffian origin in this site, such as the epoophoron or remnants of the epigenital tubules.

Aetiology

Epidemiological studies indicate that the risk of ovarian adenocarcinoma decreases with increasing parity and with prolonged use of oral contraceptives. These findings have led to the view that 'incessant' ovulation is a risk factor for ovarian adenocarcinoma and that any factor which decreases the number of ovulations during a woman's reproductive life will lessen .the risk of ovarian neoplasia. Whether 'incessant' ovulation plays its role by producing an increased number of inclusion cysts, by causing repetitive trauma to the surface epithelium or by causing the surface epithelium to be repeatedly bathed in oestrogen-rich follicular fluid is a moot point. It should be pointed out, however, that the various conditions which inhibit ovulation do not show uniform protective effects per ovulation prevented and that the evidence is conflicting as to whether some such conditions, such as late menarche, early menopause and lactation, are protective or not.

Another possible aetiological factor in ovarian adenocarcinoma is a carcinogen ascending to the ovary from the exterior by way of the reproductive passages, a factor indicated by the protective effect of hysterectomy. In this respect, talc has come under particular suspicion, partly because talc crystals have been found in ovarian adenocarcinomata (Henderson *et al.* 1979) and partly because case-control studies have shown that patients with ovarian cancer have more commonly used talc as a perineal dusting powder or on sanitary napkins than have controls (Cramer *et al.* 1982). It should be noted, however, that these studies have not shown an excess of women who had used talc on contraceptive diaphragms in the ovarian carcinoma cases and that talc has not been shown to have any carcinogenic properties (Hamilton *et al.* 1984).

That genetic factors may also be involved in ovarian carcinoma is suggested by the full documentation of over 40 families in which there has been, in several generations, a remarkably high incidence of ovarian cancer (Fox 1983a). Whether these ovarian cancer families represent an isolated phenomenon which is unrelated to apparently sporadic cases of ovarian carcinoma or whether they represent an extreme example of a more widespread familial tendency towards this disease is not yet clear.

Pathology of malignant epithelial tumours

Adenocarcinoma

Incidence

Among primary malignant epithelial tumours of the ovary, serous adenocarcinomata are the commonest form, accounting for between 40 and 50% of all cases. Endometrioid adenocarcinomata are the next commonest, though the cited proportion of adenocarcinomata which fall into this category has ranged rather widely from 16–31% (Fox & Langley 1976), this variability reflecting the application of differing criteria for the histological recognition of this type of carcinoma. Between 5 and 15% of ovarian adenocarcinomata are of the mucinous variety while 5–10% are of the clear cell type. Malignant Brenner tumours are considered as rare though their infrequency has been exaggerated.

The diagnosis of undifferentiated adenocarcinoma involves a highly subjective decision and hence the incidence of such tumours varies considerably in different series: it would, however, be a reasonable estimate that between 5 and 15% of ovarian adenocarcinomata fall into this category (Scully 1979).

Morphological features

GROSS APPEARANCES

Little point is served in attempting to describe the gross appearances of each individual type of ovarian adenocarcinoma for specific features are generally absent. The tumours are usually bulky, typically measuring between 15 and 30 cm in diameter, and may have a smooth or bosselated outer surface which can be studded with papillae. On section the neoplasm may be cystic, partially cystic or solid throughout. Cystic areas may be unilocular or, more commonly, multi-loculated and can contain either serous or mucinous fluid which may be turbid, bloodstained or frankly haemorrhagic. Fleshy or firm mural nodules may protrude into cystic tumours while, particularly but not specifically in serous adenocarcinomata, the cyst cavities may be partly or wholly filled with soft friable papillae. Solid areas may be crumbly, soft, fleshy, firm or rubbery and are commonly white, whitish-yellow or grey. Foci of haemorrhage and necrosis, often extensive, are a characteristic feature.

Histological appearances

Serous adenocarcinoma

Well differentiated serous carcinomata (Fig. 9.1) have a predominantly papillary pattern. The papillae tend to be fine, often branching and not infrequently fused at their tips. They have a delicate connective tissue support and a covering, but invading, epithelium in which the constituent cells bear an anarchic resemblance to those normally found in the tubal epithelium. A purely papillary pattern is, however, relatively uncommon and there are often a few areas showing an irregular acinar pattern, the acini tending to have slit-like lumens. Poorly dif-ferentiated serous adenocarcinomata have a predominantly solid histological pattern with sheets of small, relatively uniform cells, sometimes showing a syncytial-like appearance, admixed with poorly formed glandular acini or abortive papillae. Tumours of moderate differentiation occupy an intermediate position, often containing a melange of papillary, acinar and solid areas. Psammoma bodies, which are small laminated calcospherites, are a characteristic, but not specific, feature of serous adenocarcinomata and are seen most commonly, and most conspicuously, in well differentiated serous tumours.

Mucinous adenocarcinoma

Well differentiated mucinous carcinomata tend to show a locular and acinar pattern (Fig. 9.2), the lining epithelium being recognizably formed of columnar mucus-secreting cells which show varying degrees of multilayering, mitotic activity, and atypia. Stromal invasion is evident but it is not uncommon for well differentiated tumours, if extensively sampled, to also contain areas of benign mucinous cystadenoma or areas showing the appearances of a tumour of borderline malignancy. In less well differentiated neoplasms the loculi and acini are very irregular and partially filled by a piling-up of the markedly atypical epithelium. Poorly differentiated mucinous adenocarcinomata are formed of largely solid sheets of anaplastic cells which are interspersed with poorly formed glandular acini.

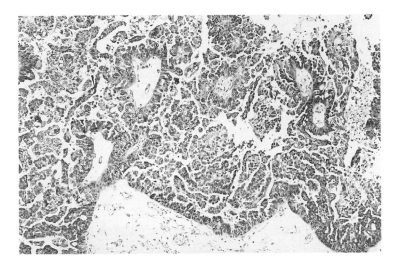

Fig. 9.1. Well differentiated serous adenocarcinoma.

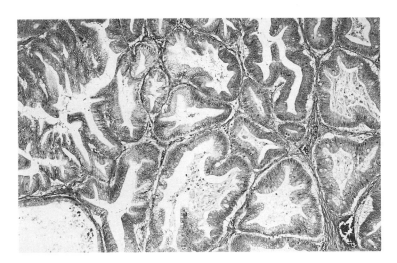

Fig. 9.2. Well differentiated mucinous adenocarcinoma.

Endometrioid adenocarcinoma

Neoplasms of this type have a histological appearance which is very similar to, indeed almost identical with, that of an endometrioid adenocarcinoma of the endometrium (Fig. 9.3). There is usually a well formed acinar pattern with the cells lining the acini often showing multilayering; the cells resemble those of the glandular epithelium of a proliferative phase endometrium but show a greater degree of pleomorphism and atypia. The stroma of the tumour resembles that of the ovary rather than that of the endometrium and stromal invasion is usually

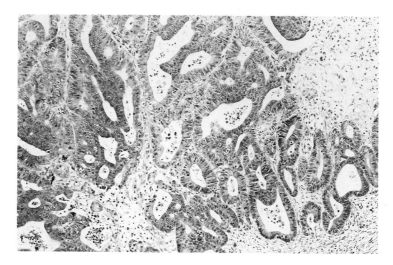

Fig. 9.3. Well differentiated endometrioid adenocarcinoma.

readily apparent. In a proportion of endometrioid adenocarcinomata a papillary pattern is evident in some areas and may even predominate: the papillae are, however, blunter than those seen in a serous adenocarcinomata and have a more abundant fibrous core. Squamous metaplasia is a common occurrence while a clear cell pattern is often focally present.

The term 'endometrioid tumour' of the ovary encompasses all the various neoplasms which may also occur in the endometrium and includes such entities as malignant Müllerian tumours of high or low grade malignancy, adenosquamous carcinoma and endometrial stromal sarcoma.

Malignant Brenner tumour

This is generally regarded as a rare neoplasm but it is probable that its infrequency has been over-emphasized by an insistence upon unnecessarily rigid and restrictive diagnostic criteria. In essence, a malignant Brenner tumour is a transitional cell carcinoma which resembles neoplasms of similar type occurring in the bladder (Fig. 9.4). The tumour may grow in a solid fashion but papillary areas can also be present; areas of squamous differentiation are common, and may predominate, while foci of adenocarcinomatous differentiation are infrequent. It is usually insisted upon that a malignant Brenner tumour cannot be diagnosed unless a transition from a benign Brenner tumour can be traced, but this implies that malignant Brenner tumours invariably originate from a previously present benign neoplasm, a view not held for any other form of ovarian adenocarcinoma. Possibly it is best to refer to malignant tumours associated with benign Brenner elements *as* a malignant Brenner tumour, and to consider those neoplasms in

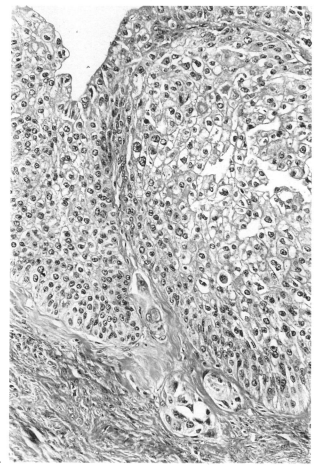

Fig. 9.4. Malignant Brenner tumour.

which a benign Brenner component cannot be identified simply as transitional
cell carcinomata (Austin & Norris 1987).

Clear cell adenocarcinoma

These tumours tend to have a complex histological pattern and contain an
admixture of tubules, glandular acini, papillae and cysts together with sheets of
cells: differing patterns may predominate in any given neoplasm. The papillae,
which may be simple or complex and sometimes have a 'glomeruloid' appearance, together with the glands and tubules have an epithelial component which is
formed either of 'hob-nail' cells or clear cells (Fig. 9.5): the former are characterized
by large prominent nuclei which occupy the bulbous tips of the cells and protrude
into the lumen whilst the latter are cuboidal or columnar cells with clear, glycogen-
rich, cytoplasm. Cystic spaces within these neoplasms may be lined by a flattened
or indifferent type of epithelium whilst some glandular acini have an endometrioid

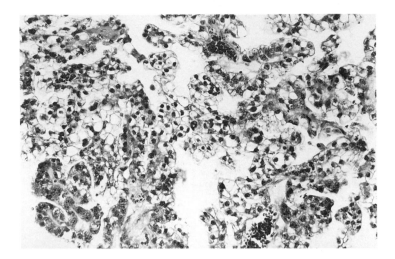

Fig. 9.5.   Clear cell adenocarcinoma.

type epithelium. Clear cells growing in solid sheets are a common, but not a constant, feature.

Spread

Bilateral involvement of the ovaries by adenocarcinoma is common and it is often far from clear whether this is due to metastatic spread or to multicentric origin. It appears highly probable, however, that spread to the contralateral ovary contributes substantially to the incidence of bilaterality, for the overall incidence of bilateral involvement increases progressively with advancing clinical stage. Possible routes of spread to the opposite ovary include transperitoneal seeding, cellular migration through the tubes and endometrial cavity and lymphatic spread via anastomoses between ovarian and uterine lymphatic vessels. The uterus is frequently involved by tumour, either because of direct extension or because of retrograde lymphatic spread, while extension to the endometrium may be either via the lymphatics or by luminal migration of tumour cells through the tube.

Transperitoneal spread is very common and is not limited to those neoplasms with external tumour excrescences, occurring with almost equal frequency in tumours with an apparently intact capsule. Direct seeding leads to implants on the pelvic peritoneum, in the pouch of Douglas and in the omentum. Deposits in the pouch of Douglas may grow through to the vagina but those in the pelvic peritoneum tend to spread over the surface, this leading to widespread adhesions. Transperitoneal spread also occurs with some frequency into the paracolic gutters (Meleka & Rafla 1975) and only within the last few years has it been recognized that involvement of the undersurface of the right leaf of the diaphragm is a common and early consequence of transperitoneal spread (Fuks 1980).

The frequency of early lymphatic spread of ovarian adenocarcinoma has also been underestimated in the past. Dissemination occurs principally to the para-aortic, iliac, obturator and hypogastric nodes and although it has been known for a long time that the para-aortic nodes contain metastatic deposits in approximately 70% of patients with advanced disease it has only relatively recently become clear that similar metastases are present in 15–20% of cases in which the tumour is still apparently at an early stage (Knapp & Friedman 1974; Fuks 1980). Mediastinal, supraclavicular and axillary nodes are sometimes involved while eventual spread via the bloodstream is mainly to the lungs and liver.

Prognosis and prognostic indices

The overall 5-year survival rate for women with ovarian adenocarcinoma is currently about 25–30%. There is little doubt that the single most important prognostic factor is the clinical, or preferably the surgicopathological, stage at the time of initial diagnosis. Nevertheless, for the individual patient staging does not give any absolute indication of prognosis, some women with stage I or II disease dying quite quickly and others with stage III or IV tumours surviving for surprisingly prolonged periods. It is therefore in the assessment of individual tumours within a given stage that histological prognostic indices are of greatest value.

Histological typing has been thought by many to be a significant prognostic factor, it being claimed that serous adenocarcinomata are associated with a particularly poor prognosis and endometrioid neoplasms with a relatively good outlook, the prognosis for mucinous and clear cell carcinomata lying somewhere between these two extremes (Kottmeier 1968; Kolstad 1986). Claims of this type ignore, however, both the tendency of many pathologists to diagnose endometrioid adenocarcinomata only if they are well differentiated and to relegate all poorly differentiated tumours into the serous category and the quite considerable interobserver variation in tumour typing (Cramer et al. 1987); furthermore, evidence for the prognostic value of histological typing has been based upon univariate analysis of the data and multivariate analysis has shown that, stage for stage and grade for grade, the histological type of an ovarian adenocarcinoma is of no prognostic significance (Sorbe et al. 1982; Malkasian et al. 1984).

The prognostic value of histological grading of ovarian carcinomata has been widely accepted (Decker 1983) but it is, in fact, far from clear how these neoplasms should be graded. The Broders' system, in which the percentage of undifferentiated cells is assessed, has been found to be prognostically useful by some (Ozols et al. 1980) but is highly subjective and is, in practice, difficult to apply in a consistent fashion. Most commonly therefore, ovarian carcinomata are graded in architectural terms as 'well', 'moderately' or 'poorly' differentiated. This system works to the extent that pathologists can easily recognize very well and very poorly differentiated tumours but the borderlines between 'well' and 'moderately' differ-

entiated tumours and between 'moderately' and 'poorly' differentiated neoplasms
have never been defined: it is therefore not surprising that there tends to be very
considerable interpathologist disagreement in ovarian tumour grading and that
individual pathologists apply a grading system in an inconsistent manner (Baak
et al. 1986a, 1987).

In recent years the introduction of the techniques of quantitative morphometry
and of DNA flow cytometry have allowed for a much more accurate, objective
and consistent approach to the problem of grading ovarian adenocarcinomata. A
number of studies have shown that the assessment of the DNA content of
ovarian tumour cell nuclei by flow cytometry is of considerable prognostic value,
aneuploid tumours being, in general, associated with a worse outlook than are
diploid neoplasms (Friedlander *et al.* 1984a; Blumenfeld *et al.* 1987; Rodenburg *et
al.* 1987). Morphometric techniques, in which morphological features are measured
with an interactive computer programme, also yield information which is of very
precise prognostic value: measurements of such parameters as the mitotic
activity index and the volume percentage of epithelium allow for the division of
ovarian adenocarcinomata, in any stage, into 'good' and 'bad' prognosis groups
(Baak *et al.* 1986a, b; Rodenburg *et al.* 1988).

Pathology of epithelial tumours of borderline malignancy

To many gynaecologists a histopathological diagnosis of ovarian epithelial tumour
of borderline malignancy is taken as being indicative of indecision on the part of
the pathologist as to whether a neoplasm is benign or malignant, an attitude
which has led to the view that 'there are no borderline tumours, only borderline
pathologists'. If this were indeed the case then the gynaecologist would have
legitimate grounds for complaint, for little point is served by elevating pathological
uncertainty into an oncological entity. Ovarian epithelial tumours of borderline
malignancy are, however, a well delineated and clearly defined group, the diagnosis of which is a positive one based upon specific histological findings (Ovarian
Tumour Panel 1983). It is true that the term 'borderline malignancy' hints at
irresolution and uncertainty, but it is marginally less objectionable than any of
the other suggested forms of nomenclature.

Definition

The World Health Organization definition of an ovarian tumour of borderline
malignancy (Serov *et al.* 1973) is 'a tumour which has some but not all of the
morphological features of malignancy: those present include, in varying combinations, stratification of epithelial cells, apparent detachment of cellular clusters
from their site of origin and mitotic figures and nuclear abnormalities intermediate
between those of clearly benign and unquestionably malignant tumours of a
similar cell type: on the other hand, obvious invasion of the stroma is lacking'.

This definition has all the characteristics, and drawbacks, of definition by a committee, evades precise answers to the difficult points raised by these neoplasms and does not sufficiently stress the prime diagnostic importance of the lack of stromal invasion. By contrast, the Ovarian Tumour Panel of the Royal College of Obstetricians and Gynaecologists (1983) has produced a clear cut and non-ambiguous definition of a borderline tumour as 'one in which the epithelial component shows some, or all, of the characteristics of malignancy but in which there is no stromal invasion'. This is a logical definition which recognizes that lack of stromal invasion is the cardinal feature of these tumours.

It is, of course, recognized that stromal invasion may be very difficult to assess: this is particularly the case with mucinous tumours and in this group of neoplasms it has been suggested that, in the absence of definite stromal invasion, a tumour should be regarded as malignant rather than as borderline if there is marked overgrowth of atypical epithelial cells (Hart & Norris 1973; Hart 1977; Colgan & Norris 1983). This view has not won wide acceptance outside the United States and as Russell (1984) has commented, 'these supplementary criteria seem to add an unnecessary complication to an already difficult area which is not justified by an increased precision of prognosis'.

Incidence

Tumours of borderline malignancy form a significant proportion of ovarian epithelial neoplasms, between 8 and 15% of serous tumours and nearly 20% of mucinous neoplasms falling into this category (Fox 1983b; Russell 1984). Endometrioid, Brenner and clear cell tumours of borderline malignancy are uncommon.

Pathological features

Serous tumours

These are nearly always papillary and most resemble a benign papillary serous cystadenoma: a suspicion that such neoplasms are not, however, fully benign may be indicated by an unusually luxuriant proliferation of fine papillae and by the presence of exophytic papillary excrescences on the outer surface of the cyst. A small proportion of serous borderline tumours are grossly similar to a benign serous papillary surface tumour but tend to have a rather more complex and dense papillary pattern.

Histologically, these neoplasms are formed of rather fine branching papillae (Fig. 9.6). In those with only minimal epithelial atypia the cellular mantle of the papillae can be clearly recognized as being of tubal type but in tumours with marked epithelial abnormalities this resemblance tends to be lost and the cells become predominantly rounded or cuboid. The epithelial component of the tumour shows a variable degree of multilayering and has a marked tendency to

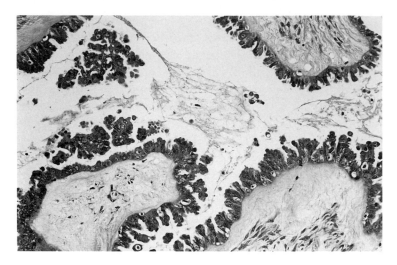

Fig. 9.6. Papillary serous tumour of borderline malignancy.

form cellular buds or tufts: these buds may break off to float freely within the cyst while fusion of the tips of adjacent epithelial buds may result in a honey-combed pattern. Nuclear crowding, atypia and hyperchromatism are of variable degree but the nucleoli are often inconspicuous: mitotic figures are uncommon and rarely atypical whilst psammoma bodies are frequently present. In most of these neoplasms there is a sharp interface between epithelium and stroma and the possibility of stromal invasion can be excluded with relative ease: in some, however, there may be epithelial invaginations into the stroma and these can cause a diagnostic difficulty which is usually resolved by serial sectioning. By and large all borderline serous tumours have a strikingly similar and characteristic appearance; furthermore, the borderline pattern tends to be consistent through-out the neoplasm, it being relatively unusual to encounter an intermingling with areas showing a benign appearance or with areas showing a focal evolution into a frank adenocarcinoma.

A notable feature of serous tumours is the high incidence, variously estimated as between 14 and 47% (Colgan & Norris 1983; Russell 1984), of bilaterality: the bilateral involvement is not always apparent to the naked eye and may only be recognized on histological examination. It is almost certain that the bilateral ovarian involvement represents the concurrent development of two primary tumours rather than the metastasis of a single primary neoplasm to the contralateral gonad.

A further, and often disconcerting, aspect of these neoplasms is the frequency, about 35%, of apparent extraovarian spread at the time of initial diagnosis, this taking the form of presumed tumour implants in the pelvic peritoneum and infracolic omentum (Aure *et al*. 1971; Katzenstein *et al*. 1978; Tasker & Langley 1985; Kliman *et al*. 1986). There has been much debate as to whether these extraovarian lesions are true metastatic implants or autochthonous lesions arising *in situ* within the subserosal mesenchymal tissues. Clinical observations would support the latter view for although some of these lesions progress, albeit usually in an indolent fashion, most will either remain stationary or regress after removal of the ovarian neoplasm (Russell 1984), a fact attested to by well documented reports of women being alive and well for many years, with no obvious evidence of tumour, despite having had peritoneal lesions for which no treatment had been given (Tasker & Langley 1985; Kliman *et al.* 1986). These clinical observations have been reinforced by histological studies which have shown that the apparent implants may show a benign, borderline or invasive pattern (McCaughey *et al.* 1984; Michael & Roth 1986; Bell *et al.* 1988). In most cases there is a simultaneous occurrence of two or three different types of lesions with various permutations of the possible combinations. The benign lesions correspond to the condition of endosalpingiosis and the admixture of benign, borderline and invasive lesions suggests that the peritoneal and omental 'implants' arise *in situ* and develop from foci of endosalpingiosis. It is unlikely, therefore, that the peritoneal and omental lesions found in women with ovarian serous tumours of borderline malignancy are, in the vast majority of cases, true metastatic implants. This is not to deny that such ovarian neoplasms can, albeit occasionally, give rise to true metastases for metastatic lesions have been described in retroperitoneal lymph nodes (Ehrmann *et al.* 1980) and in extraabdominal sites (Katzenstein *et al.* 1978; Barnhill *et al.* 1985; Kliman *et al.* 1986).

Mucinous tumours

These usually present as large multilocular cysts. The lining of the cyst is generally smooth but there may be focal areas of thickening, nodularity or endophytic papillary projections.

Borderline mucinous tumours differ significantly from their serous counterparts in that there is, commonly but by no means invariably, no uniformity of histological appearances throughout the neoplasm, some areas appearing fully benign and others showing a pattern of borderline malignancy while there may be a focal evolution into an invasive adenocarcinoma. In borderline mucinous tumours (Fig. 9.7) the epithelial component may show a complex glandular pattern but is often characterized by short papillary infoldings which give the epithelium a serrated appearance. A papillary pattern, similar to that seen in borderline serous tumours is sometimes encountered. There are varying degrees of multilayering, loss of nuclear polarity, nuclear hyperchromatism and cellular atypia whilst mitotic figures tend to be frequent but of normal type. The outpouching of the epithelium and the formation of secondary cysts or glands in many borderline mucinous neoplasms make the assessment of stromal invasion more difficult than is the case with serous tumours though this is not usually an impossible task.

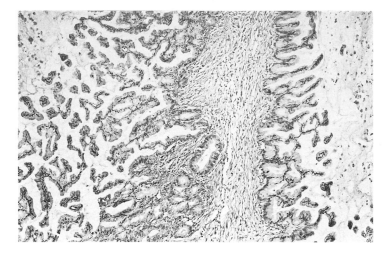

Fig. 9.7. Mucinous tumour of borderline malignancy.

In a majority of borderline mucinous tumours the epithelium is of gastro-intestinal type whilst in a smaller proportion there is an admixture of endocervical-like and intestinal type epithelium, possibly because of focal intestinal metaplasia within endocervical epithelium: in these latter neoplasms the endocervical type epithelium is often confined to benign appearing areas while the intestinal type epithelium is found in the more atypical areas. A small proportion of borderline mucinous tumours are formed solely of endocervical type epithelium and it is these that tend to have a papillary pattern very reminiscent of that seen in serous borderline tumours (Rutgers & Scully 1988).

Bilateral ovarian involvement is found in only about 5% of intestinal type borderline mucinous tumours but is more common (up to 40%) in the much rarer endocervical type neoplasms. Extraovarian spread is largely confined to the intestinal type tumours and takes the form of pseudomyxoma peritoneii, this complicating 10–15% of cases. It is not, in fact, known whether pseudomyxoma ovarii is due to true tumour implantation or to intestinal metaplasia within peritoneal tissues. Peritoneal 'implants', unassociated with pseudomyxoma ovarii peritonei, complicate a small proportion of endocervical type mucinous borderline tumours but it is highly probable that, as in the case of serous tumours, these arise *in situ* and represent a form of endocervicosis.

Endometrioid tumours

Borderline forms of this type of epithelial neoplasm are rare and present two quite different pathological pictures. One is seen in association with, and arising from, foci of endometriosis, the histological features resembling clearly those of atypical hyperplasia of the endometrium (Czernobilsky & Morris 1979). The other type is the endometrioid adenofibroma or cystadenofibroma of borderline malignancy (Fig. 9.8) in which endometrial type glands showing budding, stratification and nuclear atypia are set in, but are not invading, an abundant dense stroma (Roth *et al*. 1981; Bell & Scully 1985a).

Brenner tumours

The Brenner tumour of borderline malignancy, also known as a proliferating Brenner tumour, is usually unilateral, generally large and partly, or entirely, cystic (Roth & Sternberg 1971). Cystic areas are multilocular and, characteristically, papillary or polypoid protrusions of velvety, friable tissue extend into, and sometimes fill, the lumen. Histologically, the epithelium in the papillary areas is thrown into multilayered folds supported by delicate fibrovascular stalks (Fig. 9.9). In these areas, which may be 7−20 cell layers thick, there is an unmistakable mimicry of a grade I transitional cell carcinoma of the bladder: a variable degree of atypia and mitotic activity are seen but there is no stromal invasion.

Clear cell tumours

The borderline form of this type of neoplasm appears always to be an adeno-fibroma (Fig. 9.10) in which glandular spaces lined by hob-nail or clear cells showing varying degrees of atypia are set in an abundant stroma (Roth *et al*. 1984; Bell & Scully 1985b).

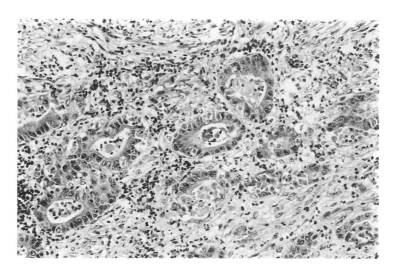

Fig. 9.8. Endometrioid adenofibroma of borderline malignancy.

A proportion of granulosa cell neoplasms are partially cystic and a few are wholly cystic, resembling a cystadenoma.

Histologically, the cells in a granulosa cell tumour are small, round or polygonal, have little cytoplasm and indistinct cell boundaries: their large, round or ovoid, pale nuclei characteristically show longitudinal grooving. The cells are arranged in a variety of patterns and although in any individual neoplasm a particular pattern may predominate there is usually an admixture of cellular arrangements. In the insular pattern the cells are arranged in compact masses or islands while in the trabecular pattern the cells form anastomosing ribbons or cords: alternatively the cells may be arranged in sheets to give a diffuse pattern. In the microfollicular pattern, granulosa cells are arranged around small spaces containing nuclear fragments, these being the Call–Exner bodies (Fig. 9.11), whilst a macrofollicular pattern is due to liquefaction within islands of granulosa cells. In cystic granulosa cell tumours the cyst lining resembles that of a Graafian follicle but usually contains microfollicles.

All granulosa cell tumours should be considered as potentially malignant though the degree of malignancy is often very low and the course pursued by the tumour is frequently extremely indolent. Recurrences or metastases tend to occur late, commonly after 5 years, not infrequently after 10 years and sometimes after 20 years. The histological pattern of the tumour is of no prognostic importance and it is indeed doubtful if there are any prognostic indicators apart from extraovarian spread. The long term survival rate for patients with this neoplasm is between 50 and 60% (Fox et al. 1975; Kolstad 1986).

Juvenile granulosa cell tumour

This is a histological variant of a granulosa cell tumour which occurs predominantly in patients aged less than 20 years though some neoplasms of this type arise in older women (Young et al. 1984). The tumours contain follicles and cysts lined by granulosa cells together with solid areas showing a haphazard admixture of granulosa and thecal cells which not uncommonly show a striking degree of luteinization (Fig. 9.12). The neoplastic cells lack the nuclear grooving character-istic of an adult type granulosa cell tumour and there is often a moderate degree of cytological atypia and mitotic activity.

About 5% of juvenile granulosa cell tumours behave in a malignant fashion: these tend to recur rapidly and disseminate widely throughout the abdominal cavity within two years of initial diagnosis, a pattern of malignant behaviour quite unlike that of an adult granulosa cell tumour.

Fibroma

Fibromata are benign but a few show increased cellularity, pleomorphism and mitotic activity; tumours showing these features to only a mild degree are classed

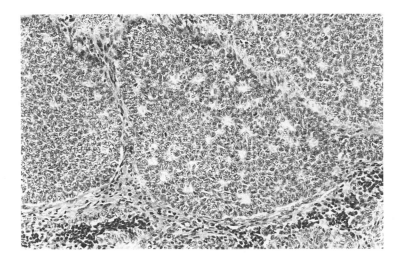

Fig. 9.11. Adult type granulosa cell tumour.

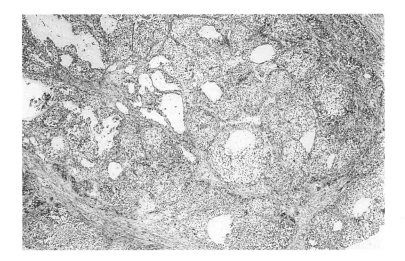

Fig. 9.12. Juvenile type granulosa cell tumour.

as cellular fibromata which will recur if incompletely removed, and those with more marked atypia and mitotic activity are categorized as fibrosarcomata, these being highly aggressive neoplasms with a poor prognosis (Prat & Scully 1981).

Androblastoma

Androblastomata are neoplasms composed of Sertoli cells, Leydig cells or a combination of the two cell types.

Pure Sertoli cell neoplasms are rare and occur as small, solid, yellowish masses. Histologically the tumours show highly differentiated tubules lined by a single layer of radially orientated Sertoli cells which commonly contain lipid droplets and are occasionally distended and vacuolated by fat. Sertoli cell neoplasms are usually benign though a Sertoli cell carcinoma has been described (Young & Scully 1984a).

Leydig cell neoplasms may arise either from stromal cells or from pre-existing hilar cells. The tumours are small, yellowish-brown and consist of Leydig cells arranged in sheets or solid cords. The cytoplasm of the Leydig cells is markedly eosinophilic whilst their nuclei are large and centrally placed. Reinke's crystals, slender rod-shaped bodies with rounded, tapering or square ends, are present in about 50% of these neoplasms but are irregularly distributed and often difficult to detect. Leydig cell tumours are nearly always benign but exceptional tumours of this type give rise to metastases, a possibility not predictable on any histological grounds.

Sertoli—Leydig cell tumours are generally solid tumours which show a wide range of histological differentiation. Well differentiated neoplasms are formed of tubules lined by Sertoli cells with variable numbers of Leydig cells between the tubules. In less well differentiated tumours the Sertoli cells are arranged in cords, solid tubules or trabeculae, these being set in a mesenchymal stroma containing clusters or nodules of Leydig cells (Fig. 9.13). Poorly differentiated Sertoli—Leydig neoplasms consist largely of sheets of spindle-shaped cells (Fig. 9.14) in which occasional irregular cord-like structures or imperfectly formed tubules may be recognized, Leydig cells also being present in small clusters.

Patterns simulating those of the rete testis are found in about 10% of Sertoli—Leydig cell tumours (Young & Scully 1983) while heterologous elements, such as intestinal epithelium, muscle or cartilage, are present in about 20% of these neoplasms (Young et al. 1982b; Prat et al. 1982).

Sertoli—Leydig cell neoplasms can occur at any age but the majority develop in women aged between 10 and 35 years. The well differentiated neoplasms always behave in a benign fashion (Young & Scully 1984b) but between 10 and 40% of the less well differentiated tumours behave in a malignant fashion, this being particularly the case for the poorly differentiated tumours (Young & Scully 1985). Recurrence or metastases, characteristically to the omentum, abdominal lymph nodes or liver, are usually apparent within one year of initial diagnosis.

Sex cord tumour with annular tubules

This uncommon, but histologically distinctive, tumour contains rounded nests in which epithelial like cells surround hyaline bodies (Fig. 9.15). The epithelial-like cells, which are thought to be immature sex cord cells, are palisaded along the periphery of the cell nests and around the hyaline bodies. About one-third of these tumours are associated with the Peutz—Jeghers syndrome and in such circumstances the lesions are usually bilateral, of microscopic size only, calcified

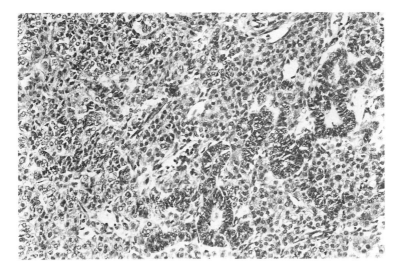

Fig. 9.13. Sertoli–Leydig cell tumour of intermediate differentiation.

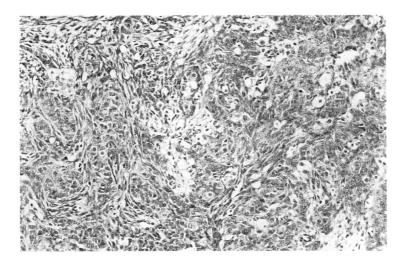

Fig. 9.14. Poorly differentiated Sertoli–Leydig cell tumour.

and benign. The tumours unassociated with the Peutz–Jeghers syndrome are unilateral, large, uncalcified, often show an overgrowth of either granulosa or Sertoli cells and behave in a malignant fashion in about 20% of cases (Young *et al*. 1982a).

Germ cell tumours

Tumours derived from germ cells may show no evidence of differentiation into either embryonic or extraembryonic tissues, can differentiate into embryonic

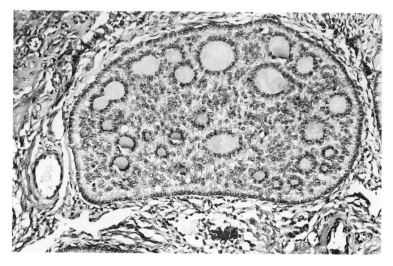

Fig. 9.15. Sex cord tumour with annular tubules.

tissues, or may differentiate along extraembryonic pathways into trophoblast or yolk sac structures.

Very little, indeed nothing, is known about the aetiology of germ cell neoplasms. Extensive studies of naturally occurring gonadal teratomata in highly inbred genetic strains of mice and of experimentally induced murine teratomata have, however, indicated that teratomata arise from parthogenetic pregnancies which undergo a short period of embryogenesis and then break up to yield a neoplasm (Fox 1987). Studies of human ovarian teratomata suggest strongly that these tumours arise in a similar manner.

Dysgerminoma

This neoplasm is formed of cells which closely resemble primordial germ cells showing no evidence of differentiation into either embryonic or extraembryonic structures: as such the tumour is identical to the seminoma of the testis (Fig. 9.16). Dysgerminomata commonly arise in patients aged between 10 and 30 years old and have a particular tendency to develop in patients with developmental abnormalities of the gonads: nevertheless the vast majority of dysgerminomata occur in otherwise fully normal individuals.

The tumours are solid, rubbery, usually measure about 15 cm in diameter and have a smooth or bosselated surface: they are bilateral in 10−20% of cases. Histologically the neoplastic cells are large, uniform, round, oval or polyhedral, with well defined limiting membranes, abundant cytoplasm and large vesicular nuclei. The cells are commonly arranged in solid nests separated by delicate fibrous septa but may form cords or strands embedded in a fibrous stroma. A lymphatic infiltration of the stroma, sometimes aggregated into follicles with

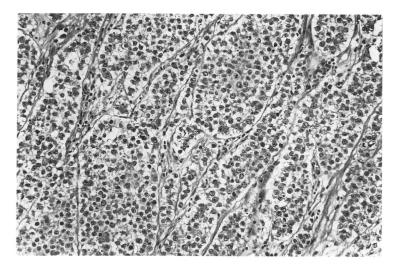

Fig. 9.16.   Dysgerminoma.

germinal centres, and small stromal granulomata are characteristic features. A small proportion of dysgerminomata contain multinucleated syncytiotrophoblastic cells.

Dysgerminomata are malignant: rupture of their enveloping 'capsule' often leads to direct implantation of tumour onto the pelvic peritoneum and omentum while lymphatic spread occurs relatively early to the para-aortic, retroperitoneal, mediastinal and supraclavicular nodes. Haematogenous spread to liver, lungs, kidney and bone occurs at a late stage. These tumours are, however, highly radiosensitive and the overall 5-year survival rate is about 90% (Nogales 1987).

Choriocarcinoma

These are germ cell tumours showing trophoblastic differentiation: they are often combined with other malignant germ cell elements but pure ovarian choriocarcinomata are occasionally encountered (Gerbie *et al*. 1975). In women of reproductive age it is usually impossible to tell whether such a neoplasm is a germ cell tumour, a metastasis from a uterine choriocarcinoma or a tumour arising from the placental tissue of an ectopic ovarian pregnancy. In premenarchal and postmenopausal patients this problem does not arise and here an origin from ovarian germ cells can be readily accepted. The tumours form large haemorrhagic masses and their histological appearances are identical to those of gestational uterine choriocarcinomata with both cytotrophoblast and syncytiotrophoblast being present. Ovarian choriocarcinomata respond poorly to the chemotherapeutic regime which is so successful for uterine gestational choriocarcinomata and they are associated with a poor prognosis (Jacobs *et al*. 1982).

Yolk sac tumours

These rare neoplasms, also known as endodermal sinus tumours, represent neo-plastic germ cell differentiation along extraembryonic lines into mesoblast and yolk sac endoderm: they share with yolk sac structures the ability to secrete alphafetoprotein (AFP).

Yolk sac tumours form large masses showing conspicuous haemorrhage, necrosis and microcystic change. Their histological appearances are very complex but there is characteristically a loose vacuolated labyrinthine network containing microcysts lined by flattened cells together with Schiller–Duval bodies, these having a mesenchymal core containing a central capillary and an epithelial investment of cuboidal or columnar cells (Fig. 9.17). A glandular pattern is often seen whilst there may be hepatoid or endodermal differentiation. Eosinophilic hyaline droplets are present in nearly all yolk sac tumours and these consist predominantly of AFP. A polyvesicular-vitelline pattern is seen in many yolk sac tumours and sometimes predominates: this is characterized by the presence of cysts lined by cuboidal or flattened cells. The cysts are separated by a spindle cell stroma and often show an eccentric constriction, simulating the conversion of the primary yolk sac to the secondary yolk sac (Nogales *et al.* 1978).

Yolk sac tumours occur predominantly in girls aged between 4 and 20 years, and are highly aggressive neoplasms which spread rapidly within the abdomen and to distant sites. Their previously apalling outlook has been much improved by the introduction of effective chemotherapy.

Teratomata

These are germ cell neoplasms showing differentiation along embryonic lines. In

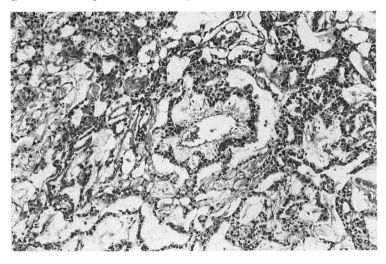

Fig. 9.17. Yolk sac tumour.

most there is a melange of tissues but in some, known as monophyletic teratomata, there is differentiation along only a single tissue pathway, e.g. solely into thyroid tissue. The terms 'benign' and 'malignant' are not truly applicable to teratomata for the prognosis of any individual neoplasm is determined not by the usual criteria of malignancy but by the degree of maturity of its constituent tissues, those in which all the components are fully mature behaving in a benign fashion and increasing degrees of tissue immaturity being associated with a progressive tendency for the neoplasm running a malignant course. Hence teratomata are classed as either 'immature' or 'mature', the term 'malignant' being reserved for those cases in which true malignant change has occurred in a mature teratoma, as, for instance, applies when a squamous cell carcinoma develops in a mature cystic teratoma.

The vast majority of ovarian teratomata are mature and cystic. A small proportion of mature teratomata are solid rather than cystic but most solid teratomata are of the immature variety (Norris et al. 1976). These latter are large, usually about 18 cm in diameter, with smooth glistening outer surfaces and occur principally during the first two decades of life. Microscopic examination of such neoplasms reveals an admixture of both mature and immature tissues although immature mesenchyme or neuroepithelium (Fig. 9.18) tend to be dominant features. Immature teratomata are graded in terms of their content of immature tissue (Thurlbeck & Scully 1960). In grade I tumours immature neural tissue is present in less than one low power field per slide while in grade II neoplasms immature neural tissue is present in 2—3 low power fields in each slide: grade III teratomata are characterized by the presence of immature neural tissue in four or more low power fields per slide. Immature teratomata behave in a malignant fashion, implanting onto pelvic peritoneum, metastasizing to retroperitoneal and

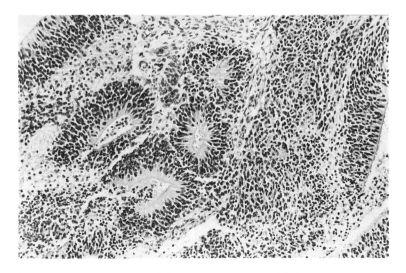

Fig. 9.18.   An immature teratoma containing immature neuroepithelium.

para-aortic lymph nodes and being disseminated via the bloodstream to the lungs and liver: the previously extremely poor prognosis of these neoplasms has been transformed by chemotherapy with approximately 80% of patients now surviving.

Monophyletic teratomata, in which differentiation is into only one tissue, are typified by the struma ovarii which consists predominantly or solely of tissue that is histologically, physiologically and pharmacologically identical to normal cervical thyroid. This ovarian thyroid tissue sometimes undergoes malignant change with a resulting thyroid adenocarcinoma which metastasizes to lymph nodes, liver and lungs (Hasleton *et al.* 1978).

Many carcinoid tumours of the ovary occur in a mature cystic teratoma, in association with gastrointestinal or respiratory type epithelium, but a few are pure and not admixed with any other tissues, these being regarded as monophyletic teratomata. Ovarian carcinoid tumours are similar to those which occur in the gastrointestinal tract, usually showing either an insular or a trabecular pattern, but are associated with a high incidence of a typical carcinoid syndrome (Robboy *et al.* 1975), this reflecting the ability of these tumours to secrete products directly into the systemic, rather than the portal, circulation. About 5% of ovarian carcinoid tumours metastasize (Talerman 1984).

A strumal carcinoid is a rare neoplasm which combines the features of a struma ovarii and a carcinoid tumour (Robboy & Scully 1980): it is thought that the carcinoid component of these neoplasms is derived from the parafollicular cells and that it is thus homologous with the medullary carcinoma of the thyroid gland.

References

Arey L.B. (1961) The origin and form of the Brenner tumor. *Am. J. Obstet. Gynecol.*, **81**, 743–51.

Aure J.C., Hoeg K. & Kolstad P. (1971) Clinical and histologic studies of ovarian carcinoma: long term follow up of 990 cases. *Obstet. Gynecol.*, **37**, 1–9.

Austin R.M. & Norris H.J. (1987) Malignant Brenner tumor and transitional cell carcinoma of the ovary: a comparison. *Int. J. Gynecol. Pathol.*, **6**, 29–39.

Baak J.P.A., Fox H., Langley F.A. & Buckley C.H. (1985) The prognostic value of morphometry in ovarian epithelial tumors of borderline malignancy. *Int. J. Gynecol. Pathol.*, **4**, 186–91.

Baak J.P.A., Langley F.A., Talerman A. & Delemarre J.F.M. (1986a) Interpathologist and intrapathologist disagreement in ovarian tumor grading and typing. *Anal. Quant. Cytol. Histol.*, **8**, 354–57.

Baak J.P.A., Langley F.A., Talerman A. & Delemarre J.F.M. (1987) The prognostic variability of ovarian tumor grading by different pathologists. *Gynecol. Oncol.*, **27**, 166–72.

Baak J.P.A., Wisse-Brekelmans E.C.M., Langley F.A., Talerman A. & Delemarre J.F.M. (1986b) Morphometric data to FIGO stage and histologic type and grade for prognosis of ovarian tumours. *J. Clin. Pathol.*, **39**, 1340–46.

Barnhill D., Heller P., Brzozowski P., Advani H., Gallup D. & Park R. (1985) Epithelial ovarian carcinoma of low malignant potential. *Obstet. Gynecol.*, **65**, 53–58.

Bell D.A. & Scully R.E. (1985a) Atypical and borderline endometrioid adenofibromas of the ovary: a report of 27 cases. *Am. J. Surg. Pathol.*, **9**, 205–14.

Bell D.A. & Scully R.E. (1985b) Benign and borderline clear cell adenofibromas of the ovary. *Cancer*, **56**, 2922–31.

Bell D.A., Weinstock M.A. & Scully R.E. (1988) Peritoneal implants of ovarian serous borderline tumors: histologic features and prognosis. *Cancer*, **62**, 2212–22.

Blaustein A. (1981) Surface (germinal) epithelium and related ovarian neoplasms. *Pathol. Ann.*, **16**, 247–94.

Blumenfeld D., Brazy P., Ben-Ezra J. & Klevecz R.R. (1987) Tumor DNA content as a prognostic feature in advanced epithelial ovarian carcinoma. *Gynecol. Oncol.*, **27**, 389–98.

Colgan T.J.B. & Norris H.J. (1983) Ovarian epithelial tumors of low malignant potential: a review. *Int. J. Gynecol. Pathol.*, **1**, 367–82.

Cramer D.W., Welch W.R., Scully R.E. & Wojchechowski C.A. (1982) Ovarian cancer and talc: a case control study. *Cancer*, **50**, 372–76.

Cramer S.F., Roth L.M., Ulbright T.M., Mazur M.T., Numez C.A., Gersell D.J., Mills S.E. & Kraus F.T. (1987) Evaluation of the reproducibility of the World Health Organization classification of common ovarian cancers. *Arch. Pathol. Lab. Med.*, **111**, 819–29.

Czernobilsky B. & Morris W.J. (1979). A histologic study of ovarian endometriosis with emphasis on hyperplastic and atypical changes. *Obstet. Gynecol.*, **53**, 318–23.

Decker D.G. (1983) Epithelial ovarian cancer. *In*: Bender H.G. & Beck L. (eds), *Carcinoma of the Ovary*. Gustav Fischer Verlag, Stuttgart, New York. pp. 137–41.

Ehrmann R.L., Federschweider J.M. & Knapp R.C. (1980) Distinguishing lymph node metastases from benign glandular inclusions in low grade ovarian carcinoma. *Am. J. Obstet. Gynecol.*, **136**, 737–46.

Fenoglio C.M. (1980) Overview article: ultrastructural features of the common epithelial tumours of the ovary. *Ultrastruct. Pathol.*, **1**, 419–44.

Fox H. (1983a) Epidemiological aspects for diagnosis and improved therapy results. *In*: Bender H.G. & Beck L. (eds), *Carcinoma of the Ovary*. Gustav Fischer Verlag, Stuttgart, New York. pp. 17–21.

Fox H. (1983b) Ovarian tumors of borderline malignancy. *In*: Morrow C.P., Bonnar J., O'Brien T.J. & Gibbons W.E. (eds), *Recent Clinical Developments in Gynecologic Oncology*. Raven Press, New York. pp. 137–50.

Fox H. (1987) Biology of teratomas. *In*: Anthony P.P. & MacSween R.P.M. (eds), *Recent Advances in Histopathology 13*. Churchill Livingstone, Edinburgh, Melbourne, New York. pp. 33–43.

Fox H. (1989) The concept of borderline malignancy in ovarian tumours: a reappraisal. *Curr. Topics Pathol.*, **78**, 111–134.

Fox H., Agrawal K. & Langley F.A. (1975) A clinicopathologic study of 92 cases of granulosa cell tumor of the ovary with special reference to the factors influencing prognosis. *Cancer*, **35**, 230–41.

Fox H. & Langley F.A. (1976) *Tumours of the Ovary*. Heinemann, London.

Friedlander M.L., Hedley D.W., Taylor I.W., Russell P., Coates A.S. & Tattersall M. (1984a) Influence of cellular DNA content on survival in advanced ovarian cancer. *Cancer Res.*, **44**, 397–400.

Friedlander M.L., Russell P., Taylor D.W. & Tattersall M.M. (1984b) Flow cytometric analysis of cellular DNA content as an adjunct to the diagnosis of ovarian tumours of borderline malignancy. *Pathology*, **16**, 301–6.

Fuks Z. (1980) Patterns of spread of ovarian carcinoma: relation to therapeutic strategies. *In*: Newman C.E., Ford C.H.J. & Jordan J.E. (eds), *Ovarian Cancer*. Pergamon, Oxford. pp. 39–51.

Gerbie M.V., Brewer J.I. & Tamimi H. (1975) Primary choriocarcinoma of the ovary. *Obstet. Gynecol.*, **46**, 720–23.

Hamilton T.C., Fox H., Buckley C.H., Henderson W.J. & Griffiths K. (1984) Effects of talc on the rat ovary. *Br. J. Exp. Path.*, **65**, 101–6.

Hart W.R. (1977) Ovarian epithelial tumors of borderline malignancy (carcinoma of low malignant potential). *Hum. Pathol.*, **8**, 541–49.

Hart W.R. & Norris H.J. (1973) Borderline and malignant mucinous tumours of the ovary: histologic criteria and clinical behaviour. *Cancer*, **31**, 1031–45.

Hasleton P.S., Keleman P., Whittaker J.S., Burslem R.W. & Turner L. (1978) Benign and malignant struma ovarii. *Arch. Pathol. Lab. Med.*, **102**, 180–84.

Henderson W.J., Evans P.M.D., Davies D.J. & Griffiths K. (1979) Talc in normal and malignant ovarian tissue, *Lancet*, **i**, 499.

Jacobs A.J., Newland J.R. & Green R.K. (1982) Pure choriocarcinoma of the ovary. *Obstet. Gynecol. Surv.*, **37**, 603–9.

Katzenstein A.A., Mazur M.T., Morgan T.E. & Kao M. (1978) Proliferative serous tumors of the ovary: histologic features and prognosis. *Am. J. Surg. Pathol.*, **2**, 339–55.

Kliman L., Rome R.M. & Fortune D.W. (1986) Low malignant potential tumors of the ovary: a study of 76 cases. *Obstet. Gynecol.*, **68**, 338−44.

Knapp R.C. & Friedman E.A. (1974) Aortic lymph node metastases in early ovarian cancer. *Am. J. Obstet. Gynecol.*, **119**, 1013−17.

Kolstad P. (1986) *Clinical Gynecologic Oncology. The Norwegian Experience*. Norwegian University Press, Oslo.

Kottmeier H.L. (1968) Surgical management — conservative: indications according to the type of the tumour. *In*: Gentil F. & Junquiera A.C. (eds), *U.I.C.C. Monograph Series Vol. II Ovarian Cancer*. Springer, Berlin. pp. 257−66.

Langley F.A. & Fox H. (1987) Ovarian tumours: classification, histogenesis and aetiology. *In*: Fox H. (ed), *Haines and Taylor: Obstetrical and Gynaecological Pathology*. Churchill Livingstone, Edinburgh. pp. 542−54.

Malkasian G.D., Melton L.J., O'Brien P.C. & Greene M.H. (1984) Prognostic significance of histological classification and grading of epithelial malignancies of the ovary. *Am. J. Obstet. Gynecol.*, **149**, 274−84.

McCaughey W.T.E., Kirk N.H., Lester W. & Dardick I. (1984) Peritoneal epithelial lesions associated with proliferative serous tumours of the ovary. *Histopathology*, **8**, 195−208.

Meleka F. & Rafla S. (1975) Variation of spread of ovarian malignancy according to site of origin. *Gynecol. Oncol.*, **3**, 108−13.

Michael H. & Roth L.M. (1986) Invasive and non-invasive implants in ovarian serous tumors of low malignant potential. *Cancer*, **57**, 1240−47.

Nogales F.F. (1987) Germ cell tumours of the ovary. *In*: Fox H. (ed), *Haines and Taylor: Obstetrical and Gynaecological Pathology*. Churchill Livingstone, Edinburgh. pp. 637−75.

Nogales F.F., Matilla A., Nogales-Oriz F. & Galera-Davidson H. (1978) Yolk sac tumors with pure and mixed polyvesicular vitelline patterns. *Hum. Pathol.*, **9**, 553−66.

Norris H.J., Zirkin R.J. & Benson W.I.. (1976) Immature (malignant) teratoma of the ovary: a clinical and pathological study of 58 cases. *Cancer*, **37**, 2359−72.

Ovarian Tumour Panel of the Royal College of Obstetricians and Gynaecologists (1983) Ovarian epithelial tumours of borderline malignancy: pathological features and current status. *Br. J. Obstet. Gynaecol.*, **90**, 743−50.

Ozols R.F., Garvin A.J., Costa J., Simon R.M. & Young R.C. (1980) Advanced ovarian cancer: correlation of histologic grade with response to therapy and survival. *Cancer*, **45**, 572−81.

Prat J. & Scully R.E. (1981) Cellular fibromas and fibrosarcomas of the ovary: a comparative clinico-pathologic analysis of seventeen cases. *Cancer*, **47**, 2663−70.

Prat J., Young R.H. & Scully R.E. (1982) Ovarian Sertoli−Leydig cell tumors with heterologous elements. (ii) Cartilage and skeletal muscle: a clinicopathological analysis of twelve cases. *Cancer*, **50**, 2465−75.

Robboy S.J., Norris H.J. & Scully R.E. (1975) Insular carcinoid primary in the ovary: a clinicopathologic analysis of 48 cases. *Cancer*, **36**, 404−18.

Robboy S.J. & Scully R.E. (1980) Strumal carcinoid of the ovary: an analysis of 50 cases of a distinctive tumor composed of thyroid tissue and carcinoid. *Cancer*, **46**, 2019−34.

Rodenburg C.J., Cornelisse C.J., Heintz A.P.M., Hermans J. & Fleuren G.J. (1987) Tumor ploidy as a major prognostic factor in advanced ovarian cancer. *Cancer*, **59**, 317−23.

Rodenburg C.J., Cornelisse C.J., Hermans J. & Fleuren G.J. (1988) DNA flow cytometry and morphometry as prognostic indicators in advanced ovarian cancer: a step forward in predicting the clinical outcome. *Gynecol. Oncol.*, **29**, 176−87.

Roth L.M., Czernobilsky B. & Langley F.A. (1981) Ovarian endometrioid adenofibromatous and cystadenofibromatous tumors: benign, proliferating and malignant. *Cancer*, **48**, 1838−45.

Roth L.M., Langley F.A., Fox H., Wheeler J.A. & Czernobilsky B. (1984) Ovarian clear cell adenofibromatous tumors: benign, of low malignant potential and associated with invasive clear cell adenocarcinoma. *Cancer*, **5**, 1156−63.

Roth L.M. & Sternberg W.H. (1971) Proliferating Brenner tumors. *Cancer*, **27**, 687−93.

Russell P. (1979) The pathological assessment of ovarian neoplasms. II. The proliferating epithelial tumours. *Pathology*, **11**, 251−82.

Russell P. (1984) Borderline epithelial tumours of the ovary: a conceptual dilemma. *Clin. Obstet. Gynaecol.*, **11**, 259−77.

Rutgers J.L. & Scully R.E. (1988) Ovarian Müllerian mucinous papillary cystadenomas of borderline malignancy: a clinicopathological analysis of 30 cases. *Cancer*, **61**, 340—48.

Scully R.E. (1979) *Atlas of Tumor Pathology, Second Series, Fascicle 16 Tumors of the Ovary and Maldeveloped Gonads*. Armed Forces Institute of Pathology, Washington D.C.

Serov S.F., Scully R.E. & Sobin L.H. (1973) *International Classification of Tumours. No. 9. Histological Typing of Ovarian Tumours*. World Health Organization, Geneva.

Sorbe B., Frankendal B. & Veress B. (1982) Importance of histological grading in the prognosis of epithelial ovarian carcinoma. *Obstet. Gynecol.*, **59**, 576—82.

Sumithran E., Susil B.J. & Looi L-M. (1988) The prognostic significance of grading in borderline mucinous tumors of the ovary. *Hum. Pathol.*, **19**, 15—18.

Talerman A. (1984) Carcinoid tumors of the ovary. *J. Cancer Res. Clin. Oncol.*, **107**, 125—35.

Tasker M. & Langley F.A. (1985) The outlook for women with borderline epithelial tumours of the ovary. *Br. J. Obstet. Gynaecol.*, **92**, 969—73.

Thurlbeck W.M. & Scully R.E. (1960) Solid teratoma of the ovary: a clinicopathological analysis of 9 cases. *Cancer*, **13**, 804—11.

Young R.H., Dickersin G.R. & Scully R.E. (1982a) Ovarian sex cord tumor with annular tubules: review of 74 cases including 27 with Peutz—Jeghers syndrome and four with adenoma malignum of the cervix. *Cancer*, **50**, 1384—1402.

Young R H., Dickersin G.R. & Scully R.E. (1984) Juvenile granulosa cell tumor of the ovary: a clinicopathologic analysis of 125 cases. *Am. J. Surg. Pathol.*, **8**, 575—96.

Young R.H., Prat J. & Scully R.E. (1982b) Ovarian Sertoli—Leydig tumors with heterologous elements. (1) Gastrointestinal epithelium and carcinoids: a clinicopathologic analysis of thirty six cases. *Cancer*, **50**, 2248—56.

Young R.H. & Scully R.E. (1983) Ovarian Sertoli—Leydig cell tumors with a retiform pattern: a problem in histopathologic diagnosis: a report of twenty-five cases. *Am. J. Surg. Pathol.*, **7**, 755—71.

Young R.H. & Scully R.E. (1984a) Ovarian Sertoli cell tumors: a report of ten cases. *Int. J. Gynecol. Pathol.*, **2**, 349—63.

Young R.H. & Scully R.E. (1984b) Well differentiated ovarian Sertoli—Leydig cell tumors: a clinico-pathological analysis of 23 cases. *Am. J. Surg. Pathol.*, **3**, 277—90.

Young R.H. & Scully R E. (1985) Ovarian Sertoli—Leydig cell tumors: a clinicopathological analysis of 207 cases. *Am. J. Surg. Pathol.*, **9**, 543—69.

10

Surgical Management of Ovarian Cancer

JOHN H. SHEPHERD

Ovarian cancer remains an enigmatic disease often presenting at an advanced stage with little in the way of symptoms to warn either the patient or the doctor of its onset. Until recently the prognosis had changed little over the previous 30 years and was poor in the vast majority of cases. Patients with abdominal distension, mild discomfort, vague masses or acute obstruction were explored by a variety of different surgical specialists including gynaecologists, general surgeons and urologists. At laparotomy, widespread carcinomatosis would often be found with ascites and the situation deemed hopeless. A biopsy would be taken and then the abdomen closed with no further treatment given. Today, this approach has been altered due to a greater understanding of the disease and its natural history with an awareness leading to a more accurate preoperative diagnosis and preparation for surgery utilizing a multidisciplinary approach. This encompasses many specialists including gynaecological surgeons, medical oncologists and radiotherapists as well as anaesthetists, histopathologists, radiologists and general physicians.

At last improving results in overall management are becoming evident in large centres, although ultimately the majority of patients still die of their disease. However, an improvement in median survival and disease free interval before relapse justifies this more positive approach and gives realistic hope for the future.

Incidence

It is predominantly a disease of the upper and middle classes (Cohart 1955) occurring primarily in westernized countries. The last office of population and census surveys report (1986) indicated that 4473 ovarian tumours occurred in England and Wales that year. Including other adnexal and miscellaneous tumours of undetermined origin (29) and fallopian tube carcinomata (37) the total number of adnexal/ovarian tumours was 4539. 3635 died, thus confirming that the majority (over 80%) of patients still die from their disease (deaths, OPCS 1984; survey, OPCS 1986).

This gives an incidence of 14 per 100 000 women affected in England as compared with 21 per 100 000 in Scandinavia and 3 per 100 000 in Japan (Kolstad & Beecham 1975).

Although the peak incidence of the disease is in the seventh and eighth decade of life, it should be remembered that this cancer does occur in a younger age group (Fig. 10.1). Between 90 and 100 women below the age of 40 die from the disease per year in England and Wales alone.

Natural history

While the rarer tumours of ovarian origin, namely those of gonadostromal and of a germ cell origin, spread by accepted lymphatic and blood vessel routes as well as by transperitoneal spread, epithelial tumours predominantly metastasize by widespread transcoelomic dissemination. Understanding this natural history is important when deciding upon the management of such patients. Initial tumour volume may be indirectly proportional to individual host survival; the disease, however, may be relatively noninvasive with minimal destruction of vital and extraovarian organs. As the tumour increases in size, metastases establish themselves and spread. Physiological and anatomical effects then occur which will compromise the gastrointestinal tract especially. This may lead to a mechanical obstruction resulting in malabsorption and a biochemical disorder.

Women at risk of ovarian cancer

Early detection of these tumours is difficult, but in retrospect it is realized that there is an 'at risk' woman for developing such an ovarian cancer. Typically, she may be nulliparous or infertile, and will have had some form of ovarian dysfunction leading to premenstrual tension, breast swelling, or dysmenorrhoea. She

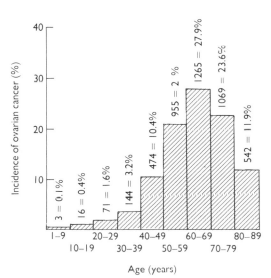

Fig. 10.1. Age distribution of ovarian cancer. 4539 patients with ovarian and adnexal ovarian-like tumours (England and Wales) (OPCS 1984).

may have had an early menopause. Although there is a remarkable lack of symptomatology, quite often there may have been complaints of vague abdominal discomfort, pelvic pressure, dyspepsia, urinary frequency, low back pain or constipation. Such symptoms should arouse suspicions to alert the gynaecologist or medical practitioner. As this disease predominantly affects postmenopausal women, any patient who is found to have a palpable postmenopausal ovary should be regarded as having a malignancy until proved otherwise (Barber & Graber 1971). The normal ovary decreases gradually in size with inactivity so that 2–3 years after menopause it is barely 1 cm in diameter.

The combined oral contraceptive pill may exert a protective effect on the ovary as may multiple pregnancies. Thus it is possible that incessant ovulation predisposes to cancer. There is an increasing incidence of familial ovarian cancer being reported (Piver et al. 1984). It has to be questioned, however, whether this is the same disease entity or in fact a mesothelial malignancy with incidental ovarian involvement. One has to be wary before advising prophylactic oophorectomy with castration and its inevitable consequences of osteoporosis, risk of heart disease and postmenopausal symptoms. Such drastic measures do not appear necessarily to prevent the onset of so-called 'ovarian cancer' which in some instances may have arisen in other mesothelial tissues (Tobacman et al. 1982).

Preliminary results from the familial ovarian cancer study at the Institute of Cancer Research and Royal Marsden Hospital suggest that ovarian cancer shows a significant familial clustering. Most of this is accounted for by a small number of families at very high risk. It is estimated that a woman aged 30 who has an affected mother and sister has a risk of approximately 1% per year or 40% by the age of 40 years. There are about 2000 women aged 25–40 in England and Wales who fall into this category and they will suffer roughly 500 ovarian cancer deaths by the age of 60 (personal communication, Ponder et al. 1989)

Recent changes in outlook and management

Treatment of ovarian cancer has undergone dramatic changes over the last few years. The rarer germ cell and gonadostromal tumours which previously carried an appalling prognosis and often affected young women, are now potentially curable with current chemotherapeutic measures. This also allows more conservative surgery and the possibility of future childbearing having achieved a cure.

Not so with epithelial tumours, however, which still represent the majority of cases (Table 10.1). They present a great therapeutic challenge to those dealing with them. Surgery remains the cornerstone of therapy but its exact role has altered. The patients present with surgical problems, either related to distension, vomiting, obstruction, pain or simply a palpable mass. Not only does surgery often become necessary to make a diagnosis, but it allows a thorough exploration

Table 10.1. Histopathology of 403 surgically treated cases of ovarian cancer (SBH & RMH 1981−88)

		No.	%
Epithelial	Serous	187	47
	Mucinous	80	20
	Endometrioid	45	11
	Undifferentiated	29	7
	Mesonephroid	19	5
	Adenosquamous	1	<1
	Brenner	0	0
	Carcino sarcoma	0	0
		361	90
Germ cell	Teratoma	6	
	Dysgerminoma	5	
	Endodermal sinus	3	
	Embryonal carcinoma	2	
	Choriocarcinoma	0	
	Gonadoblastoma	0	
Gonadal stromal	Granulosa cell	4	
	Thecoma	2	
	Sertoli−Leydig tumour	1	
	Lipid cell tumour	0	
		23	5
Non-specific	Fibroma	0	
mesenchymal	Leiomyoma	0	
	Lymphoma	0	
	Sarcoma	0	
Secondary	Breast	10	
	Colon	4	
	Stomach	3	
	Lymphoma	1	
	Endometrial	1	
		19	5

of the abdomen so that the disease is precisely staged by a thorough surgical and histopathological evaluation. Regrettably, surgical staging is still inaccurate and at least one-third of cases need to be 'up-staged' on reassessment prior to commencing further treatment (Young *et al*. 1983).

The initial tumour bulk is relevant with regard to host survival, but more importantly the postoperative tumour volume has a direct relationship with survival (Parker *et al*. 1970; Aure *et al*. 1971). If no palpable tumour remains after surgery, then the prognosis and survival are far better than if disease remains (Declos & Quinlan 1969; Griffiths *et al*. 1972). This is irrespective of further treatment or what form it may take (Griffiths 1975; Wharton & Herson 1981).

If chemotherapy is to be effective then it is essential for as much of the disease as possible to be removed by surgical extirpation prior to aggressive drug therapy. The principles of tumour kinetics determine that chemotherapy is more likely to be successful if only micrometastases remain (Schabel 1969). A tumour mass 1 kg in weight may contain 10^{12} cells: 1 g of residual tumour has 10^9 cells remaining. The theoretical advantage of striving to reduce the residual disease to less than 5 mm is in fact dubious from the kinetic standpoint (Van Lindert *et al*. 1983). The Goldie–Coldman hypothesis suggests, however, that large tumours may be resistant to chemotherapy unless the entire mass is removed. The spontaneous mutation rate is high and may be associated with phenotypic drug resistance due to an innate property of the tumour (Goldie & Goldman 1979).

It is not always possible to obey the basic rules of cancer surgery when dealing with widespread ovarian carcinomatosis. Although the aim is to resect a tumour mass with clear margins of resection, on occasions, due to the way that this tumour spreads a degree of macroscopic peritoneal disease or smaller microscopic disease will remain. It was Meigs who first suggested that as much tumour as possible should be removed so that the effect of postoperative irradiation was enhanced (Meigs 1935). The concept of a maximal surgical effort was conceived initially by Munnell (1968). He reported an overall increase in survival of patients with ovarian cancer from 28–40% and indicated that this was due to a more complete and successful surgical reduction of tumour bulk prior to postoperative irradiation. Subsequently, Griffiths quantified this theory, indicating that remaining tumour nodules should be less than 1.5 cm in diameter (Griffiths 1975) in order to give a better chance for response with adjuvant therapy and longer term survival. This was confirmed by Hacker *et al*. (1983) and Van Lindert *et al*. (1983).

More recently, radioimmunoscintigraphy has been shown to be of great value in the diagnosis and assessment of ovarian cancer with an accuracy of diagnosis and detection of primary and metastatic malignant disease of 95% when correlating preoperative radioimmunoscintigraphy findings at exploratory laparotomy. This procedure is minimally invasive without apparent side effects. It offers additional opportunity for tumour detection which is an alternative to existing methods (Shepherd *et al*. 1987).

Preoperative investigations

Patients who present with a pelvic mass or ascites and a likely diagnosis of ovarian carcinoma need to be fully evaluated before undergoing exploratory laparotomy. A chest X-ray is essential to exclude pulmonary spread or an effusion. Although ultrasound scan and computerized axial tomography (CT scans) are useful for monitoring tumour response during therapy, if measurable disease is present, they add little to the initial preoperative management or assessment from the surgeon's standpoint. Using laparotomy as the yardstick, both ultrasound and CT scanning may be accurate for assessing masses in the pelvis and ultrasound is useful for excluding liver secondaries, but neither are reliable enough in the abdomen (Cosgrove *et al.* 1980). Small disease less than one centimetre in diameter is difficult to detect with present equipment and limitations in resolution. With developing technology and nuclear magnetic resonance this will improve in the future. The value, however, of an intravenous urogram to outline the ureters and also a barium enema to visualize the colon is regrettably too often forgotten. These allow preoperative planning so that the surgeon is prepared for the appropriate surgery before embarking on a procedure. It also excludes the possibility of a colonic primary with Krukenberg secondary deposits on the ovaries. Similarly, if there are significant upper gastrointestinal symptoms or dyspepsia then a barium meal with a possible follow through would be indicated. Lymphangiography may be of value especially to visualize the para-aortic nodes but unfortunately there is a high incidence of false negative and false positive results with this procedure.

New imaging techniques are desperately needed not only for preoperative assessment of ovarian cancer but also for monitoring progress or response. With development in ultrasound using the sector scanner, ovarian morphology can be studied more closely. This may be used as a screening procedure as well as for studying suspicious ovaries on examination (Campbell *et al.* 1982; Oram & Jacobs 1987). The use of radiolabelled monoclonal antibodies has also recently yielded useful results highlighting metastatic disease prior to an initial exploratory laparotomy in patients with ovarian cancer (Epenetos *et al.* 1982) and also prior to second look procedures following treatment (Granowsra *et al.* 1985).

Needless to say, prior to any surgery full haematological and biochemical assessment is important. Blood for tumour marker assays may be of value especially in young women with pelvic masses of unknown origin. Serum should always be kept in the young age group for retrospective assessment of beta-human chorionic gonadotrophin (β-HCG), alphafetoprotein (AFP) and chorioembryonic antigen (CEA), even if these are not available prior to surgery. If a germ cell or gonadostromal tumour is found a preoperative value of what might prove to be a useful tumour marker is then available. Regrettably the same does not apply to the more common epithelial tumours although these may be present in many nonspecifically (Donaldson *et al.* 1980). The detection of other antigens such as CA 125 is proving to be useful as an index for recurrent or progressive disease. This particular antigen has been credited with an especially high sensitivity and a specificity of 90–94% (Bast *et al.* 1983). An alternative approach is to use a combination of tumour markers in monitoring patients with ovarian cancer. Statistical models have shown that the predicted value of simultaneous determinations of such antigens as chorioembryonic antigen (CEA), tissue polypectoid antigen (TPA), feretin and cancer antigen (CA 125) is 91.7% in reflecting the clinical course of the disease (Lahousen *et al.* 1987). Such monitoring at this time is impractical in the majority of centres but needs further consideration in the future.

Preparation of patients for surgery

With a diagnosis of suspected ovarian cancer, the patient should be prepared for major surgery. Any underlying medical disorders such as diabetes mellitis, hypertension, anaemia, cardiac or pulmonary disease should be corrected and treated accordingly. A large number of these patients may be cachectic and already in negative nitrogen balance which will continue for some time following an operation. If the patient is obstructed or requires a bowel resection for other reasons then intravenous hyperalimentation should be considered. This may then be continued postoperatively. However, with the patient taking fluids sufficiently by mouth, the enteral route may be used and the patient given an elemental diet with a high calorie, high protein and very low roughage intake. The bowel may thus be adequately prepared while at the same time improving the metabolic status of the patient. Suitable aperients such as magnesium sulphate should be given to empty the bowel at the same time. Antibiotics are also given as part of the bowel preparation. Neomycin or kanamycin may be given 48 h preoperatively. An enema the night before surgery will also clear the lower bowel. Prophylactic antibiotics with a broad spectrum of cover should be given starting with the premedication and continued for 24–48 h postoperatively. This has been shown to reduce postoperative infections in extensive gynaecological surgery (Creasman et al. 1982) and should be considered in any category of surgery with high risk of febrile morbidity (Cartwright et al. 1984). Similarly, subcutaneous heparin for prophylactic anticoagulation is advisable as with any patient undergoing radical pelvic surgery who has a large pelvic mass that may be obstructing pelvic veins causing thrombosis which is often present prior to surgery in the first place. On occasions with huge masses, it may be necessary at the time of laparotomy to gently elevate the abdominopelvic mass that may be occluding the inferior vena cava and consider placing an occlusive clip across this to prevent either recurrent small pulmonary emboli or a large thrombus shifting and embolizing during the operative procedure. In these cases there will be considerable collateral blood supply and venous drainage evident. Anticoagulation would be continued until the patient is completely mobilized to reduce the risk of fatal pulmonary embolism and further venous thrombosis. The use of compression stockings and early mobilization with postoperative physiotherapy is recommended.

Surgical exploration and tumour resection

The aim of primary surgery should be to explore the abdomen thoroughly in order to obtain a satisfactory diagnosis and confirmation of the primary tumour site. Thereafter, the disease must be accurately staged. This may only be satisfactorily performed by a vertical incision which may be extended to above the umbilicus if necessary. Adequate exposure of not only the pelvis but of the upper abdomen also and subdiaphragmatic regions is thus obtained. At the same time the posterior abdominal wall, lesser sac and para-aortic regions are accessible for explorations and if necessary surgical resection (Piver & Barlow 1976). It cannot be stressed forcefully enough how important it is to have an adequate exposure for not only a complete examination of all parts of the abdomen and pelvis but also for the most optimal and appropriate surgical procedure to be performed. A dilemma arises when inoperable ovarian cancer is found unexpectedly at laparotomy in a woman undergoing hysterectomy for an assumed benign mass such as fibroids. Extensive surgery might then be difficult if not dangerous through a low transverse incision. Such a case may require re-exploration at a later date through a more appropriate incision though some might advocate closing the cosmetic incision and reopening the abdomen vertically. This problem should not arise with elderly women who have a pelvic mass, as clearly a Pfannensteil incision would be inadvisable if there is a high chance of neoplasia. With younger patients, in their 20s and 30s, however, this may not be so clear cut.

Intra-abdominal assessment

Once the abdomen is open, prior to handling the tumour and performing an exploration, any ascites or free fluid which may be present should be aspirated and sent for cytological examination. If there is no free fluid, then peritoneal washings should be taken by instilling 300 cc of normal saline into the abdomen and then aspirating this fluid from the pelvis, paracolic gutters and subdiaphragmatic areas. If a pelvic mass appears to be contained with no abdominal spread, then apart from the washings it may be useful to take smears from the subdiaphragmatic peritoneum using either a sterile Ayre spatula to scrape it or a scalpel handle.

Operability

Once the abdomen has been explored then a decision has to be taken as to the extent of surgery that is either possible or practical. Ideally, the aim should be to reduce the bulk of tumour as much as possible, and optimal cytoreductive surgery would involve leaving no residual disease greater than 1 cm in diameter (Griffiths 1975; Wharton & Herson 1981). A radical oophorectomy procedure is carried out which comprises an extended total abdominal hysterectomy with bilateral salpingo-oophorectomy, omentectomy, appendicectomy and resection of any involved segments of the gastrointestinal or genitourinary tracts which are grossly involved (Figs 10.2 and 10.3). The para-aortic nodes should be carefully palpated and if these are involved or suspicious, they should be biopsied by selective sampling, remembering that the ovarian lymph drainage is to the para-aortic lymph nodes at the level of the renal vessels.

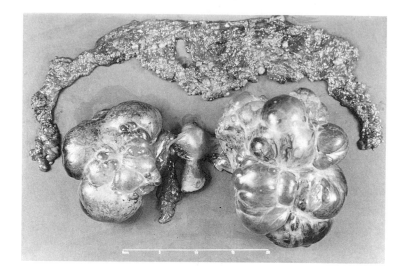

Fig. 10.2. Typical specimen from a patient with ovarian cancer comprising large bilateral semi-solid serous tumours as well as disease in the pelvic peritoneum. The omentum contains multiple small areas of metastatic spread.

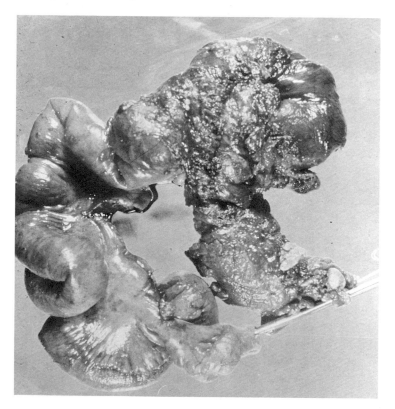

Fig. 10.3. Extensive metastatic disease involving terminal ileum and caecum necessitating a right hemi-colectomy.

This procedure is not difficult if adequate exposure is obtained by incising the posterior parietal peritoneum over the bifurcation of the aorta. The incision is extended superiorly as far as the third part of the duodenum and the fat pad of tissue containing lymph nodes is removed from this region so that a specimen of 5–6 cm is obtained. This is especially important as a staging procedure when trying to decide which stage a particular patient should be placed into (see Table 10.2). It should be emphasized that this is carried out, therefore, as a diagnostic procedure rather than with any therapeutic intent. The degree to which an individual case may be optimally 'debulked' depends not only on the patient and her particular tumour, but also the surgeon and particular centre where the procedure is being carried out. In centres where there is a particular interest and expertise in ovarian cancer surgery, optimal cytoreduction is possible in about 85% of patients (Chen & Bonner 1985; Heintz et al. 1986; Griffiths 1987). The feasibility of a successful optimal procedure clearly rests with the experience of the surgical team. Regrettably, it has to be concluded that most patients with advanced ovarian cancer do not have the opportunity of aggressive tumour reduction surgery. This has been clearly shown by three national co-operative ovarian cancer trials. An Italian study of 531 patients indicated that only 31% had optimal cytoreduction (Gruppo Inter-regional co-operativo Oncologico Gynaecologia 1987). The Clinical Oncology Society of Australia in 1986 showed that only 45% of 284 patients benefited from appropriate radical surgery and in a Dutch study (Neijt et al. 1987) 48% of 191 patients were optimally debulked. Although these studies do indicate the difficulty in making a preoperative diagnosis of ovarian cancer in some patients, they also show that there is a degree of uncertainty regarding the need and place for extensive radical surgery in these cases. Often it may take time to decide whether the disease is resectable but careful exploration and mobilization often reveals that so-called inoperable disease is in fact not so. The retroperitoneal approach may be required, starting high at the pelvic brim. If the rectosigmoid is included in the tumour mass, as not infrequently happens, so that the pouch of Douglas is completely obliterated with the uterus, fallopian tubes and ovaries buried, then this should be included as part of the resection (Hudson 1973). If possible, when the bowel is resected, primary end to end anastomosis should be performed; hence the bowel preparation preoperatively. If the large bowel is resected, then a defunctioning colostomy or temporary caecostomy may be of value. Prophylactic colostomy for future obstruction has little place in the management of this disease although on occasions, as an emergency procedure for complete intestinal obstruction, a colostomy may be required. Approximately 25% of cases explored may require a non-gynaecological procedure including bowel resection, splenectomy or ureteric reanastomosis.

Table 10.2. Staging of ovarian cancer (FIGO 1988)

Stage I		Growth limited to the ovaries
	Ia	Growth limited to one ovary; no ascites
		No tumour on the external surface; capsule intact
	Ib	Growth limited to both ovaries; no ascites
		No tumour on the external surfaces; capsule intact
	Ic*	Tumour either stage Ia or Ib, but with tumour on surface of one or both ovaries; or with capsule ruptured; or with ascites present containing malignant cells or with positive peritoneal washings
Stage II		Growth involving one or both ovaries with pelvic extension
	IIa	Extension and/or metastases to the uterus and/or tubes
	IIb	Extension to other pelvic tissues
	IIc*	Tumour either stage IIa or IIb but with tumour on surface of one or both ovaries; or with capsule(s) ruptured; or with ascites present containing malignant cells or with positive peritoneal washings
Stage III		Tumour involving one or both ovaries with peritoneal implants outside the pelvis and/or positive retroperitoneal or inguinal nodes. Superficial liver metastasis equals stage III
		Tumour is limited to the true pelvis but with histologically proven malignant extension to small bowel or omentum
	IIIa	Tumour grossly limited to the true pelvis with negative nodes but with histologically confirmed microscopic seeding of abdominal peritoneal surfaces
	IIIb	Tumour involving one or both ovaries with histologically confirmed implants of abdominal peritoneal surfaces none exceeding 2 cm in diameter
		Nodes are negative
	IIIc	Abdominal implants greater than 2 cm in diameter and/or positive retroperitoneal or inguinal nodes
Stage IV		Growth involving one or both ovaries with distant metastases. If pleural effusion present, there must be positive cytology to allot a case to stage IV
		Parenchymal liver metastasis equals stage IV

* In order to evaluate the impact on prognosis of the different criteria for allotting cases to stage Ic or IIc it would be of value to know if the source of malignant cells was (1) peritoneal washings or (2) ascites and if rupture of the capsule was (a) spontaneous or (b) caused by the surgeon.

Secondary spread

The pelvic peritoneum is the commonest site for secondary spread beyond the female genital organs and the omentum is the next most common. The appendix and the mesentery as well as the serosal aspect of the small and large bowel and paracolic gutters are often involved and if the tumour size is such that it is more than 1–2 cm then these nodules should be excised. Although it is not necessary to remove multiple small deposits that may be scattered throughout the abdominal cavity and into the pelvis, the larger nodules must be resected. If the parenchyma of the liver is grossly involved and the patient has pleural effusions of positive cytology, then clearly the prognosis is not as good. Under these circumstances it may not be practical to carry out extensive tumour reduction surgery, but certainly any bulk disease should be removed. This will make the patient more comfortable and hopefully prevent the accumulation of any ascites and delay complications such as gastrointestinal obstruction. It is important that any residual disease should be mapped out and recorded so that this may be monitored during further therapy. Also, diagnostic 'second look' operative procedures such as laparotomy, or laparoscopy, may be directed to these sites.

A number of cases will be explored and deemed inoperable: the definition of this may vary from surgeon to surgeon. Operability in strict surgical terminology applies to curability by total extirpation of disease with adequate and clear margins of resection including channels of potential lymphatic spread in the *en bloc* specimen. This, of course, does not apply to ovarian cancer with its different and varied natural history and mode of spread. Resectability as opposed to operability might be a more appropriate term applied to the removal of large bulk disease whilst at the same time microscopic or minute 1–2 mm nodules may remain.

Inoperability

If surgical resection is not possible, a biopsy will be taken and the abdomen closed. It is most important that if this is the case, the primary site should be determined as far as possible. On occasions, such patients will require re-exploration by more experienced surgeons in order to reduce the tumour bulk as described above. This, however, is not always practical and under these circumstances, it is reasonable for chemotherapy to commence in an attempt to render disease more operable so that definitive surgery may be undertaken later. Although there is little evidence to suggest that preoperative chemotherapy actually changes the resectability of a tumour, this approach has had gratifying results in some patients. Maximal tumour reductive surgery has been possible at a later date either when the patient has been transferred to a specialist unit, or if she is re-explored by a more experienced surgeon. This appears to be especially so in

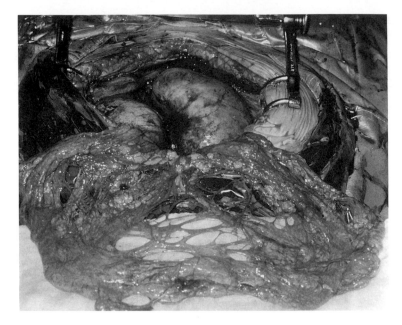

Fig. 10.4. Laparotomy appearance of a previously inoperable tumour when re-explored 3 months later having had two courses of combination chemotherapy including platinum.

younger patients and may be due in part to a chemical peritonitis that develops in response to many tumours resulting in a tremendous inflammatory reaction. With the passage of time, antibiotics and even chemotherapy, this picture may change and apparently non-operable tumours become resectable (Fig. 10.4).

Staging of ovarian cancer

The initial aim of an exploratory laparotomy is to stage the patient as a diagnostic procedure as well as gain histopathological confirmation of the diagnosis. The International Federation of Obstetrics and Gynaecology (FIGO) recommended surgical staging for ovarian cancer is as shown in Table 10.2. At the FIGO Meeting in Rio de Janeiro in November 1988 minor changes were made in the ovarian cancer staging but the basic outlines are the same as previously accepted. By placing an individual patient into a particular stage it is possible to give not only a prognosis but also decide on the next therapeutic option and in particular whether adjuvant therapy is indicated or not. At the same time, reporting and recording of such cases on a world-wide basis is facilitated.

Radical oophorectomy: optimal surgery

A radical oophorectomy procedure, debulking the tumour in an optimal way, may take 3–4 hours and therefore the operating list must be arranged accordingly.

There is little place for such surgery at the end of a long and busy routine theatre session or by an inexperienced junior surgeon in the middle of the night. When patients present as an emergency, in obstruction for example, or with an acute abdomen, the aetiology of the problem should be determined as far as possible preoperatively. This will enable the appropriate surgical team to be best prepared for whatever surgery is necessary. Clearly palliative intestinal bypass or diversion may be all that is possible under these circumstances, but the same rules should apply at laparotomy as would if this were an elective procedure.

Conservative surgery

More than three-quarters of patients will be in an advanced stage at presentation and as such will require radical surgery. Table 10.3 indicates the surgical staging at presentation as reported on a world-wide basis to FIGO (1988); 55.4% of patients presented at an advanced stage. However, individual units attracting a specific specialist referral of pelvic cancer cases may have a higher percentage of advanced cases referred as reflected in the figures shown. Hence, at the combined gynaecological oncology unit at St Bartholomew's and the Royal Marsden Hospital, 80% of surgically explored cases are in fact advanced stage III or IV disease. A comparatively small number of early stage tumours are seen and this may also be a reflection of more accurate staging according to the criteria laid down earlier. However, a certain number may be stage I and of these a proportion will be young women. Under some circumstances conservative surgery consisting of the unilateral salpingo-oophorectomy may be performed rather than a radical oophorectomy procedure. However, there should be strict criteria for a patient undergoing conservative management with epithelial ovarian cancer. The criteria should include a stage IA tumour which is well differentiated in a young woman of low parity. The pelvis should otherwise be completely normal and the tumour well encapsulated and free of adhesions. There should be no invasion of the capsule, lymphatics of the mesovarium and the peritoneal washings should be negative. The opposite ovary should be biopsied along with the omentum and this should appear macroscopically free of disease at laparotomy. Close follow up of all such patients is vital but if all these criteria are fulfilled then unilateral

Table 10.3. Surgical staging at presentation (FIGO 1988)

Stage	World-wide (%)	SBH & RMH (%)
I	26.1	12
II	15.4	8
III	39.1	56
IV	16.3	24
No stage	3.1	—

oophorectomy may be performed. At a later date, after childbearing, the question as to whether the opposite ovary should be removed and the pelvis cleared arises. Present practice differs on opposite sides of the Atlantic. It should be remembered that up to 15% of ovarian tumours may be stage I. There are certain poor prognostic factors which would allow this stage to have only a 60–70% chance of survival. These poor prognostic factors include extracystic excrescences, ruptured cysts, an adherence of the tumour to the pelvis, or other gynaecological organs. Clearly, if both ovaries are solid and papilliferous, there is no place for conservative surgery, as would be the case also with any evidence of extraovarian spread (Table 10.4).

In cases where there may be doubt of the diagnosis, frozen section examination by the pathologist may help to distinguish a benign tumour or inflammatory mass from a malignant cyst when evidence of extrapelvic disease is absent. Nevertheless, certain cases may undergo conservative and therefore less than adequate surgical removal as judged by the final pathology report once this becomes available. If necessary, further surgery may be performed under these circumstances. This may be to complete an accurate surgical staging or to complete definitive surgical extirpation as a radical oophorectomy procedure. Clearly this would depend on the exact circumstances, pathology, extent of previous surgery, surgical staging and age of the patient.

The role of lymphadenectomy

It must be remembered that an important route of spread and metastasis from ovarian cancer is the retroperitoneal embolization of tumour via the lymphatic system. The ovaries primarily drain to the para-aortic region along the gonadal vessels. In 1974 Knapp & Friedman showed that a significant number of patients with stage I ovarian cancer do in fact have positive para-aortic lymph nodes (Chen & Lee 1983). It was subsequently found that 37.7% of patients with ovarian cancer had positive para-aortic lymph nodes whereas only 14.8% had

Table 10.4. Conservative surgery in epithelial carcinoma — criteria required for unilateral salpingo-oophorectomy

---

Stage IA
Young woman of low parity desiring children
Well differentiated tumour
Encapsulated and freely mobile
Other pelvic organs normal
No invasion of capsule, hilar lymphatics or other vessels
Peritoneal washings negative cytologically
Omental biopsy negative
Biopsy of other ovary normal
Close follow up essential
Careful consideration of completing pelvic clearance after childbearing finished

---

pelvic node involvement. At the same time, Burghardt *et al.* (1984) emphasized the importance of a retroperitoneal lymph node dissection from both the diagnostic and therapeutic point of view. An argument could be made for debulking large and involved lymph nodes in order to give a better chance for chemotherapy to be effective. At the same time, the surgical interruption of lymphatic channels, which would allow microembolic metastases to occur, could also be argued. However, the blatant removal of an extensive number of otherwise normal lymph nodes cannot be encouraged or justified from an immunological point of view. There is a certain morbidity to the procedure although in experienced hands this is minimal. Although practised in central Europe, with an apparent improvement in overall survival, this has to be seen in the context of better chemotherapy being used as adjunctive treatment, especially platinum compounds, as well as a more thorough and aggressive surgical debulking policy in general (Burghardt *et al.* 1987). At present the policy in this country is to reserve lymphadenectomy for diagnostic purposes and in particular to be able to place patients in either stage I or stage III (see Table 10.2).

Aims of surgery

The exact extent of surgery has to be an individual decision taken by each surgeon on exploring the patient concerned. The arguments for radical surgery with tumour bulk reduction are predominantly fourfold.

1 To improve tumour response to further therapy, either chemotherapy or radiotherapy. Undoubtedly it is the first surgical clearance that has the best chance of achieving a cure or at the least improving the survival of the patient. In a comparative study of 1292 patients treated surgically and reported from the M.D. Anderson Hospital, the diameter of the largest residual tumour mass was the single most important prognostic factor (see Table 10.5). Patients with stage III disease with no macroscopic tumour remaining after surgery have a 63% 5-year survival compared with a 3% chance of survival if more than 10 cm diameter of tumour remains. Forty-one percent of those with disease of less than 1 cm will survive (Smith & Day 1979). Optimal cytoreductive surgery is most effective in prolonging survival in patients first seen without clinical ascites or large metastatic disease (Hacker *et al.* 1983). If radiotherapy has a role it is in those with either no disease or only minimal residual disease remaining after surgery. Whole abdominopelvic irradiation may increase patient survival in these circumstances (Dembo *et al.* 1979).

2 Such surgery will delay or prevent inevitable complications from the disease occurring. These will predominantly involve the formation of ascites with abdominal distension, intestinal obstruction, and on occasions, urinary tract obstruction.

3 To alter the immunological status of the patient, reverse immunosuppression and immunologic enhancement in such a way that the patient would be able to

Table 10.5. Residual tumour size correlated with survival rates

Tumour size (cm)	No. of patients	Survival rates %	
		2 year	5 year
Stage II			
None	120	74	52
0–1	60	71	53
1–2	18	67	17
3–6	23	47	22
7–9	6	33	0
10+	15	53	30
Stage III			
None	31	80	63
1–2	84	70	41
3–6	144	28	8
7–9	36	16	0
10+	273	16	3
Stage IV			
None	6	50	50
0–1	10	20	20
1–2	14	14	0
3–6	67	12	0
7–9	13	0	0
10+	68	5	0

mobilize her own response to the disease more easily. The immunogenicity of ovarian cancer has been demonstrated *in vivo* (Disaia *et al*. 1972; Chan *et al*. 1973; Levin *et al*. 1975; Mitchell & Kohorn 1976). A question that must be asked is whether chemotherapy or even radiotherapy ever completely reduces the number of malignant cells present to zero. More likely, with chemotherapy, is that repeated 'log kill' of cells occurs but a low level or plateau is reached so that the patient herself may then mobilize her own immune system to deal with remaining disease, or live with it in symbiosis.

4   Finally, it should not be forgotten that there is a tremendous psychological effect and benefit from removing a large abdominopelvic mass which the patient may feel and see. If she knows that this is a malignancy, then removing it will encourage her, especially when she is undergoing further therapy which in itself may not be very pleasant. To merely open the patient's abdomen and then close it having left a large mass present can only further depress her, so that she automatically thinks that she is doomed when the word 'cancer' is either mentioned or even suggested. In such patients, both chemotherapy and radiotherapy are much more likely to be effective to smaller areas of disease rather than large masses with necrotic centres and consequent hypoxia which will not respond as well to therapy.

Morbidity associated with surgical management

With careful preparation and continuing postoperative supervision, an aggressive surgical approach is associated with a remarkably low morbidity. Assuming that the greater majority of patients with advanced disease would die if left alone within 6–12 months (and many sooner) a severe complication rate of 7% is highly acceptable (see Table 10.6). To this list may be added the occasional incisional hernia in the rather extended incision (4%). However, this rarely needs repairing and only once in the reported author's series in an athletic young lady who cycled from John O'Groats to Lands End and herniated on the way!

The question of psychological suitability for aggressive management, both surgical and especially chemotherapeutic, has to be carefully considered. The patient must be carefully assessed as to her ability to cope with the stresses of treatment by a sympathetic team. Elderly patients may become confused and any hypoxia or even chest infection can precipitate this and may lead to an acute psychotic episode. An inability to cope with the diagnosis and its overall management without adequate support, especially at home, can on occasions lead to suicide.

Clearly, patients who have large abdominopelvic masses compressing pelvic veins and on occasions the inferior vena cava are at risk of developing not only pelvic and deep venous thrombosis but also pulmonary emboli. Care must be given to the surgical elevation of large and heavy masses compressing the inferior vena cava as well as the pelvic veins. Prophylactic anticoagulation is important under these circumstances.

It should be clearly understood that if patients with advanced ovarian disease are to be cured, then it is the chemotherapy that they receive after surgery that is going to cure them. However, such patients, in order to be cured, must be

Table 10.6. Morbidity associated with surgical management of 403 patients (SBH & RMH 1981–88)

Death within 28 days	5
Pulmonary embolus	5
Axillary vein thrombosis	2
Deep venous thrombosis	2
Fistula — gastrointestinal	2
Fistula — urological	1
Dehiscence	1
Haemorrhage	2
Bowel obstruction	2
Ileus (7 days)	2
Schizophrenia/acute psychosis	2
Suicide	1
Cardiac disease	2
Total	29 = 7%

correctly prepared by optimal surgical extirpation and tumour bulk reduction prior to commencement of such therapy. Objective response rates in the range of 60–95% have been reported with the current available chemotherapy both as single agents and in combination (Schwartz & Smith 1980). Some patients have now been cured of their advanced disease but the question arises as to how long such chemotherapy should be continued as these agents are associated with short and long term complications which might be lethal. These include, on the one hand, myelosuppression and anaemia, and on the other acute lymphoblastic leukaemia. There is evidence to show that the greater the number of courses of single agent chemotherapy (Melphalan) prior to a second look procedure, the greater the chance of no residual disease being found. This may not be the case with more aggressive regimes, either in combination or as a high dose single agent therapy. It is interesting that although histological grade has made a substantial difference when single alkylating agents have been administered (Wharton & Herson 1981) this does not appear to be so with multiple combination therapy including platinum (Jacobs *et al.* 1982).

Second look surgical reassessment

This involves a complete reassessment of the abdomen after optimal primary surgery and suitable adjuvant chemotherapy. The patient should be clinically disease free and in complete remission. Radiological assessment by chest X-ray, ultrasound and computerized axial tomography scan of the abdomen and pelvis, intravenous urogram and barium enema should also be negative.

The second look procedure was first suggested in order to identify recurrent bowel carcinomas before becoming clinically apparent (Wangensteen *et al.* 1957). This procedure is highly applicable to ovarian carcinoma (Rutledge & Burns 1966). However, it should be understood that there is a difference between second look surgery to either assess response to treatment or detect recurrent disease especially in early stage tumours, and re-exploration of the abdomen. The latter procedure may be carried out if only a minimal procedure had been possible at the initial laparotomy or if progression of disease is detected and complications occur necessitating surgical intervention. Under these circumstances, a tumour bulk reduction procedure will be necessary in order once more to render the patient not only more comfortable, but also more suitable for further therapy. However, the most important factors associated with recurrent cancer appear to be the volume of residual disease following initial surgery and the amount of chemotherapy prior to the second look procedure (Schwartz & Smith 1980). This implies that the later one does the second look procedure, the better the chances of a prolonged survival. However, this may represent a tortology in that the longer a patient survives in complete remission following chemotherapy, the more likely she is to have had a complete clearance due to the drugs.

Laparoscopy is of limited value as a second look procedure. It is questionable if it is accurate enough to definitively rule out residual disease, especially in the retroperitoneal tissues of the pelvis and also the para-aortic nodes (Creasman *et al*. 1978). However, it may be useful to complete the staging of an ovarian tumour which had been unexpectedly found at laparotomy performed via a low transverse incision thus making thorough exploration of the upper abdomen including the liver and subdiaphragmatic areas impossible. The laparoscope allows an excellent view of these areas to be obtained, whilst at the same time the paracolic gutters, pelvic and serosal aspects of the bowel and omentum may be visualized in part. However, it is not possible to visualize or palpate the retroperitoneal tissues, especially the pelvic or para-aortic lymph nodes. Taking peritoneal washings as evidence of persisting microscopic disease is not enough as has been shown by a false negative rate of 50% in patients with microscopic disease only at second look laparotomy (Shepherd *et al*. 1984). In these patients the disease tends to be retroperitoneal and therefore hidden from view.

'Second look' surgery

In order to determine the exact status of the disease following a complete course of chemotherapy, a full laparotomy will enable not only peritoneal washings to be taken on opening the abdomen but also multiple biopsies from any suspicious areas. There is a limit to what may be performed safely via the laparoscope. Any adhesions that are present should be excised and sent for histological examination. Obvious nodules may be present beneath the diaphragm and on the serosal aspect of the colon. These may be sampled or smears taken from the diaphragm if it is not obviously involved. If the omentum had not been removed at the first operation, then it should be at this stage as a diagnostic procedure; this may be therapeutic if it were to be macroscopically diseased. Para-aortic nodes should be explored and sampled selectively. The pelvic peritoneum should also be opened to expose the infundibulo—pelvic ligament and stump where the ovarian pedicles had been ligated originally. This area should be excised and examined. Similarly, the vault of the vagina may contain microscopic disease, and this will only be detected on opening the pelvic peritoneum in the posthysterectomy pouch of Douglas. On average 20—30 specimens will be obtained at such a second look procedure allowing a complete histopathological assessment of response to treatment and evaluation of intra-abdominal disease. Such a complete assessment is not possible laparoscopically.

Although second look surgery is relatively safe, it is by no means 100% accurate. Approximately 30% of patients deemed negative at a second look laparotomy recur either within the abdominal cavity or the retroperitoneal space (Podratz *et al*. 1988). With such a high false negative rate one must also question whether second look laparotomy for ovarian cancer is indeed justified (Sounendecker 1988). Practices have differed on both sides of the Atlantic with a second look procedure becoming established as routine in the USA, but not so in the UK and Europe, where the procedure has been reserved for therapeutic trials (Oram & Jacobs 1987). Looked at in a randomized clinical trial prospectively, there is no evidence to show that the procedure of a second look laparotomy in fact confers any survival benefit on patients with epithelial ovarian cancer (Luesley *et al.* 1988). At this time, therefore, the value of diagnosing or confirming remission is purely academic and acceptable in a trial situation when assessing the efficacy of a particular drug regime or protocol. The theoretical knowledge that may be obtained is of practical use only if there are further therapeutic options left for the patient, remembering that second and third line chemotherapy or alternative treatment is not as effective as the first attack. Nevertheless, this approach with initial aggressive surgery followed by chemotherapy either in combination or as a single agent, preferably with a platinum compound, has allowed great improvement in not only response rates but also 5-year survival (Fig. 10.5). Patients who have no residual tumour following initial surgery have a 65–70% negative second look procedure (Schwartz & Smith 1980; Curry *et al.* 1981). In those patients who have less than 2 cm residual tumour remaining following their initial surgery, it is possible to achieve 72% negative second look assessment (Wharton & Herson 1981). Even with disease greater than 3 cm, between 10 and 33% of patients may be cured of disease when reassessed (Curry *et al.* 1981; Greco *et al.* 1981).

If one looks at survival after a second look operation in those patients with no evidence of disease, there is a 75% chance of a 5-year survival. If there has been regression and only microscopic disease is present at the second look procedure, the 5-year survival is approximately 40%. When there has been little change following therapy, the 5-year survival consequently decreases to approximately 15% (Schwartz & Smith 1980). Up to 30% of patients may develop recurrent cancer following a negative second look operation. The most important factors associated with a recurrence appear to be the volume of persistent tumour remaining at the end of the initial procedure and the amount of chemotherapy that is given prior to performing the second look assessment. If recurrence occurs following the second look operation, it is usually obvious within 12 months.

Re-exploration and secondary reductive surgery

Perhaps the most debatable point is what should be done if persistent cancer at a second look operation is found. There is evidence to show that the long term survival is affected by the volume of cancer left after this procedure also. When all macroscopic tumour is removed at the second look procedure, the 5-year survival may still be 27% (Fig. 10.6). In terms of tumour size, patients with residual tumour of less than 2 cm in diameter may have a survival of 29% and patients with tumour greater than 2 cm, a 5-year survival of only 9% (Schwartz & Smith 1980). Other authors have similarly shown that when optimal secondary resection of tumour is performed, the patient's survival (20 months) is significantly

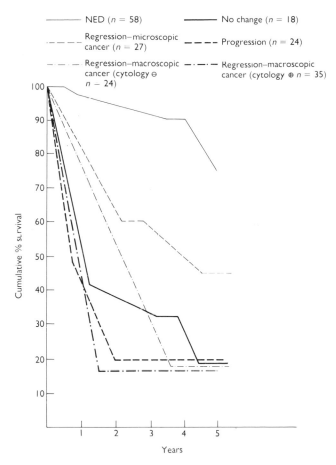

Fig. 10.5. Survival rate after second look operation. n = number of patients. ⊖ = no malignant cells in peritoneal washings. ⊕ = malignant cells in peritoneal washings (Schwartz & Smith 1980, reproduced with permission).

better than those in a non-optimal group (5 months) (Berek *et al.* 1983). These authors concluded that a secondary attempt at bulk removal of tumour is justifiable in patients who had incomplete responses to primary chemotherapy and who have no clinical evidence of ascites. This is in conflict with previous evidence that suggested that removal of all macroscopic disease at second look operations did not improve survival expectancy (Raju *et al.* 1982; Luesley *et al.* 1984). Unless an optimal and complete surgical excision is achieved either primarily or secondarily the chances for increased longevity of life are clearly small.

Borderline tumours

With individualization of patients and their histopathology it is possible to carry

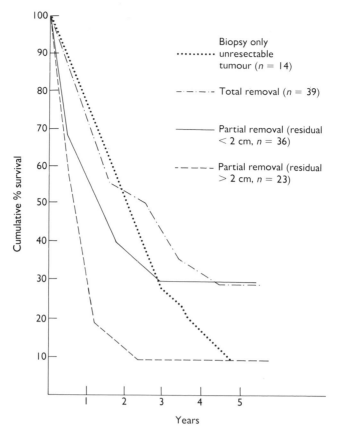

Fig. 10.6. Survival rate after second look operation as determined by the maximum diameter of the largest residual tumour mass upon completion of the operation. n = number of patients (Schwartz & Smith 1980, reproduced with permission).

out conservative surgery (unilateral oophorectomy or salpingo-oophorectomy) in some patients who have borderline epithelial tumours. This would apply to younger patients wishing to retain their childbearing potential.

If there is a high index of suspicion at initial surgery it is important that frozen section facilities are available for immediate diagnosis. Stage I disease may be adequately treated by unilateral oophorectomy as long as the other ovary is biopsied, and further staging laparotomy samples are taken. A full laparotomy is required with adequate samples taken from suspicious areas and continuous follow up even at 10−15 years is important as a significant number of recurrences seem to occur at that time.

Assessment of the cases operated on at St Bartholomew's Hospital has indicated that mucinous tumours appear to be commoner (10% of all mucinous tumours) than serous tumours, 3% of which are borderline. Serous tumours appear to occur at a younger age (a mean of 35 years) as compared to mucinous tumours (mean age 50 years).

Most borderline tumours present at stage I diagnosis (80%). Bilaterality was commoner in serous tumours (57%) and did not appear to occur with mucinous tumours. The overall response to further adjunctive therapy (chemotherapy using accepted protocols) is good with no patients dying of their disease to date.

The collated 5-year survival figure for serous tumours of borderline malignancy is 90–95% (Colgan & Norris 1983) with a 10-year survival of 75–90% (Julian & Woodruff 1987). Mucinous borderline tumours have a 5-year survival of 81% (Nikrui 1981) and a 10-year survival of 95% (Hart & Norris 1973). Fifteen-year survival falls to 73% with mucinous tumours and 57% with serous tumours (Nikrui 1981). It is thus important that follow up should continue to at least this time (see also Chapter 9).

Salvage surgery

There is a small group of patients who may be suitable for extensive salvage surgery. These are patients who may have been deemed to have inoperable disease at an initial or even second laparotomy and have subsequently received numerous courses of chemotherapy. There may have been a limited response but if a considerable bulk of tumour remains, especially with symptoms of recurring subacute obstruction, abdominal pain and distension, and on occasions ureteric compression and renal compromise, then consideration should be given to a further exploratory laparotomy with radical resection of the tumour. There are certain patients who may appear to follow their tumour into the clinic in that the tumour bulk is so enormous, filling the whole abdomen. Twenty-five such patients were assessed following extensive previous treatment by chemotherapy but unsuccessful previous surgery prior to referral to the Royal Marsden Hospital (Wiltshaw & Shepherd 1987). By carrying out a further laparotomy it was possible to clear all macroscopic disease which mainly consisted of large tumour masses, but at the same time, to relieve sites of obstruction. These were inevitably lengthy procedures requiring extensive surgical resection.

When this group was compared with other patients referred in whom such surgery was not deemed to be feasible, it was found that median survival of the patients undergoing salvage surgery was 2 years 10 months as compared to 9 months for the inoperable group. Close inspection of the characteristics of these 25 patients submitted to salvage surgery are shown in Table 10.7. The fact that such surgery is possible may partly be a characteristic of the tumour itself. The patient may in fact have operable, albeit difficult and aggressive, disease which despite this has not yet killed her. It may be that the tumour has partially responded to the chemotherapy in that most of these patients do not have ascites or residual small microscopic disease at the time of laparotomy. As would be expected, the residual disease remaining at the end of salvage surgery makes a considerable difference and usually, with large tumour masses that are relatively discrete, it is possible to remove all the tumour macroscopically. This situation is

Table 10.7. Characteristics of patients surviving 1 year or more following salvage surgery

Characteristic		% surviving one year or more
Age at diagnosis	<55.years	50
	55 years or more	33
Survival before salvage surgery	>12 months	86
	12 months or less	37.5
WHO performance status	0−1	58
before salvage surgery	2−3	14
Surgeon	Specialist	58
	Generalist	36
Residual disease at end of	0−2 cm	61.5
salvage surgery	>2 cm	30

different to other types of ovarian cancer which may spread extensively retro-peritoneally or with multiple small macroscopic disease involving all parietal surfaces. The fact that a specialist gynaecological oncologist performs this surgery with apparent better results than a generalist indicates that there is a place for referral to specialist units when extensive ovarian cancer surgery is contemplated (see Fig. 10.7).

Non-epithelial ovarian tumours

Early stage disease may be surgically treated less radically by conserving the contralateral ovary and uterus if these are normal. These tumours will occur in the younger age group and it is mandatory that a patient undergoing a laparotomy when this diagnosis is possible should have serum taken for tumour marker estimation of beta-HCG, AFP and also CA 125. This serum can be saved until after the histopathology is available for retrospective analysis but will be invaluable as a baseline for follow up, especially if chemotherapy is required in the future (see Chapter 12).

If there is a question about diagnosis then frozen section facilities must be available and if it is not possible to obtain a definitive answer at that time then removal of the presenting pelvic mass should be carried out and the final histopathology awaited before proceeding to any further surgical resection. It is always possible to re-explore the patient at a later date if necessary. A thorough exploratory laparotomy is mandatory, then combination chemotherapy should be given. More advanced disease needs aggressive surgery and pelvic clearance prior to chemotherapy. If tumour markers are raised, then these may be followed postoperatively and noninvasive methods used to visualize abdominal and pelvic disease. Re-exploration is only indicated in the presence of plateauing or rising tumour marker levels or in masses detected clinically.

During chemotherapy, after conservative surgery, menstruation may be affected

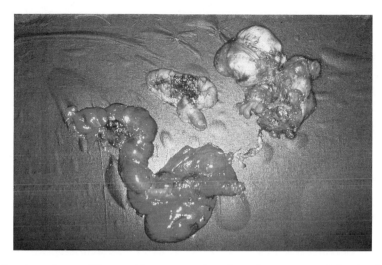

Fig. 10.7. Specimen from a 39-year-old woman undergoing salvage surgery following initial laparotomy with biopsy and caecostomy formation followed by twelve courses of combination chemotherapy. The specimen includes the caecum and ascending colon with hepatic flexure, a portion of terminal ileum, the appendix, and a large abdominopelvic mass consisting of the rectosigmoid, both fallopian tubes and ovaries including the primary site of her cancer and the uterus buried within the pelvic mass. This woman is alive and well with a manageable colostomy 3 years following surgery and no recurrent disease at present.

leading to secondary amenorrhea. This usually reverts spontaneously after therapy and providing complete remission is obtained then pregnancy may be considered after a suitable disease-free time interval, such as 2 years.

Conclusion

The advice George Bernard Shaw gave in his *Doctor's Dilemma*, to avoid using drug treatment was to 'stimulate the phagocytes'. This was very sound but he was wrong. The place of surgery in ovarian cancer is undisputed. On the one hand one still may aim to achieve a surgical cure in early stage disease, but it is becoming increasingly evident that adjunctive therapy is required to achieve this. Earlier diagnosis, and more sophisticated methods may in future increase the number of patients who present before the disease has spread beyond the pelvis. In these patients, careful assessment by a second look procedure in order to know whether to continue or stop therapy is of theoretical value but of questionable benefit to the individual patient at present. Re-exploration with further bulk reduction of tumour may have a beneficial role providing therapeutic options remain feasible.

In the past, ovarian cancer has been an enigma and carried an appalling prognosis. However, this altered approach combining radical surgery with aggressive chemotherapy is at last beginning to give a ray of hope and raise the possibility of curing such patients. Evidence is now becoming available to show that over the last 20 years results in selected centres that treat many patients with ovarian cancer are showing a significant improvement in survival. The overall survival of patients with ovarian cancer has improved from 25 to 30% over the last 25 years at the Royal Marsden Hospital. More importantly, stage III disease now has a 5-year survival that has improved from 10 to 25%. Even stage IV is now not as desperate as it used to be. Twenty years ago the 5-year survival was zero but now 10% of patients will survive to 5 years. The results of stage I and II, however, remain much as before with 75—80% survival of stage I and 50% of stage II. This improvement in survival may be attributed to the overall change in approach to the treatment of the disease not only in terms of more radical surgery striving for complete tumour removal but also more effective and aggressive chemotherapy especially using platinum-based compounds. The situation in the future must surely continue to improve.

References

Aure J.C., Joag K. & Kolstad P. (1971) Clinical and histologic studies of ovarian carcinoma. *Obstet. Gynecol.*, **27**, 1—9.

Barber H.R.K. & Graber E.A. (1971) The P.M.P.O. (post menopausal palpable ovary syndrome). *Obstet. Gynecol.*, **38**, 921—23.

Bast R.C., King T.L., St John E. *et al.* (1983) A radio-immuno assay using a monoclonal antibody to monitor the course of epithelial ovarian cancer. *New Engl. J. Med.*, **309**, 883—87.

Berek J.S., Hacker N.F., Lagasse L.D. *et al.* (1983) Survival of patients following secondary cytoreductive surgery in ovarian cancer. *Obstet. Gynecol.*, **61**, 189—93.

Burghardt E., Lahousen M. & Stettner H. (1987) The role of lymphadenectomy in the treatment of ovarian cancer. *In*: Sharpe F. & Soutter W.P. (eds) *Ovarian Cancer—The Way Ahead*. Chameleon Press, London. pp. 257—67.

Burghardt E., Pickel H. & Stettner H. (1984) Management of advanced ovarian cancer. *Eur. J. Gynecol. Oncol.*, **3**, 155—59.

Campbell S., Goessens L., Goswamy R. *et al.* (1982) Real-time ultrasonography for determination of ovarian morphology and volume. A positive early screening test of ovarian cancer? *Lancet*, **i**, 425.

Cartwright P.S. Pittaway D.E., Jones III H.W. *et al.* (1984) The use of prophylactic antibiotics in obstetrics and gynaecology. A review. *Obstet. Gynecol. Surv.*, **39**, 537.

Chan S., Koffler D. & Cohen C.J. (1973) Cell-mediated immunity in patients with ovarian cancer. *Am. J. Obstet. Gynecol.*, **115** 467—70.

Chen S.S. & Bonner R. (1985) Assessment of morbidity and mortality in primary cytoreductive surgery for advanced carcinoma. *Gynecol. Oncol.*, **20**, 190.

Chen S.S. & Lee L. (1983) Incidence of para-aortic and pelvic lymph node metastases in epithelial carcinoma of the ovary. *Gynecol. Oncol.*, **16**, 95—100.

Clinical Oncology Society of Australia (1986) Chemotherapy for advanced ovarian adenocarcinoma; a randomized comparison of continuation versus sequential therapy using Chlorambucil and Cisplatin. *Gynecol. Oncol.*, **23**, 1.

Cohart E.M. (1955) Socio-economic distribution of cancer of female sex organ in New Haven. *Cancer*, **8**, 3.

Colgan T.J.B. & Norris H.J. (1983) Ovarian epithelial tumours of low malignant potential; a review. *Int. J. Gynecol. Pathol.*, **1**, 367—87.

Cosgrove D.O., Barker G.H., Husband V.R. *et al.* (1980) Carcinoma of the ovary; an evaluation of the role of ultrasound and CT scanning in its management. *Proceedings of the 4th World Federation of Ultrasound in Medicine and Biology*.

Creasman W.T., Abu-Ghazaleh S. & Schmidt H.J. (1978) Retro-peritoneal metastatic spread of ovarian cancer. *Gynecol. Oncol.*, **6** (5), 447−50.

Creasman W.T., Hill G.B., Weed J.C. Jr *et al.* (1982) A trial of prophylactic Cefamandole in extended gynaecological surgery. *Obstet. Gynecol.*, **59** (3), 309−14.

Curry S.L., Zembo M.M., Nahhas W.A. *et al.* (1981) Second look laparotomy for ovarian cancer. *Gynecol. Oncol.*, **11** (1), 114−18.

Declos L. & Quinlan E.J. (1969) Malignant tumours of the ovary managed with post operative mega voltage irradiation. *Radiation*, **93**, 659−63.

Dembo A.J., Bush R.S., Beale F.A. *et al.* (1979) Ovarian carcinoma; improved survival following abdominopelvic irradiation in patients with a complete pelvic operation. *Am. J. Obstet. Gynecol.*, **134**, 793−800.

Disaia P.J., Sinkovics J.G., Rutledge F.N. *et al.* (1972) Cell mediated immunity to human malignant cells. *Am. J. Obstet. Gynecol.*, **114**, 979−89.

Donaldson E.S., Van Nagell J.R. Jr, Pursell S. *et al.* (1980) Multiple biochemical markers in patients with gynaecologic malignancies. *Cancer*, **45**, 948−53.

Epenetos A.A., Briton K.E., Shepherd J.H. *et al.* (1982) Targeting of iodine 123-labelled tumour associated monoclonal antibodies, ovarian, breast and gastrointestinal tumours. *Lancet*, **ii**, 999.

Goldie J.H. & Goldman A.J. (1979) A mathematical model for relating the drug sensitivity of tumours to their spontaneous mutation rate. *Cancer Treat Rep.*, **63**, 1727−33.

Granowsra M., Britton K., Shepherd J.H. *et al.* (1985) A prospective study of ^{123}I labelled monoclonal antibody imaging in ovarian cancer. *J. Clin. Oncol.*, **4**, 730−6.

Greco F.A., Julian C.G., Richardson R.C. *et al.* (1981) Advanced ovarian cancer; brief intensive chemotherapy and second look operations. *Obstet. Gynecol.*, **58** (2), 199−2−5.

Griffiths C.T. (1975) Surgical resection of tumour bulk in the primary treatment of ovarian carcinoma. Symposium on ovarian carcinoma. National Cancer Institute. *Monograph*, **42**, 101−4.

Griffiths C.T. (1987) Carcinoma of the ovary; surgical objectives. *In*: Sharp F. & Soutter W.P. (eds), *Ovarian Cancer; the Way Ahead*. Chameleon Press, London. pp. 235−44.

Griffiths C.T., Grogan R.H. & Hall T.C. (1972) Advanced ovarian cancer. Primary treatment with surgery, radiotherapy and chemotherapy. *Cancer*, **29**, 1−7.

Gruppo (Inter-regionale co-operatio Oncologico Gynecologico) (1987) Randomised comparison of Cisplatin with Cyclophosphamide/Cisplatin and with Cyclophosphamide/Doxorubicin/Cisplatinum in advanced ovarian cancer. *Lancet*, **ii**, 353.

Hacker N.F., Berek J.S., Lagasse L.D. *et al.* (1983) Primary cytoreductive surgery for epithelial ovarian cancer. *Obstet. Gynecol.*, **61**, 413−20.

Hart W.R. & Norris H.J. (1973) Borderline and mucinous tumours of the ovary; histologic criteria and clinical behaviour. *Cancer*, **31**, 1031−1−45.

Heintz A.P.M., Hacker N.F., Berek J.S. *et al.* (1986) Cytoreductive surgery in ovarian carcinoma; feasibility and morbidity. *Obstet. Gynecol.*, **67**, 783.

Hudson C.N. (1973) Surgical treatment of ovarian cancer. *Gynecol. Oncol.*, **1**, 4.

Jacobs A.J., Deliodisch L. & Cohen C.J. (1982) Histologic correlates of virulence in ovarian adenocarcinoma. *Am. J. Obstet. Gynecol.*, **143** (5), 574−80.

Julian C.G. & Woodruff J.D. (1987) The biological behaviour of low grade papillary serous carcinoma of the ovary. *Obstet. Gynecol.*, **40**, 860−67.

Knapp R.C. & Friedman E.A. (1974) Aortic lymph node metastasis in early ovarian cancer. *Am. J. Obstet. Gynecol.*, **119**, 1013−17.

Kolstad P. & Beecham J.C. (1975) Epidemiology of ovarian neoplasia. *Amsterdam Excerpta Medica ICS*, **364**.

Lahousen M., Stettner T., Pickel H. *et al.* (1987) The predictive value of a combination of tumour markers in monitoring patients with ovarian cancer. *Cancer*, **60**, 2228−32.

Levin L., McHardy J.E., Curling O. *et al.* (1975) Tumour antigenicity in ovarian cancer. *Br J Cancer*, **32**, 152−59.

Luesley D., Blackledge G., Kelly K., Wade-Evans T., Lawton F., Hilton C., Rollason T., Jordan J., Lateef T. & Chan K.K. (1988) Failure of second-look laparotomy to influence survival in epithelial ovarian cancer. *Lancet*, **2**, 599−603.

Luesley D.M., Chan K.K., Fielding J.W.L. *et al.* (1984) Second look laparotomy in the management of epithelial ovarian carcinoma. An evaluation of fifty cases. *Obstet. Gynecol.*, **64**, 421−26.

Meigs J.V. (1935) *Tumours of the Female Pelvic Organs*. McMillan, New York.

Mitchell M.S. & Kohorn E.I. (1976) Cell mediated immunity and blocking factor in ovarian cancer. *Obstet. Gynecol.*, **48**, 590–97.

Munnell E.W. (1968) The changing prognosis and treatment in cancer of the ovary. *Am. J. Obstet. Gynecol.*, **100**, 790.

Neijt J.P. Burrel R., Huinink W., Van Der Berg *et al.* (1987) Randomized trial comparing two combination chemotherapy regimes (CHAPS v. CP) in advanced ovarian carcinoma. *J. Clin. Oncol.*, **5**, 1157.

Nikrui N. (1981) Survey of clinical behaviour of patients with borderline epithelial tumours of the ovary. *Gynecol. Oncol.*, **12**, 107–119.

Oram D. & Jacobs I. (1987) Improving the prognosis in ovarian cancer. *In*: Studd J. (ed.), *Progress in Obstetrics and Gynecology*. Churchill Livingstone, Edinburgh. Vol. 6, pp. 399–432.

Parker R.T., Parker C.H. & Wilbanks G.D. (1970) Cancer of the ovary. *Am. J. Obstet.*, **108**, 878–88.

Piver M.S. & Barlow J.J. (1976) Pre-operative and intra operative evaluation in ovarian malignancy. *Obstet. Gynecol.*, **478** (3), 312–15.

Piver M.S., Mettlin C.J., Tsukada Y. *et al.* (1984) Familial cancer registry. *Obstet. Gynecol.*, **64**, 195.

Podratz K.C., Malkasian G.D., Wieland H.S., Chen S.S., Lee R.A. Stanhope C.R. & Williams T.J. (1988) Recurrent disease after negative second look laparotomy in Stage III and IV ovarian carcinoma. *Gynecol. Oncol.*, **29**, 274–82.

Podratz K.E., Schray M.F., Wieland H.S. *et al.* (1988) Evaluation of treatment and survival after positive second look laparotomy. *Gynecol. Oncol.*, **31**, 9–21.

Ponder B., Hodgson S. & Easton D. (1989) Personal communication. Protocol for studies of familial ovarian cancer. Preliminary results.

Raju K.S., McKinna J.A., Barker G.H. *et al.* (1982) Second look operations in the planned management of advanced ovarian carcinoma. *Am. J. Obstet. Gynecol.*, **144**, 650–54.

Rutledge F. & Burns B.C. (1966) Chemotherapy for advanced cancer. *Am. J. Obstet. Gynecol.*, **96**, 761–72.

Schabel F.M. Jr (1969) The use of tumour growth kinetics in planning 'curative' chemotherapy of advanced solid tumours. *Cancer*, **29**, 2384–89.

Schwartz P.F. & Smith J.P. (1980) Second look operations in ovarian cancer. *Am. J. Obstet. Gynecol.*, **138** (8), 1124–30.

Shepherd J.H., Epenetos A. & Britton K. (1983) Radioimmune diagnosis of ovarian carcinoma using tumour associated monoclonal antibodies. *Gynecol. Oncol.*, **15**, 134.

Shepherd J.H., Granowska M., Birtton K.E., Mathers K., Epenetos A., Ward B. & Slevin M. (1987) Tumour associated monoclonal antibodies for the diagnosis and treatment of ovarian cancer. *Br. J. Obstet. Gynaecol.*, **94**, 160–67.

Shepherd J.H. & Ward B.G. (1984) Personal communication.

Smith J.P. & Day T.G. Jr (1979) Review of ovarian cancer at the University of Texas Systems Cancer Centre, M.D. Anderson Hospital and Tumour Institute. *Am. J. Obstet. Gynecol.*, **135**, 984–90.

Sounendecker E.W.W. (1988) Is routine second look laparotomy for ovarian cancer justified? *Gynecol. Oncol.*, **31**, 249–55.

Tobacman J.K., Greene M.H., Tucker M.A. *et al.* (1982) Intra-abdominal carcinomatosis after prophylactic oophorectomy in ovarian cancer prone families. *Lancet*, **ii**, 795–97.

Van Lindert A.C.M., Alsbach G.P.J., Barents J. *et al.* (1983) The abdominal radical tumour reductions procedure. *In*: Heintz A.P.M., Griffiths C.T. & Trimbos J.B. (eds), *Surgery in Gynaecological Oncology*. Martinus Nijhoff, The Netherlands.

Wangensteen O.H., Lewis F.J. & Tongen L.A. (1957) The 'second look' in the cancer surgery. Patient with colic cancer and unsolved lymph node negative on 'sixth look'. *Lancet*, **ii**, 303–13.

Wharton J.T. & Herson J. (1981) Surgery for common epithelial tumours of the ovary. *Cancer*, **48** (2 suppl), 582–89.

Young R.C., Decker D.G. & Wharton J.T. (1983) Staging laparotomy in early ovarian cancer. *J. Am. Med. Ass.*, **250**, 3072.

11

Cancer of the Fallopian Tube

JOHN H. SHEPHERD

Fallopian tube cancer is an extremely rare tumour accounting for less than 0.5% of all gynaecological cancers. It is rarely diagnosed preoperatively but should always be remembered as a possibility in patients with unexplained postmenopausal bleeding. The vast majority of cases are discovered at laparotomy for an adnexal mass (McGoldrick *et al.* 1945).

Incidence

Approximately 1000 cases have been reported in the world literature. Less than 40 occur annually in England and Wales and in the author's institution the ratio of ovarian cancer to fallopian tube carcinoma is 150:1. During 1986, 37 cases were reported (OPCS 1986) with 17 deaths (OPCS 1984), representing 0.9% of all gynaecological malignancies (Harrison *et al.* 1989).

Pathology

Both benign and malignant tumours can affect the fallopian tube and of the latter the majority will be secondary tumours from other pelvic malignancies (see Table 11.1). More common than any of these are conditions which enlarge and affect the fallopian tubes, namely, endometriosis, ectopic pregnancy and pelvic sepsis, with either a tubo-ovarian abscess or hydrosalpinx. The rarity of malignant tumours makes any of these a highly *unlikely aetiological factor*.

Most malignant tumours are adenocarcinomas of which these varieties are described (Hu *et al.* 1950):
1 Papillary
2 Papillary alveolar (Fig. 11.1)
3 Alveolar medullary (Fig. 11.2)

Natural history

The papillary adenocarcinoma is the most common and characteristic. The papillary alveolar pattern probably results from fusion of adjoining papillae giving a

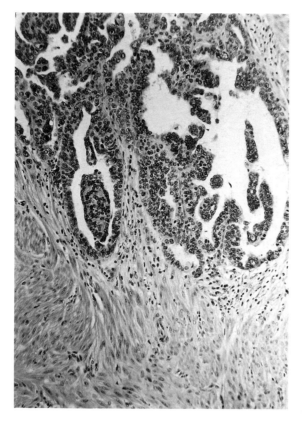

Fig. 11.3. Papillary adenocarcinoma of the fallopian tube invading myometrium. (Reproduced by kind permission of Mr J.M. Monaghan.)

The classical triad of profuse vaginal discharge, pain and an adnexal mass was described as *hydrops tubae profluens* by Latzko in 1910. Although said to be pathognomonic of fallopian tube cancer, it is in fact uncommon in most reported cases. Nevertheless, when unexplained and recurrent postmenopausal bleeding or discharge occurs, this possibility must be excluded. Laparotomy with subsequent pan-hysterectomy may be necessary if repeatedly negative uterine curettages occur following persistent postmenopausal bleeding. An ultrasound scan of the pelvis may be of value to visualize a tubal enlargement prior to surgery. Occasionally bizarre presenting symptoms such as exfoliation dermatitis may occur (Axelrod *et al*. 1988) but usually the tumour will develop insidiously as does ovarian carcinoma.

Staging

Although there is no official FIGO staging, the most useful classification is a modification of that applicable to ovarian cancer (see Table 11.2). The majority of tumours present, as with ovarian carcinoma, either as stage III or IV; about one-fifth are stage I.

Table 11.2. Staging classification of fallopian tube carcinoma (modified FIGO)

Stage 0	Carcinoma *in situ* limited to tubal mucosa
I	Growth limited to the tube
IA	Growth limited to one tube, no ascites. Tumour extending into the submucosal or muscularis but not penetrating to the serosal surface of the fallopian tube
IB	Growth limited to both tubes, no ascites. Tumour extending into the submucosal or muscularis but not penetrating to the serosal surface of the fallopian tube
IC	Growth limited to one or both tubes, ascites, or tumour extending to the serosal aspect of the fallopian tube
II	Growth involving one or both tubes with pelvic extension
IIA	Extension and/or metastasis to the ovary or uterus
IIB	Extension to the other pelvic tissues
III	Growth involving one or both tubes with widespread intraperitoneal metastasis to the abdomen (the omentum, the small intestine and its mesentery)
IV	Growth involving one or both tubes with distant metastasis outside the peritoneal cavity

Treatment

The optimum management of this disease is not immediately obvious due to the lack of sufficient numbers in any single series. Surgery clearly is the mainstay of treatment: diagnosis and staging are established by laparotomy. Postoperative radiotherapy and chemotherapy have been administered with variable results. Because of certain similarities with ovarian carcinoma, due to the often widespread and small size of metastases, it is not unreasonable to treat this disease as for an ovarian cancer. A significant number will metastasize to the retroperitoneum and para-aortic region (Peters *et al.* 1989).

Surgery

Following a thorough exploratory laparotomy along the lines of that required prior to a radical oophorectomy procedure for ovarian carcinoma, a pan-hysterectomy (total abdominal hysterectomy with bilateral salpingo-oophorectomy) with resection of as much tumour bulk as possible should be performed. Omentectomy is also carried out as both a diagnostic procedure in early stage disease and for therapeutic reasons, when macroscopic metastases are evident. Selective sampling of any suspicious lymph nodes in either the para-aortic or pelvic regions is important for a complete assessment.

Radiotherapy

Analysis of postoperative radiotherapy is difficult due to variability in dosage and types of radiotherapy employed (Phelps & Chapman 1974). Widespread disease does not benefit from abdominal or pelvic radiotherapy. Morbidity from small bowel and adjacent tissue damage may be considerable. In early stage disease, however, intraperitoneal radioactive phosphorus (^{32}P) may have a role if no residual disease remains macroscopically. The use of postoperative pelvic irradiation does not improve survival in early stage disease (Roberts & Lifshitz 1982).

Chemotherapy

A logical adjuvant to surgery is the use of chemotherapy (Peters et al. 1989). Most large centres recommended treatment along the lines of ovarian cancer, either using single alkylating agents (Boronow 1973) or combination therapy (Deppe et al. 1980; Harrison et al. 1989). Progestogens have also been added but not with any clear evidence of value. The majority of reports encourage the use of either single agent platinum or combinations especially platinum, doxorubicin or cyclophosphamide.

Sarcomas

These are extremely rare and occur in adolescence as well as the elderly. Primary surgery followed by chemotherapy consisting of either doxorubicin or ifosfamide may be appropriate.

Choriocarcinoma

These may follow as a consequence of trophoblastic disease arising within an ectopic pregnancy. Management following diagnosis would proceed as with the intrauterine disease.

Prognosis

The stage of disease at the time of diagnosis is the most important factor regarding prognosis of fallopian tube cancer. Of the four stages, stage I has a 60% 5-year survival, stage II 25%, stage III 10% and stage IV 5%. The histological grade and differentiation of the tumour also have a bearing on survival. Those with a grade I or papillary tumour have a 34% 5-year survival. Those with papillary alveolar tumours have a 35% 5-year survival and those with an alveolar medullary tumour a 24% chance of survival (Green & Scully 1962).

Conclusion

This unusual tumour should be considered when patients present with symptoms of gynaecological pathology that cannot be easily explained. Once diagnosed a logical approach is to undertake surgical extirpation and then to follow this with appropriate chemotherapy. This would now consist of an alkylating agent such as melphalan or chlorambucil or a combination regimen including a platinum compound (cisplatin or an analogue such as JM8). Close follow up may be helped by second look reassessment if therapeutic options for treatment remain feasible.

References

Axelrod J.H., Herbold D.R., Freel J.H. & Palmer S.M. (1988) Exfoliative dermatitis; presenting sign of fallopian tube carcinoma. *Obstet. Gynecol.*, **71** (6:2), 1045–47.

Boronow E.C. (1973) Chemotherapy for disseminated tubal cancer. *Obstet. Gynecol.*, **42**, 62.

Deppe G., Brucknar H.W. & Cohen C.J. (1980) Combination chemotherapy for advanced carcinoma of the fallopian tube. *Obstet. Gynecol.*, **56**, 530.

Eddy G.L., Copeland L.J., Gershenson D.M., Atkinson E.N., Wharton J.T. & Rutledge F.N. (1984) Fallopian tube carcinoma. *Obstet. Gynecol.*, **64** (4), 546–52.

Fogh I. (1969) Primary carcinoma of the fallopian tube. *Cancer*, **23**, 1332.

Green T.H. & Scully R.E. (1962) Tumours of the fallopian tube. *Clin. Obstet. Gynaecol.*, **5**, 886.

Harrison C.R., Averette H.E., Jarrell M.A., Penalver M.A., Donato D. & Sevin B.U. (1989) Carcinoma of the fallopian tube; clinical management. *Gynecol. Oncol.*, **32** (3), 331–35.

Hu C.Y., Taymor M.L. & Hertig A.T. (1950) Primary carcinoma of the fallopian tube. *Am. J. Obstet. Gynecol.*, **50**, 58.

McGoldrick J.C., Strauss H. & Rao J. (1945) Primary carcinoma of the fallopian tube. *Am. J. Surg.*, **59**, 559.

Peters W.A., Anderson W. & Hopkins M.P. (1989) Results of chemotherapy in advanced carcinoma of the fallopian tube. *Cancer*, **63** (5), 836–38.

Phelps H.M. & Chapman K.E. (1974) Role of radiation therapy in treatment of primary carcinoma of the fallopian tube. *Obstet. Gynecol.*, **43**, 669.

Roberts J.A. & Lifshitz (1982) Primary adenocarcinoma of the fallopian tube. *Gynecol. Oncol.*, **13**, 301.

Sedlis A. (1961) Primary carcinoma of the fallopian tube. *Obstet. Gynecol. Surv.*, **16**, 209.

Yoonessi M. (1979) Carcinoma of the fallopian tube. *Obstet. Gynecol. Surv.*, **34**, 257.

12

Chemotherapy of Ovarian Cancer

EVE WILTSHAW

In 1983 there were over 4500 new cases of ovarian cancer in England and Wales, making it the most common malignancy of the genital tract. During the last 70 years the death rate has doubled while deaths from other female genital tract tumours have fallen. Attempts to screen patients for ovarian cancer are still in their infancy and methods of prevention are little understood, thus we must continue to hope that treatment will improve the outcome in this challenging group of patients.

Treatment programmes have lengthened short term survival in patients who still tend to present late in the course of their disease (stage III is commonest) and cure seems as far away as it was 20 years ago. At the same time management has become more complex and therapeutic morbidity has risen. It is important, therefore, that therapists are aware of what can be achieved and what cannot. They must also have knowledge of the best use of drugs to produce the best ratio of efficacy to morbidity. Treatment must be tailored to the individual, bearing in mind all the circumstances of her disease, other clinical problems she may have and her overall life expectancy as well as her own wishes. Overtreatment for the sake of 'trying to do something' should be resisted, for although this may make the physician/surgeon and relatives feel better cytotoxic drugs are too dangerous and too unpleasant to give virtually as a placebo. It is also important not to undertreat because whatever benefits chemotherapy has to offer may be lost while the patient is exposed to inadequate therapy. Good management is a fine balance of multiple judgements of what will be of greatest benefit in a particular case.

This chapter offers guidance only on the medical management of various ovarian malignancies but in all cases the best management is likely to be given by the specialist rather than the enthusiastic amateur. The details of individual care cannot be conveyed in a few pages. Ask yourself who you would like to treat you or your wife in the circumstances that your patient finds herself in and how would you want to be treated, if at all.

Epithelial ovarian cancer

Stage I

The primary treatment for stage I ovarian epithelial carcinoma is surgical removal of the involved ovary; usually bilateral salpingo-oophorectomy and hysterectomy are advocated. Indeed surgery is the only modality which has proven value in terms of cure. For stage Ia, Ib grade I tumours most surgeons now believe that unilateral oophorectomy is sufficient particularly in young women who wish to bear children, although many advocate removal of the remaining ovary and uterus when childbearing is completed. In these very early cases postoperative treatment is not indicated and 100% 5-year survival is to be expected. Nevertheless, long term follow up should be undertaken including repeated pelvic examination, CA 125, ultrasound and perhaps CT scanning.

For patients with higher grade tumours and all stage Ic cases most clinicians recommend postoperative treatment of some kind. Unfortunately data to support the use of postoperative treatment are still lacking. Such a study would probably require at least 600 patients in each arm and primary surgical staging would have to be uniform. In the meantime, most patients are given either abdominopelvic radiotherapy, oral melphalan or, in a few centres, cisplatin alone or in some combination. All these treatments have toxicities both short and long term, including the risk of a second malignancy (melphalan), bowel damage (radiotherapy) and renal damage or long standing neuropathy (cisplatin). These risks must be taken into account when deciding on postoperative treatment for any stage I case. This is especially important in the absence of positive evidence of long term benefit for any of the treatments advocated. Indeed, one retrospective analysis of 656 patients with early stage disease entered into prospective clinical trials showed no benefit for postoperative therapy (Guthrie et al. 1983). In our own hospital patients with stage Ia−Ic, grade I−III ovarian carcinoma have been given no postoperative therapy since 1979. So far there has been no apparent detriment as a result of the policy and survival at 5 years is 91%, disease free survival 79% (Fig. 12.1) (Wiltshaw et al. 1987). These figures compare well with the world literature where postoperative treatment is given with melphalan or abdomino-pelvic radiotherapy. It is important to note that there were no tumours of low malignant potential (borderline) in this series. However, this watch and wait policy cannot improve the survival of stage I ovarian cancer patients and the question remains: can chemotherapy at relapse still be curative?

In a summary of several US trials in 'early ovarian cancer' Piver (1989) concluded that since cisplatin is the most effective agent in late stage ovarian cancer it should be used in early stage disease 'except those not needing treatment, completely staged with stage Ia, Ib with gI or gII tumours'. This author believes that if chemotherapy is chosen for a stage I case postoperatively then cisplatin should be given at 100 mg/m^2 for a total of five courses at monthly intervals.

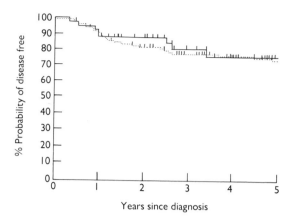

Fig. 12.1. Five-year survival of stage Ia– Ic cases without postoperative treatment (——, n=44) compared to similar cases given postoperative treatment with abdominopelvic radiotherapy or pelvic radiotherapy plus chlorambucil (· · · · ·, n=113) over the years 1979–84 at the Royal Marsden Hospital.

Patients at greatest risk of recurrence usually have poorly differentiated tumours and/or tumours with a mesonephroid histology.

Stages II, III and IV

Once an ovarian cancer has spread postoperative treatment is essential. Relative survival figures in the USA even at 5 years show that while 85% of stage I cases are alive this figure drops to 58% for stage II and to 20% for stages III and IV combined (Sondik *et al.* 1985).

The most common sites for initial spread of tumour are pelvic and abdominal peritoneal surfaces especially the paracolic gutters and undersurface of the diaphragm. Omental appendiceal and mesenteric deposits are also common. Initially nodal disease is para-aortic and pelvic, with occasional inguinal and supraclavicular node involvement. It is believed that clinical ascites is caused by tumour tissue blocking lymphatic channels draining the peritoneum but the cause of the frequently seen pleural effusion especially on the right is less clear. Later or with more aggressive tumours parenchymal liver deposits develop and more rarely brain and even bone metastases have been reported.

Survival of patients appears to be dependent on the following.

1 The operability of the tumour at initial surgery—that is, can the surgeon remove all visible tumour without endangering life? This is more a measure of the expertise and tenacity of the surgeon, rather than the infiltrative qualities of the tumour.

2 The presence of larger masses, peritoneal deposits and ascites at first surgery or, to put it another way, the total tumour burden at diagnosis (Heintz *et al.* 1988).

3 The sensitivity of the tumour to cytotoxic chemotherapy. It is probable that only 60–70% of tumours are sensitive to currently available anticancer drugs and it is also apparent that with time the majority of those develop resistance— what is less certain is which are the best drugs or combination of drugs to be used.

There have been a plethora of studies in recent years comparing one chemotherapy cocktail with another and arguments as to whether combinations are essential for best results or indeed whether single agent treatment with melphalan or chlorambucil is sufficient for initial therapy.

Studies prior to the advent of cisplatin showed that oral alkylating agents such as chlorambucil (Wiltshaw 1965) and melphalan (Omura et al. 1983) did produce responses in patients with overt disease of about 40% with up to 15% complete responses (CR). However, these responses were short lived (median 7 months) and when no useful second line agent was available 50% of stage III and IV patients were dead within 13 months and few survived 3 years. More recently, studies have been more difficult to interpret since virtually all patients failing to respond, or relapsing after alkylating agent therapy, have then been given cisplatin with the probability of further response in up to 50% of them.

This phenomenon was clearly demonstrated by Lambert & Berry (1985) in a comparative study of cisplatin versus cyclophosphamide where all patients failing on cyclophosphamide were changed to cisplatin. This study showed a better initial response rate for cisplatin and longer disease free survival but overall survivals were similar due to salvage by second line cisplatin therapy in relapsed cases initially given cyclophosphamide. Thus in comparing single agent or combination therapy it is best to look at the survival up to the point when relapse or second treatment was offered.

What seems to be emerging is that of the single agents cisplatin is clearly the most active, this activity being dependent on dose (Wiltshaw et al. 1986) and dose intensity (Levin & Hryniuk 1987).

Nevertheless, combination chemotherapy remains popular especially in the USA. This popularity is based on the success of combination chemotherapy in Hodgkin's disease, lymphoma and leukaemia and on the theory put forward by Goldie & Coldman (1979) that most mammalian cells start with intrinsic sensitivity to anticancer drugs but develop spontaneous resistance at a variable rate. The theory implies that single agent therapy is likely to fail rapidly because of the emergent resistant clones, but that the use of multiple agents will reduce the likelihood of these clones surviving. Fortunately in recent years a series of trials have been done to test whether combination chemotherapy, including the most popular agents, are of greater benefit than single agent cisplatin.

The first important study showed that the combination known as hexa-CAF (hexamethylmelamine, cyclophosphamide, adriamycin and 5-fluorouracil) was less effective than CHAP-5 (cyclophosphamide, hexamethylmelamine, adriamycin and cisplatin given over 5 days) both in terms of complete remission rate (79% vs. 50%) and prolonged progression free survival (19.5 months vs. 6.8 months). Indeed in this study the overall survival was also better, CHAP-5 attaining a median of 26.1 months and hexa-CAF 19.6 months (Neijt et al. 1984).

The next interesting study came from Italy comparing cyclophosphamide, adriamycin and cisplatin (CAP) with cyclophosphamide and cisplatin (CP) and cisplatin alone (P). The complete response rates were 26%, 20% and 20%, respectively, at second look operation but there was no significant difference in disease free or overall survival. It should be noted that doses of cisplatin were the same in each arm of the study (Gruppo 1987).

Following on from these studies the Dutch compared the CHAP regimen with cisplatin and cyclophosphamide (PC) and found that the response rates and survival were similar (Neijt *et al.* 1985), and finally there have been several studies showing lack of additional benefit from doxorubicin (Barker & Wiltshaw 1981; Omura *et al.* 1983) in randomized trials.

The favoured regimen now in the USA appears to be a combination of cisplatin and cyclophosphamide (CP) while in the UK it is believed that single agent cisplatin given at a dose of 100 mg/m^2 is comparable with the CP regimen where 50–75 mg is given together with cyclophosphamide 500–1000 mg/m^2 (Table 12.1).

Whichever regimen is chosen, if it contains cisplatin then certain unpleasant side effects and toxicities are to be expected, including nausea and vomiting with diarrhoea in some cases; renal toxicity; ototoxicity including tinnitus and high tone hearing loss and neuropathy. If cisplatin 100 mg/m^2 is given then five courses at monthly intervals are recommended if serious neuropathy and renal damage are to be avoided. It is also necessary to give intravenous hydration before and after the cisplatin and to maintain a good fluid excretion of drug, if necessary by the addition of mannitol.

Because of the severe, often irreversible, toxicities for cisplatin other platinum analogues have been developed in an attempt to reduce the morbidity of treatment. The best of those tested so far is carboplatin (JM8) and the drug is now on the market in Europe and recently has been approved by the FDA for sale in the USA as a 'second line therapy' in ovarian cancer. Studies have shown that carboplatin is active in ovarian cancer after tumours have already responded to cisplatin (Evans *et al.* 1983) and that toxicity is minimal except for nausea and vomiting and thrombocytopenia at doses of 300–400 mg/m^2 (Table 12.2). Studies have also shown that carboplatin can be used with other drugs with some

Table 12.1. Recommended chemotherapy regimens for stage II–IV epithelial ovarian cancer

Cisplatin	100 mg/m^2 i.v. bolus with 24-hour pre- and post-i.v. hydration with normal saline + 20% KCl every 4 weeks for five courses
Carboplatin	400 mg/m^2 i.v. in 200 ml of 5% dextrose over 30 min every 4 weeks for six courses (AUC 4–5 is approximately equivalent to 400 mg/m^2 in the average woman with GFR 70–100 ml/min)
Cisplatin + cyclophosphamide	Cisplatin 75 mg/m^2 i.v. bolus with 24-hour pre- and post-i.v. hydration with normal saline + 20% KCl *plus* Cyclophosphamide 600 mg/m^2 i.v. bolus Both to be given on day 1 and repeated every 4 weeks for six courses

Table 12.2. Toxicity comparison between cisplatin 100 mg/m^2 and carboplatin 400 mg/m^2

Toxicity	Carboplatin	Cisplatin
Nausea and vomiting	++	+++
Leucocytes	+	±
Platelets	+++	±
Transfusion requirements	++	++
Fall in EDTA clearance	±	+++
Audiographic hearing loss	−ˎ	+++
Neuropathy	−	++
Alopecia	±	±

activity in ovarian cancer. A summary of these and other similar studies are reported in Multimodal Treatment of Ovarian Cancer (Piver 1989).

In summary, the best therapy for ovarian cancer patients with stage II to IV disease is with a platinum-based compound. If combination chemotherapy is preferred then additional cyclophosphamide is the drug of choice. In choosing the appropriate platinum compound for first line therapy the best drug is undoubtedly carboplatin, but the present cost of this compound has deterred many from choosing it in all cases.

Table 12.1 shows recommended regimens and it should be noted that whereas cisplatin is toxic to the kidneys its toxicity does not depend on renal function. On the other hand carboplatin toxicity does depend on its efficient excretion although the drug itself is rarely renally toxic. It is important that in all future studies carboplatin dose should be based on renal clearance rather than on mg/m^2 and in this regard EDTA clearance is much more accurate than creatinine clearance. Indeed if cisplatin has been given, creatinine clearance will not accurately measure glomerular filtration rate especially in those patients who have experienced major weight loss (Daugaard et al. 1988).

The dose of carboplatin given on the basis of glomerular filtration rate (GFR) can be easily calculated using the formula dose in mg = AUC factor × (GFR + 25) (Calvert et al. 1989).

When the area under the curve (AUC) is equal in all patients the toxicities are predictable and efficacy more accurately defined.

Length of chemotherapy and long term results

There is increasing evidence that continuing chemotherapy longer than 6 months is of little avail although there are no prospective randomized studies to prove this. One recent report compared patients treated with PAC for six or nine courses and the chosen length of treatment was on the basis of at which centre they were treated. However, the cases seemed to be reasonably comparable and second looks were performed on 21/39 after six courses and 15/41 after nine courses. There was gross residual disease in 67% and 53%, respectively, and microscopic disease in 33% and 47%. There was no statistical difference between the two groups in this regard nor in terms of survival (Watring *et al.* 1989).

While longer term chemotherapy is probably not indicated many workers have attempted to prolong disease free survival in responding patients (i.e. those who at second look operation have no residual or minimal residual disease) by giving alternative treatment. The majority of reporters have used whole abdominal and pelvic radiotherapy or intraperitoneal radioisotopes but none have shown useful benefits, although increased morbidity is to be expected.

Another attempt to improve survival by the use of BCG together with chemotherapy also failed to improve survival even in responding tumours (Alberts *et al.* 1989).

It is perhaps not surprising that 6 months treatment with cytotoxic drugs will not cure patients with a large load of tumour such as is present in many stage III and IV cases but, unfortunately, present data suggest that death from later stage disease continues exponentially and that cure by drugs remains a rarity. One study has followed all patients to death or for 10 years, and of 56 patients, all given PAC therapy and prospectively followed, the survival and disease free survival were 32% and 18% at 5 years; this had dropped to 9% and 7% by 10 years follow up. The authors conclude that the rate of relapse decreases at 5 years but does not cease and cure does not seem likely (Sutton *et al.* 1989). A similar result was seen in a retrospective review of 429 patients with stage III and IV disease entered into single agent and combination chemotherapy trials by Wharton *et al.* (1984). Survival for the single agent series was 19% at 4 years. The combination chemotherapy patients had a 31% 4-year survival. In this series only 22/236 patients had cisplatin as a single agent and only 46/159 contained cisplatin in a combination scheme as first line therapy. There are, as yet, no data on survival for stage II patients given platinum based chemotherapy but oral melphalan does not appear to improve survival.

Second line treatment

Second line treatment is usually tried in two situations:
1 When the tumour proves resistant to initial chemotherapy.
2 When the tumour relapses after partial or complete response to first line drugs.

In this situation many new and old drugs have been tested for their usefulness. Unfortunately there are no orthodox or new drugs which will produce regular responses in cases resistant to initial platinum compound chemotherapy, although in a large retrospective study in the Royal Marsden Hospital we found that 8% of cases would respond to an analogue (Gore *et al.* 1989). Alkylating agents are useless here as well as combinations of drugs such as hexa-CAF. Indeed this is a situation where experimental treatment should be tried as soon as resistance is established.

Where patients have already responded and later relapsed from chemotherapy second options are available. These are to give a platinum compound again and in this situation cisplatin 100 mg/m^2 or carboplatin 400 mg/m^2 (or its equivalent based on AUC) will produce a response rate between 30−60% depending on the length of the initial remission. The longer that remission the greater the chance of a further response (Gore et al. 1990).

Another possible approach is to try hexamethylmelamine (HMM). This drug, which has doubtful additional effect in combination chemotherapy, has been looked at again recently as a single agent. Manetta et al. (1989) report that of 52 patients treated 50 had already received cisplatin. Nevertheless they noted a 15% CR rate which is very encouraging, and indicated that at a dose of 400 mg orally on a daily basis for 14 days every month the drug was well tolerated. This result needs confirmation.

Assessment of response and benefits

When treating patients it is essential to carefully monitor whether they are benefiting from therapy both in terms of symptomatic relief or regression of tumour, and today there are many ways of looking at this. First, the patient should be listened to regarding symptoms due to disease and symptoms due to toxicity and an assessment of their physical quality of life should be made. This is usually called performance status, and although a very crude estimate of quality of life, it is one of the most important factors in measuring the usefulness of therapy against its morbidity (Table 12.3). It is essential to also enquire about side effects of treatment and to record them in some detail.

Measures for assessment of regression of tumour are CA 125 blood levels, ultrasound, particularly of the pelvis, and computed tomography of the abdomen and pelvis. CA 125 measurements in patients with high levels when treatment

Table 12.3. WHO performance status

Grade	Performance status
0	Able to carry out all normal activity without restriction
1	Restricted in physically strenuous activity but ambulatory and able to carry out light work
2	Ambulatory and capable of all self-care but unable to carry out any work; up and about more than 50% of waking hours
3	Capable of only limited self-care; confined to bed or chair more than 50% of waking hours
4	Completely disabled; cannot carry out any self-care; totally confined to bed or chair

begins are a very good guide to tumour regression and, indeed, to prognosis. If the CA 125 level falls to T1/2 at <20 days then the prognosis is much better than if that T1/2 is longer than 20 days (Fig. 12.2) (Van der Burg *et al.* 1988). If CA 125 rises on therapy then treatment should be changed or abandoned, since although a fall in levels to normal does not always correlate with complete clinical or surgical regression, a rising or steady level of CA 125 is always associated with the presence of resistant tumour.

Ultrasound and CT scans are also helpful in measuring response or recurrence of tumour but tests must always be used for the benefit of patients and by this it is meant that if a positive test cannot be followed by useful treatment, then tests for the sake of information alone may well increase anxiety to no good purpose.

Second look operation (SLO) has been very popular in recent years and is still the most accurate measure of the degree of regression of tumour. Unfortunately, since further therapy after SLO has not proved useful so far and since even pathologically documented CR is not indicative of cure it is only of value in the research setting where new treatments can be tried after orthodox treatment has failed.

Intraperitoneal therapy

While intraperitoneal (IP) radioactive isotope therapy has been popular intermittently for the last 25 years it is only recently that IP chemotherapy has been actively pursued. Studies usually take the form of experimental treatments after initial partial response to systemic treatment and various cytotoxic drugs have been used, especially high doses of cisplatin and adriamycin and lower relative doses of melphalan and bleomycin, as well as combinations of drugs. A Tenchkoff catheter or Port-a-cath is usually put in place during second surgery and the drugs then instilled on a once-a-month basis leaving the catheter in place.

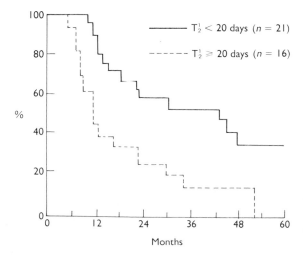

Fig. 12.2. Survival related to the rate of fall of CA 125 blood levels (Van der Burg *et al., Gynecol. Oncol.*, **30**, 307 (1988) with kind permission).

Undoubtedly there have been some regressions with these treatments, particularly those patients who started with small nodules (<2 mm disease), but there have also been problems including deaths from myelosuppression, septicaemia and bowel perforation.

Another theoretically interesting approach is the use of radioactive ^{131}I labelled monoclonal antibodies but so far results have been rather disappointing probably because the antibodies may be less specific than is necessary for effective targeting. Lastly, biological response modifiers such as interferon, interleukins and tumour necrosis factor have all been tried in this context.

All these approaches remain experimental and should only be undertaken as part of a scientific study. So far there are no comparative studies and no evidence for prolongation of survival. These treatments are not suitable for patients with more than tiny nodules of tumour.

High dose chemotherapy

Because of the relatively effective chemotherapy of ovarian cancer with cytotoxic drugs, the failure to show the kind of increased survival and cures seen in some more sensitive tumours (e.g. germ cell tumours and some haematological malignancies), together with the theory that the log cell kill for most drugs is based on dose, and lastly that in many studies dose intensity (i.e. drug delivered/time) is important to best results, some researchers have become increasingly interested in giving exceptionally high doses of single or multiple drugs. This high dose therapy is sometimes associated with autologous bone marrow infusion in an attempt to reduce the severe myelosuppressive effects.

Ozols *et al.* (1985) reported that with the use of very high dose cisplatin, 40 mg/m^2 daily for 5 days, a 32% response rate was seen in 19 patients; in 1987 the same authors reported that of 30 patients treated with carboplatin (800 mg/m^2) every 35 days, 27% responded. Unfortunately no patient whose tumour was resistant to initial orthodox chemotherapy had a remission. It is also disappointing to note that a response rate of 30% for patients relapsing after cisplatin based treatment is no higher than would be expected with 100 mg/m^2 or carboplatin at 400 mg/m^2. This suggests that resistance is not overcome by relatively small changes in peak blood levels of the platinum compounds.

Our own studies using carboplatin at 1000 mg/m^2 show that even in chemotherapy naïve cases (FIGO stage IV) the response rate is no higher than would be expected for the conventional doses (approximately 60%), although the number of clinically complete responders is increased from 10—15% in historical controls to 30% with high doses (unpublished data)

Should these kind of studies prove of lasting value to patients with very large amounts of tumour then very high doses of drugs should be tested in earlier stage disease (FIGO II and stage III minimal residual disease) if cures are to be achieved.

postoperative combination chemotherapy (Gershenson & Silva 1989). The recommendation is based on a retrospective look at 82 patients treated between 1956 and 1985 with a variety of chemotherapy. While the overall survival of patients was excellent (median >120 months), the authors claim that the 5-year survival of patients on combination chemotherapy of '94% is significantly better ($P = 0.01$) than 87% for those who had single agent chemotherapy'. Bearing in mind the retrospective nature of the study and the fact that only 24 patients received combination treatment this recommendation should be viewed with caution at present. Indeed, the possible survival of these patients without chemotherapy cannot be judged in this context.

In the present state of knowledge it is recommended that borderline cases stage II–IV should be followed closely, without therapy, using every possible clinical means of assessing tumour growth so that more can be learned about the natural history. In the event of symptomatic or progressive disease then cytotoxic drugs may be used although no particular agent or agents can be recommended, and especially careful monitoring of tumour size should continue and results be reported in the literature. No patient with borderline tumour should be entered into studies of frank ovarian epithelial carcinoma.

Germ cell tumours

Germ cell tumours constitute about 5% of all ovarian malignancies in Western countries and about 15% in oriental and black societies. However, they are a very important group in that about 70% of them occur in females under the age of 30 years. Their importance has increased greatly over the last 10 years since the use of combination chemotherapy has been followed by a dramatic change in survival. The success of present day therapy has been associated also with a reduction in surgical excision so that many young patients may expect to retain fertility as well as expect cure.

Investigation and staging

Any young woman presenting with a palpable adnexal mass should be investigated carefully with ultrasound because if the lesion is solid or a mixture of solid and cystic components then a neoplasm is likely and malignancy possible. Indeed adnexal masses >2 cm in diameter in premenarchal females or greater than 8 cm in premenopausal women probably all require surgical exploration. In a young woman further investigation is advisable; in particular a blood sample should be taken to measure AFP and β-hCG levels which are frequently raised in germ cell tumours. Ultrasound and computed tomography can also greatly help in assessing the extent of tumour in the abdominopelvic cavity as well as showing small amounts of ascitic fluid, pelvic and para-aortic lymphadenopathy and liver parenchymal metastases.

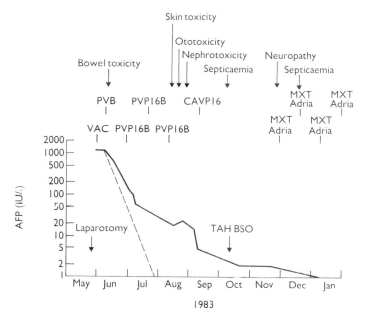

Fig. 12.3. Graph showing the intensity of chemotherapy sometimes required to produce a complete remission of tumour in a case of germ cell tumour of the ovary (stage III). (——), level of AFP; (· · ·), fall of AFP at the rate of half-life = 5 days. The figure also shows the toxicities engendered by chemotherapy. This patient remains well and in complete remission.

Provided that the patient is fit enough it is essential for accurate diagnosis and staging to proceed to laparotomy and a midline adequate incision should be made. The extent of tumour and a histological diagnosis can thus be made by removal of the tumour bearing ovary and biopsy of any other involved area. If no obvious tumour is seen outside the ovary an omentectomy and several biopsies of peritoneum should be performed as for epithelial ovarian cancer. Even if there is quite extensive metastic spread, however, there is no evidence that extensive surgery is beneficial and it is very important to leave the other ovary and uterus intact if possible, so that childbearing potential is retained. In cases of stage I disease surgical excision other than a unilateral oophorectomy and biopsy of the other ovary should not be performed.

Postoperative therapy

Dysgerminoma is the only germ cell tumour where radiotherapy can be curative, but recently doubts have been raised as to whether it should be abandoned in favour of chemotherapy on the basis that cure is as good with drugs and the toxicity of treatment is less. For stage I dysgerminoma surgery is often curative although second tumours do arise in the other ovary (about 15%) and some arise in a gonadoblastoma, a benign tumour seen in phenotypic females with abnormal

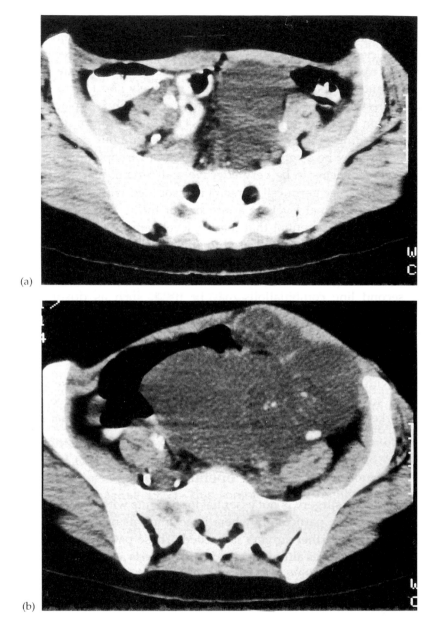

Fig. 12.4. (a) CT scan of the pelvis showing a rapid growth in size of a metastatic germ cell mass while the patient underwent chemotherapy. During this time the AFP fell to normal and the patient was well. (b) At laparotomy in June 1988 the mass was removed intact and showed only well differentiated teratomatous elements, but part of the colon which was also involved in the mass had to be excised.

Now cure rates approaching 100% are achievable in stage I germ cell tumours of all histologies and in stage II or more disease cures of up to 80% are now being reported though the prognosis is less good for the older patient (over 30 years) and for patients with high levels of AFP (>500 IU/l) or β-hCG (>50 000 IU/l) (Figs 12.5, 12.6).

Fertility

There are now several reports of successful pregnancies after completion of chemotherapy. The first normal pregnancy following chemotherapy was reported by Duncan & Young (1980) and in the author's series two normal pregnancies have occurred. One of these patients conceived only 2 months after stopping cytotoxic drugs. Recently a large series of germ cell tumours were reported by Bianchi et al. (1989), of which 61/80 had conservative surgery, and five patients have attempted pregnancy following PVB therapy, four being successful.

Carcinoid, struma ovarii, gonadoblastoma

Carcinoids rarely occur in the ovary, are usually unilateral and only a very few have been known to metastasize. Thus the treatment of choice is unilateral salpingo-oophorectomy only.

Struma ovarii also is a rare tumour; less than 5% are malignant. It usually presents as stage I disease and unilateral salpingo-oophorectomy is recommended for younger patients. The effect of chemotherapy on metastatic disease is not yet established.

Gonadoblastoma usually arises in a phenotypic female who has a male 46XY karyotype or a mosaic (45XY/46XY). Their malignant potential results from an overgrowth of the germ cell element, usually a dysgerminoma, but occasionally

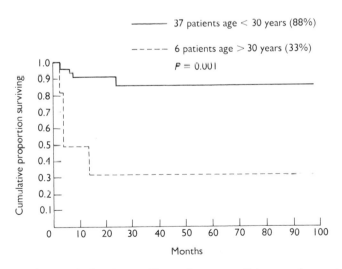

Fig. 12.5. Analysis of survival of patients with ovarian germ cell tumours by age > or <30 years (1977–86) (Newlands et al. (1988), In Williams et al. (eds), Textbook of Uncommon Cancer. Wiley, Chichester, with kind permission).

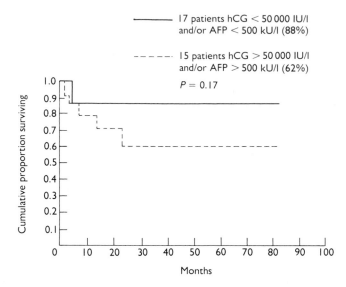

Fig. 12.6. Analysis of survival of patients with ovarian germ cell tumours by the initial serum concentration of human chorionic gonadotrophin (hCG) and alphafetoprotein (AFP) (1979–86) (Newlands *et al.* (1988), *In* Williams *et al.* (eds), *Textbook of Uncommon Cancer.* Wiley, Chichester, with kind permission).

endodermal sinus or other germ cell tumours may be found. Since they arise in abnormal gonads both should be removed and if a malignant germ cell tumour is present adjuvant chemotherapy should then be given.

Dermoid cyst with squamous carcinoma

Very occasionally a dermoid cyst shows partial conversion to carcinoma. The malignancy is usually of squamous type and there is some evidence that these arise from epidermal tissue (Ribeiro *et al.* 1988).

The tumours are highly malignant and rapidly recur despite radical surgery. With recurrence there is frequently an associated hypercalcaemia of uncertain aetiology. The author has recently attempted to treat recurrent disease with the PVB regimen but with no effect. All the patients died within 17 months of diagnosis although some stage I patients in the literature do apparently survive the disease; cure seems likely if the patient has no evidence of recurrence more than 2 years after diagnosis (Ribeiro *et al.* 1988).

Other rare malignant tumours

Granulosa cell tumour

Confusion over the management of this rare tumour arises because, in general, its malignant potential is relatively low and recurrence may occur a long time after initial diagnosis (Norris & Taylor 1968; Stenwig *et al.* 1979). Over a 20-year period about 20% recur and most of these patients die of their disease.

It is important to distinguish between the juvenile and adult types, especially in management terms, since the juvenile type almost always presents as stage I and in patients less than 30 years old. Late recurrences have not been recorded but the tumour does occasionally occur in both gonads (about 3%). Thus after surgery no further treatment is required.

In the adult form of the disease many present with stage I disease (50–90% in larger series) but recurrences up to >20 years later have been reported. Prognosis is affected by the stage at presentation as well as the size of tumour. In one series tumours larger than 15 cm had a 53% 10-year survival and 100% for tumours which were 15 cm or less (Fox *et al.* 1975). This was confirmed by Bjorkholm & Silversward (1981) where in stage I cases there was a 4% mortality for tumours of less than 5 cm and 20% in tumours of 5 cm or more. On the basis of these data postoperative therapy may be considered reasonable in granulosa cell tumours with this poor prognostic factor. Unfortunately there is, as yet, no firm information on which to base a reasonable management plan. Patients with overt disease do respond well to radiotherapy but are not cured even by adjuvant abdomino pelvic radiotherapy; similarly, response to chemotherapy is frequently seen but most are short lived and the optimal choice of drugs is not yet defined.

A review of the literature suggests that the best agents are cisplatin and an alkylating agent such as cyclophosphamide and possibly doxorubicin. Recently the EORTC has reported on a phase II study of combination chemotherapy using cisplatin, vinblastine and bleomycin in recurrent granulosa cell tumour. Of 32 patients entered only 13 are fully evaluable but 12/13 responded with 7 CRs. Toxicity has been severe but six patients are disease free at between 8 and 47 months (Pecorelli *et al.* 1989).

An excellent review of the present position of this tumour and its management has been made by Malkasian (1988).

Sertoli–Leydig cell tumours

It seems that pure Sertoli cell tumours are benign and cured by oophorectomy and Leydig cell tumours are similarly curable in the majority of cases. However, rarely these and the mixed tumours may metastasize and prove fatal in just 2 years. Poorer prognosis is associated with a high mitotic rate (>10 mitoses/10 HPF) and at recurrence palliative therapy may be useful, but the chemotherapy of choice is uncertain, there being anecdotal reports of response to the VAC regimen and to PEB.

Sarcomas

Rarely a mixed Müllerian tumour of the ovary is diagnosed; such tumours have an even worse prognosis than similar lesions arising in the uterus. About 50% of patients are dead within 6 months and very few patients with more than stage I disease survive longer than a year. There is some indirect evidence that postoperative radiotherapy may reduce local recurrence but does not affect survival, so an effective chemotherapy regimen is essential to improving prognosis. In this regard the rarity of the tumour has been a handicap to advancement but a few relatively large series suggest that doxorubicin alone is of little benefit (Morrow *et al.* 1986) and that VAC given with radiotherapy can produce good regressions but may be very toxic (Carlson *et al.* 1983). Most recently Plaxe *et al.* (1989) reported a series of 11 patients completing treatment with cisplatin 50 mg/m^2 plus doxorubicin 50 mg/m^2 'in addition to cyclophosphamide, etoposide and hexamethylmelamine'. Eight patients had a CR (73%). When the details of this study are published in full a proper trial of this combination may be needed.

Lymphoma

Primary lymphoma of the ovary is very rare although secondary involvement is not uncommon. Only in Birkett's lymphoma are primary bilateral tumours seen and this may be curable with intensive chemotherapy. For other lymphomatous tumours unilateral ovarian lymphoma may be cured by surgery but only if this is the solitary site of disease. When the diagnosis is made lymphography and bone marrow examination are essential to stage the case accurately and if tumour is found elsewhere chemotherapy appropriate to high grade lymphoma must be given. Cure may then be expected in the majority of cases. These patients should be treated by a medical oncologist with experience in the management of lymphomas and since chemotherapy in this area is continually improving the best current combination treatment can then be applied.

Small cell carcinoma

Dickersin *et al.* (1982) first defined this tumour histologically. They described 11 young women with the pathology and hypercalcaemia was noted in most of them postoperatively. They did not discuss therapy although they noted that the prognosis was uniformly bad. So far few new cases have been reported and none have responded to agents commonly used in ovarian cancer. These patients need to be treated urgently postoperatively with experimental drugs if we are to reverse their usual rapid downhill course.

Second tumours following chemotherapy

It has always been expected that cytotoxic drugs would prove carcinogenic and leukaemogenic if enough patients survived their original tumour for long periods. Until recently these figures were not available but now survival has improved for certain types of patients and second malignancies are being reported, particularly in patients treated for Hodgkin's disease and ovarian cancer. Some second tumours would be expected to arise spontaneously in such populations but the reported incidence suggests an added factor due to previous chemotherapy. This is particularly true of acute leukaemia, usually of the myelomonocytic type, which seems to occur two or more years after diagnosis and first chemotherapy. In ovarian cancer the risk has been estimated at 5 to 10% in any 10-year survivors following alkylating agent chemotherapy (Reimer 1982) and seems to occur most often following long term melphalan treatment (Greene *et al.* 1982), although other drugs (e.g. cyclophosphamide, busulphan, treosulfan and chlorambucil) have been implicated.

Other tumours which may develop after cytotoxic chemotherapy are bladder cancer (particularly after cyclophosphamide) (Schmahl *et al.* 1982); in the case of ovarian cancer there seems to be an increased risk of several different tumours and Reimer (1982) believes that some of these, including bladder cancer and lymphoma, were related to chemotherapy while others (endometrium, colon and breast) were not.

Long term effects of cisplatin in this regard are not yet known, but the risks of second tumours in good prognosis cases are probably best avoided by keeping alkylating agent therapy to a maximum of 9 months.

Fortunately, there seems to be no indication that other tumours or, indeed, acute leukaemia, are increased in young patients treated successfully for germ cell tumours.

References

Alberts D.S., Mason-Liddil N., O'Toble R.V. *et al.* (1989) Randomized phase III trial of chemoimmunotherapy in patients with previously untreated stages III and IV suboptimal disease ovarian cancer: a SWOG study. *Gynecol. Oncol.*, **32**, 8–15.

Aure J.C., Hoeg K. & Kolstad P. (1971) Clinical and histological studies of ovarian carcinoma: long term follow-up of 790 cases. *Obstet. Gynecol.*, **37**, 1–9.

Barker G. & Wiltshaw E. (1981) Randomised trial comparing low-dose cisplatin and chlorambucil with low dose cisplatin, chlorambucil and doxorubicin in advanced ovarian carcinoma. *Lancet*, **ii**, 747–50.

Bianchi U.A., Pecorelli S., Bini S. *et al.* (1989) Conservative treatment in non-epithelial ovarian cancer. Abstract No. 58, 20th Annual Meeting Soc. Gynecol. Oncol. in *Gynecol. Oncol.*, **32**, 108.

Bjorkholm E. & Silversward C. (1981) Prognostic factors in granulosa cell tumors. *Gynecol. Oncol.*, **11**, 261–74.

Calvert A.H., Newell D.R., Gumbrell L.A. *et al.* (1989) Carboplatin dosage: prospective valuation of a simple formula based on renal function. *J. Clin. Oncol.*, **7**, 1748–56.

Carlson J.A., Edwards C., Wharton J.T., Gallager H.S., Declos L. & Rutledge F. (1983) Mixed mesodermal sarcoma of the ovary. *Cancer*, **52**, 1473–77.

Chen K.T.K. & Flam M.S. (1986) Peritoneal papillary serous carcinoma with long term survival. *Cancer*, **58**, 1371–73.

Daugaard G., Rossing N. & Rorth M. (1988) Effects of cisplatin on different measures of glomerular function in the human kidney with special emphasis on high-dose. *Ca. Chemother. Pharmacol.*, **21**, 63–167.

Dickersin G.R., Kline I.W. & Scully R.E. (1982) Small cell carcinoma of the ovary with hypercalcemia. *Cancer*, **49**, 188–97.

Duncan I.D. & Young J.L. (1980) Endodermal sinus tumour of the ovary: serum AFP levels before and after treatment and during pregnancy. *Br. J. Obstet. Gynaecol.*, **87**, 535−38.

Einhorn L.H. & Donahue J. (1977) Cis-diammine dichloroplatinum, vinblastine & bleomycin combination chemotherapy in disseminated testicular cancer. *Ann. Int. Med.*, **87**, 293−98.

Evans B.D., Raju K.S., Calvert A.H., Harland S.J. & Wiltshaw E. (1983) Phase II study of JM8, a new platinum analog, in advanced ovarian carcinoma. *Ca. Treatment Rep.*, **67**, 997−1000.

Fox H., Agrawal K. & Langley F.A. (1975) A clinicopathological study of 92 cases of granulosa cell tumor of the ovary with special reference to the factors influencing prognosis. *Cancer*, **35**, 231−41.

Fox H. & Langley F.A. (1976) *Tumours of the Ovary*. Heinemann, London.

Fromm G., Gershenson D. & Silva E. (1989) Papillary serous carcinoma of the peritoneum. Abstract 119, 20th Annual Meeting of the Soc. Gynecol. Oncol. in *Gynecol. Oncol.*, **32**, 122.

Gerhadry R., Parmely L. & Woodruff J.D. (1977) The origin and clinical behaviour of ten paraovarian tumours. *Am. J. Obstet. Gynecol.*, **129**, 873−80.

Gershenson D. & Silva E. (1989) Metastatic serous ovarian tumors of low malignant potential. Abstract 145, 20th Annual Meeting Soc. Gynecol. Oncol. in *Gynecol. Oncol.*, **32**, 128.

Goldie J.H. & Coldman A.J. (1979) A mathematic model for relating the drug sensitivity of tumors to their spontaneous mutation rate. *Ca. Treatment Rep.*, **63**, 1727−33.

Gore M.E., Fryatt I., Wiltshaw E. & Dawson T. (1990) Treatment of relapsed carcinoma of the ovary with cisplatin or carboplatin following initial treatment with these compounds. *Gynecol. Oncol.*, **36**, 207−11.

Gore M.E., Wiltshaw E., Dawson T., Fryatt I.J. & Robinson B. (1987) Non-cross resistance between cisplatin and carboplatin in ovarian cancer. *Proc. Am. Soc. Clin. Oncol.*, **6**, A460.

Greene M.H., Boice J.D., Greer B.E. *et al.* (1982) Acute nonlymphocytic leukaemia after therapy with alkylating agents for ovarian cancer. *New Engl. J. Med.*, **307**, 1416−21.

Gruppo Interegionale Cooperative Oncologico Ginecologia (1987) Randomised comparison of cisplatin with cyclophosphamide/cisplatin and with cyclophosphamide/doxorubicin/cisplatin in advanced ovarian cancer. *Lancet*, **ii**, 353−59.

Guthrie D., Davey M.L.J. & Phillips P.R. (1983) Study of 656 patients with 'early' ovarian cancer. *Gynecol. Oncol.*, **17**, 363.

Hart W.R. & Norris H.J. (1973) Borderline and malignant mucinous tumours of the ovary: histologic criteria and clinical behaviour. *Cancer*, **31**, 1031−45.

Heintz A.P.M., Van Oosterom A.T., Baptist J., Trimbos M.C., Schaberg A., Van der Velde E.A. & Nooy M. (1988) The treatment of advanced ovarian carcinoma (I): clinical variables associated with prognosis. *Gynecol. Oncol.*, **30**, 347−58.

Hudson C.N. (1985) *Ovarian Cancer*. Oxford University Press, London.

Julian C.G. & Woodruff J.D. (1972) The biological behaviour of low-grade papillary serous carcinoma of the ovary. *Obstet. Gynecol.*, **40**, 860−67.

Katzenstein A.A., Mazur M.T., Morgan T.E. & Kao M. (1978) Proliferative serous tumors of the ovary: histologic features and prognosis. *Am. J. Surg. Pathol.*, **2**, 339−55.

Kliman L., Rome R.M. & Fortune D.W. (1986) Low malignant potential tumors of the ovary: a study of 76 cases. *Obstet. Gynecol.*, **68**, 338−44.

Lambert H.E. & Berry R.J. (1985) High dose cisplatin compared with high dose cyclophosphamide in the management of advanced epithelial ovarian cancer (FIGO stages III and IV). Report from the North West Thames Cooperative Group. *Br. Med. J.*, **290**, 889−93.

Levin L. & Hryniuk W.M. (1987) Dose intensity analysis of chemotherapy regimens in ovarian carcinoma. *J. Clin. Oncol.*, **5**, 756−67.

Malkasian G.D. (1988) Tumours of granulosa−theca cell derivation. *In*: C.J. Williams *et al.* (ed), *Textbook of Uncommon Cancer*. Wiley, Chichester.

Manetta C., MacNeill J., Lyter B. *et al.* (1989) Hexamethylmelamine (HMM) for advanced ovarian cancer. Abstract 1988, 20th Annual Meeting of the Soc. Gynecol. Oncol. in *Gynecol. Oncol.*, **32**, 115.

Morrow C.P., Bundy B.N., Hoffman J., Sutton G. & Homesley H. (1986) Adriamycin chemotherapy for malignant mixed mesodermal tumor of the ovary. *Am. J. Clin. Oncol.*, **9**, 24−26.

Neijt J.P., Bokkel Huinink W.W., Van der Burg M. *et al.* (1985) Combination chemotherapy with CHAP-5 and CP in advanced ovarian carcinoma: a randomized trial of the Netherlands joint study group for ovarian cancer. *Proc. Am. Soc. Clin. Oncol.*, **4**, C442.

Neijt J.P., Van der Burg M.E.L., Vriesendorp R., Van Lindert A.C.M., Van Lent M. *et al.* (1984) Randomized trial comparing two combination chemotherapy regimens (Hexa-CAF vs CHAP-5) in advanced ovarian carcinoma. *Lancet*, **ii**, 594–600.

Newlands E.S., Southall P.J., Paradinas F.J. & Holden L. (1988) Management of ovarian germ cell tumours. *In*: C.J. Williams *et al.* (ed), *Textbook of Uncommon Cancer*. Wiley, Chichester.

Nikrui N. (1981) Survey of clinical behaviour of patients with borderline epithelial tumors of the ovary. *Gynecol. Oncol.*, **12**, 107–19.

Norris H.J. & Taylor H.B. (1968) Prognosis of granulosa–theca tumors of the ovary. *Cancer*, **21**, 255–63.

Omura G.A., Morrow C.P., Blessing J.A., Miller A., Buchsbaum H.J., Holmesley H.D. & Leone L. (1983) A randomized comparison of melphalan versus melphalan plus hexamethylmelamine versus adriamycin plus cyclophosphamide in ovarian carcinoma. *Cancer*, **51**, 783–89.

Ozols R.F., Ostchega Y., Curt G. & Young R.C. (1987) High dose carboplatin in refractory ovarian cancer patients. *J. Clin. Oncol.*, **5**, 197–201.

Ozols R F., Ostchega Y., Myers C.E. *et al.* (1985) Cisplatin in hypertonic saline in refractory ovarian cancer. *J. Clin. Oncol.*, **3**, 1246–50.

Pecorelli S., Wagener C., Bonazzi C. *et al.* (1989) Cisplatin (P), vinblastine (V) and bleomycin (B) combination chemotherapy in recurrent or advanced granulosa cell tumor of the ovary (GCTO): an EORTC gynecology cancer cooperative group study. Abstract 68, 20th Annual Meeting of the Soc. Gynecol. Oncol. in *Gynecol. Oncol.*, **32**, 110.

Piver M.S. (1989) Multimodality treatment in early ovarian cancer: the US experience. *In*: Conte *et al.* (eds), *Multimodal Treatment of Ovarian Cancer*. New York, Raven Press.

Plaxe S., Dottino P., Goodman H., Deligdische L., Idelson M. & Cohen C. (1989) Treatment of advanced ovarian mixed mesodermal tumors with post operative doxorubicin and cisplatin based chemotherapy. Abstract 155, 20th Annual Meeting of the Soc. Gynecol. Oncol. in *Gynecol. Oncol.*, **32**, 130.

Reimer R.R. (1982) The risk of second malignancy related to the use of cytotoxic chemotherapy. *CAA Cancer Journal for Clinicians*, **32**, 286–92.

Ribeiro G., Hughesdon P. & Wiltshaw E. (1988) Squamous carcinoma arising in dermoid cysts and associated with hypercalcemia—a clinicopathologic study of six cases *Gynecol. Oncol.*, **29**, 222–30.

Schmahl D., Habs M., Lorenz M. & Wagner I. (1982) Occurrence of second tumours in man after anticancer drug treatment. *Cancer Treat Rev.*, **9**, 167–94.

Serov S.F., Scully R.E. & Sobin L.H. (1973) Histological typing of ovarian tumours. *International Classification of Tumours No. 9*, World Health Organization, Geneva.

Smith J.P. & Rutledge F. (1975) Advances in chemotherapy of gynecologic cancer. *Cancer*, **36**, 669–74.

Sondik E.J., Young J.L., Horm J.W. & Gloeckler L.A. (1985) *Annual Cancer Statistics Review*. NIH Publication 86–2789.

Stenwig J.T., Hazekamp J.T. & Beecham J.B. (1979) Granulosa cell tumors of the ovary: a clinicopathologic study of 118 cases with long term follow up. *Gynecol. Oncol.*, **7**, 669–74.

Sutton G., Bundy B., Omura G., Yordan E. & Beecham J. (1989) Stage III ovarian tumours of low malignant potential (LMP) treated with cisplatin combination therapy. Abstract 35, 20th Annual Meeting Soc. Gynecol. Oncol. in *Gynecol. Oncol.*, **32**, 102.

Sutton G.P., Stehman F.B., Einhorn L.H., Roth L.M., Blessing J.A. & Eherlich C.E. (1989) Ten year follow-up of patients receiving cisplatin, doxorubicin and cyclophosphamide chemotherapy for advanced epithelial ovarian carcinoma. *J. Clin. Oncol.*, **7**, 223–29.

Van der Burg M.E.L., Lammes F.B., Van Putten W.L.J. & Stoter G. (1988) Ovarian cancer: the prognostic value of the serum half-life of CA125 during induction chemotherapy. *Gynecol. Oncol.*, **30**, 307–12.

Watring W., Semrad N., Alaverdian V., Latino F. & Pretorius G. (1989) Second-look procedures in ovarian cancer patients receiving six vs nine courses of platinum, adriamycin, cytoxan (pAc) chemotherapy: the SCPMG experience 1982–1985. *Gynecol. Oncol.*, **32**, 245–47.

Wharton J.T., Edwards C.L. & Rutledge F.N. (1984) Long term survival after chemotherapy for advanced epithelial ovarian carcinoma. *Am. J. Obstet. Gynecol.*, **136**, 997–1005.

Williams S., Blessing J., Adcock C. & Homesberg H. (1984) Treatment of ovarian germ cell tumours with cisplatin, vinblastine and bleomycin (PVB). *Proc. Am. Soc. Clin. Oncol.*, **3**, 175.

Wiltshaw E. (1965) Chlorambucil in the treatment of primary adenocarcinoma of the ovary. *J. Obstet. Gynaecol. Brit. Commonwealth*, **72**, 586—94.

Wiltshaw E., Evans B., Rustin G., Gilbey E., Baker J. & Barker G. (1986) A prospective randomized trial comparing high-dose cisplatin with low-dose cisplatin and chlorambucil in advanced ovarian carcinoma. *J. Clin. Oncol.*, **4**, 722—29.

Wiltshaw E., Osborne J. & Gallagher C. (1987) Laparoscopic follow-up of early ovarian cancer. *In*: F. Sharp & W.P. Soutter (eds) *Ovarian Cancer — the Way Ahead*. Royal College of Obstetricians & Gynaecologists, London.

Wiltshaw E., Stuart-Harris R., Barker G.H. *et al.* (1982) Chemotherapy of endodermal sinus tumour (yolk sac tumour) of the ovary: preliminary communication. *J. Roy. Soc. Med.*, **75**, 888—92.

13

Chemotherapy in Gynaecological Malignancies other than Ovarian Cancer and Gestational Trophoblastic Tumours

JOHN BUXTON & GEORGE BLACKLEDGE

Modern chemotherapy has radically altered the outlook for some women with gynaecological malignancies. The prognosis for women with gestational trophoblastic and nonepithelial ovarian tumours has been dramatically improved by effective chemotherapy monitored by accurate tumour markers. In epithelial ovarian cancer cisplatin based chemotherapy regimens produce high response rates and possibly improve survival. Progress in other gynaecological tumours has been less dramatic. Nevertheless potentially important developments are being made in these diseases.

Gynaecological tumours are potentially curable if detected and treated at an early stage but a significant proportion of women with early stage disease and a far greater proportion with locally advanced or metastatic disease develop recurrence within 5 years of primary treatment. This implies that radical radiotherapy and surgery do not constitute the optimal therapeutic approach. Since the only realistic chance of achieving a cure is with the primary treatment clinicians must explore new therapeutic avenues if improvements in the results of treatment are to be achieved. Treatment failures occur either because the disease extends outside the treatment field (directly or by metastases) at the time of presentation or because the disease is resistant to treatment. For these reasons systemic chemotherapy may be useful either as adjuvant or as neoadjuvant therapy.

The activity of cytotoxics is usually tested in patients who present with recurrent disease. This group of patients are often symptomatic and have traditionally been treated with palliative chemotherapy. Significant relief of disease related symptoms may be achieved in these patients but the duration of remission is usually short. The potential benefits of treatment must, therefore, be balanced against the considerable toxicity that some combinations produce. Few studies have addressed this problem directly and further research in this area is required.

Thus there are a number of potentially useful applications for systemic chemotherapy in tumours other than gestational trophoblastic tumours and ovarian cancer. In this chapter the present status of chemotherapy in the treatment of these diseases will be reviewed.

Cervical cancer

Around 4000 new cases of this disease are diagnosed annually in England and Wales (OPCS 1988). Although overall survival has improved in the last two decades stage specific survival figures for treated women remain unchanged implying that there have been no improvements in treatment. Around 45% of all patients who develop this disease have relapsed and died within 5 years of primary treatment.

The majority of these tumours are squamous in origin (Kavanagh *et al.* 1987) but it has become apparent that a significant number of what would previously have been described as squamous carcinomas do in fact have adenomatous components when stained for mucin. Very few studies have reported specifically on chemotherapy in non-squamous cervical cancer (Slayton *et al.* 1984; Homesley *et al.* 1986; Thigpen *et al.* 1986c; Kavanagh *et al.* 1987). At present there are not sufficient data to show whether these tumours behave differently in their response to chemotherapy although cisplatin and piperazinedione appear to have activity (Thigpen *et al.* 1986c) and Kavanagh *et al.* reported a response rate of 42% in 24 patients treated with cisplatin, doxorubicin and 5-fluorouracil (Kavanagh *et al.* 1987).

As in most gynaecological malignancies the role of chemotherapy naturally divides into two areas; first, in recurrent disease, the traditional role of systemic chemotherapy for the palliation of symptomatic recurrence and secondly in primary disease where the potential for adjuvant and neoadjuvant chemotherapy is being explored.

Recurrent disease

A number of single agents have demonstrated activity in recurrent disease (Table 13.1). The results of many studies are difficult to interpret because the sample size is not adequate to give narrow confidence limits for response rates. Patient selection may also be important in determining the likelihood of observing response (Bonomi *et al.* 1988). For example, selection of patients who have either been heavily pretreated with chemotherapy or who have a poor performance status, for a phase II study, is likely to produce a response rate inferior to that seen in previously untreated patients. Many if not all patients entered in these studies will have been previously treated with pelvic radiotherapy which disrupts pelvic vasculature and may select resistant disease. This may influence the assessment of drug activity since the majority of patients present with pelvic recurrence. A further problem with studies in recurrent disease is assessing response. Assessment of response in these circumstances may be hampered by the almost inevitable postradiation fibrosis that is found. This mandates careful assessment of response by both clinical and radiographic methods.

Most notable among the single agents have been cisplatin and ifosfamide, an

Table 13.1. Single agents in cervical cancer

		Response/cases	Response rate (%)	95% CI
Cyclophosphamide	(Malkasian et al. 1977)	2/40	5	0–12
	(Omura et al. 1981)	2/30	7	0–16
Ifosfamide	(Coleman et al. 1986)	12/30	40	22–58
	(Meanwell et al. 1986)	10/30	33	16–50
Cisplatin (50 mg/m^2)	(Bonomi et al. 1985)	31/150	21	14–28
	(Thigpen et al. 1987)	27/164	16	11–23
Cisplatin (100 mg/m^2)	(Bonomi et al. 1985)	52/166	31	24–38
Carboplatin	(McGuire et al. 1988)	29/176	14	9–19
Iproplatin	(McGuire et al. 1988)	19/176	11	6–16
Methotrexate	(De Palo et al. 1973)	3/23	13	0–27
(+vincristine)	(Hakes et al. 1979)	5/31	17	4–30
Bleomycin	(De Palo et al. 1973)	3/23	13	0–27
	(Krakoff et al. 1977)	10/32	30	14–46
Vincristine	(Hreschchyshyn 1963)	9/31	29	13–45
Vindesine	(Rhomberg 1986)	6/20	30	10–50
	(Vermorken et al. 1984)	5/21	24	6–42
Vinblastine	(Kavanagh et al. 1985)	2/20	10	0–23
Adriamycin	(Wallace et al. 1978)	12/61	20	10–30
5-Fluorouracil	(Malkasian et al. 1977)	20/208	10	6–14
Mitoxantrone	(Hording et al. 1986)	0/17	0	0–20
CCNU	(Omura et al. 1978)	2/58	3	0–7
MeCCNU	(Omura et al. 1978)	3/62	5	0–10
Porfiromycin	(Panattiere 1976)	9/34	26	11–41

95% CI = 95% confidence intervals for observed response rate.

oxazophosphorene derivative and structural analogue of cyclophosphamide. Cisplatin has been extensively evaluated in this disease but although initial early reports showed high response rates, studies including larger numbers have shown response rates of between 17–27%. There is some evidence that a dose response relationship exists with this drug. In a randomized phase II study of three different schedules with two different doses conducted by the Gynecologic Oncology Group (GOG), the overall response rates for 50 mg and 100 mg/m^2 were 23% and 27%, respectively (Bonomi et al. 1985). In one arm of the study patients received 100 mg/m^2 fractionated over five days. The response rate in this group was the same as that in the arm that received 50 mg/m^2. The higher response rate demonstrated for 100 mg/m^2 as a bolus, reflected an increase in the number of partial responses (13/122 as opposed to 22/138) with no increase in the number of complete responses that were seen (12%). Whether cisplatin is given as a slow bolus or as a 24-h infusion appears to make no difference to response rates or toxicity (Thigpen et al. 1986d).

In phase II studies of ifosfamide, either as a 24-h infusion (5 g/m^2) or fractionated over five days (7.5 g/m^2), in recurrent and advanced disease objective response rates of between 33–40% have been observed (Coleman et al. 1986; Meanwell et al. 1986). In one of these studies a significantly lower response rate was observed for sites of disease in areas that had previously been irradiated compared to sites in previously non-irradiated areas (Meanwell et al. 1986). This has important implications for the use of this drug in primary disease. Although a much lower response rate of 11% (3/27) was seen in a study reported by the GOG, with all of the responses being partial responses, this observation must be interpreted with caution, since all but one of the patients had previously received platinum based therapy (Sutton 1988, personal communication).

There have been a number of reports of highly active combinations in recurrent disease (Table 13.2). The highest response rates reported are for the combinations of cisplatin, vinblastine, bleomycin (PVB) and cisplatin, ifosfamide, bleomycin (BIP) which have shown response rates of 66% and 69%, respectively, with comparatively high rates of complete responders (18% and 20%) (Friedlander et al. 1983; Buxton et al. 1989). Other cisplatin combinations have been less impressive although in combination either with bleomycin, adriamycin, cyclophosphamide or methotrexate response rates of 56% and 57% have been reported (Bezwoda et al. 1986; Edmonson et al. 1988). Another potentially interesting combination is that of cisplatin and 5-fluorouracil which in a small series reported by the GOG showed a response rate of 50% (Rotmensch et al. 1988). The significance of this regimen is discussed further in the section on radiosensitizers. Combinations of cisplatin and mitomycin C have been popular but are probably no better than single agent cisplatin (Alberts et al. 1987). A number of studies using mitomycin C combinations particularly with bleomycin have been reported. Occasionally response rates in excess of 80% have been reported for this combination (Miyamoto et al. 1978) but the majority of studies have shown response rates in the

Table 13.2. Combination chemotherapy in cervical cancer

		Response/cases	Response rate (%)	95% CI
Adr/Cyclo	(Wallace et al. 1978)	7/39	18	6–30
Adr/Vincr	(Wallace et al. 1978)	9/54	17	7–27
Adr/Vincr/5FU	(Omura et al. 1981)	3/31	10	1–21
Adr/Vincr/5FU/Cyclo	(Chan et al. 1982)	19/31	58	41–75
Adr/methylCCNU	(Day et al. 1978)	14/31	45	27–63
Adr/Mtx	(Papavasiliou et al. 1978)	7/24	29	11–47
	(Trope et al. 1980)	5/24	21	5–37
Bleo/MMC	(Leichman et al. 1980)	3/19	16	0–32
	(Trope et al. 1983)	12/23	36	16–56
DDP/Mtx	(Bezwoda et al. 1986)	21/37	57	41–73
DDP/5FU	(Rotmensch et al. 1988)	12/24	50	30–70
DDP/Cytarabine	(Keeney et al. 1985)	7/32	22	8–36
DDP/MMC	(Alberts et al. 1987)	13/51	25	13–37
DDP/Bleo	(Edmonson et al. 1988)	8/25	32	14–50
DDP/Bleo/Vinbl	(Friedlander et al. 1983)	21/33	66	50–82
DDP/Bleo/MMC	(Picozzi et al. 1985)	6/28	21	6–36
DDP/Cyclo/Adr	(Hoffman et al. 1988)	6/28	21	6–36
	(De Murua et al. 1987)	3/30	10	0–21
DDP/Bleo/Cyclo/Adr	(Edmonson et al. 1988)	15/27	56	37–75
DDP/Bleo/MMC/Vincr	(Alberts et al. 1987)	12/54	22	11–33
	(Lahousen et al. 1987)	20/39	51	35–67
DDP/Bleo/MMC/Vind	(Vermorken et al. 1987)	28/48	58	44–72
DDP/Ifos/Bleo	(Buxton et al. 1989)	34/49	69	56–82

Adr:	Adriamycin	Mtx:	Methotrexate	Vinbl:	Vinblastine
Cyclo:	Cyclophosphamide	MMC:	Mitomycin C	Vind:	Vindesine
Vincr:	Vincristine	DDP:	Cisplatin	Ifos:	Ifosfamide
5FU:	5-Fluorouracil	Bleo:	Bleomycin		

95% CI = 95% confidence intervals for observed response rate.

order of 16−36% (Leichman *et al.* 1980; Trope *et al.* 1983). Bleomycin pulmonary toxicity can be a problem if high doses are given. In one series three patients were affected one of whom died (Trope *et al.* 1983).

Although some combinations produce high response rates, responses are seldom durable and rarely last longer than 6 months. The main benefit from chemotherapy is the relief of disease related symptoms such as pelvic pain. High activity regimens have considerable toxicity and evidence to confirm that combinations are superior to single agents in terms of the trade off between toxicity and relief of disease related symptoms is lacking. Randomized trials are required to answer this question. Since there is little evidence to suggest that chemotherapy produces a survival advantage in these women there seems little to be gained by treating asymptomatic recurrence. In symptomatic patients the results of treatment should be monitored carefully and if there is no evidence of response within two or three cycles of treatment alternative strategies to control symptoms should be considered.

Neoadjuvant chemotherapy

Failure to cure inoperable cervical cancer may result from suboptimal treatment of the pelvic disease or the existence of metastatic disease outside the treatment fields at the time of diagnosis. In treatment planning the volume of pelvic disease is one of the most important factors, larger lesions requiring higher doses of radiation to achieve similar rates of central control to those achieved with lower doses in small volume disease. This principle applies to both central and metastatic disease and is supported by clinical data (Thar *et al.* 1982).

The incidence of extrapelvic metastatic spread also correlates with both the size and stage of the primary tumour (Morgan & Nelson 1982). Irradiation of para-aortic lymph nodes with effective doses of radiation is associated with unacceptable treatment related morbidity and mortality and multiple metastatic sites are not amenable to radiotherapy (Piver & Barlow 1977). Neoadjuvant chemotherapy (i.e. systemic treatment prior to radical local radiotherapy) offers potential; first for cytoreducing bulky pelvic disease which may improve local control rates and secondly for sterilizing sites of metastatic disease.

To be useful in this setting chemotherapy must be highly active since potentially curative conventional therapy is delayed, it must produce response rapidly to avoid excessive toxicity which combined with radiotherapy toxicity might limit delivery of a radical dose of radiation, it should not enhance the acute or long term toxicity from radiation and it should at the very least improve rates of central disease control but preferably also confer a survival advantage.

This approach has been tested in a number of phase II pilot studies. Symonds *et al.* treated 30 patients (23 stage III and 7 stage IVa) with two cycles of cisplatin, vincristine and bleomycin prior to radical local radiotherapy (Symonds *et al.* 1987). Seventeen patients (57%) achieved a partial response to the chemotherapy with 25/30 patients disease free three months after completing radiotherapy.

Local control in this group was excellent with 71% free of pelvic disease at death or last follow-up. The actuarial survival at 30 months was 66% and there was no evidence that acute or late radiotherapy toxic effects in normal tissues were enhanced. Kirsten *et al.* treated 31 patients with stage IIb—IV and 16 patients with stage Ib—IIa disease, with cisplatin, vinblastine and bleomycin prior to radical local radiotherapy or radical surgery (Kirsten *et al.* 1987). Thirty-one patients had evidence of tumour regression after chemotherapy with only three showing evidence of tumour progression during treatment. Median survival in this series was 22 months and there was a significant difference in survival between those patients who responded to chemotherapy and those that did not. Radiotherapy toxicity was not enhanced by prior treatment with cytotoxics. Benedetti *et al.* reported on 33 patients with bulky stage Ib/IIa (six cases) or stage IIb—IIIb disease treated with cisplatin, bleomycin and methotrexate prior to radical surgery (Benedetti *et al.* 1988). Twenty-five patients responded to chemotherapy with a low incidence of involved pelvic nodes (16%) at eventual laparotomy. Buxton *et al.* reported response in 11/14 patients (79%) with advanced primary disease treated with cisplatin, ifosfamide and bleomycin (Buxton *et al.* 1988). Cisplatin, bleomycin, vincristine and mitomycin C have been used as neoadjuvant therapy prior to radiotherapy in a number of studies and have confirmed that radiotherapy toxicity is not increased (Van der Berg *et al.* 1984) and that response rates are high (Lipsztein *et al.* 1987; Weiner *et al.* 1988).

These studies have confirmed that neoadjuvant chemotherapy is a feasible approach in the treatment of advanced stage disease. Acute radiation toxicity does not appear to be enhanced by giving chemotherapy prior to radiotherapy and the activity of most regimens is similar to that seen in phase II studies in recurrent disease. Some groups have reported a small number of patients whose disease progresses through chemotherapy and it has been suggested on the basis of data presented from some centres that chemotherapy may be acting as a marker for radiosensitive disease (Kirsten *et al.* 1987). This hypothesis is based upon the observation that patients with disease which is static during chemotherapy or who have disease progression rarely respond to subsequent radiotherapy whereas those who respond to chemotherapy are very likely to achieve a good response to subsequent radiotherapy.

The major questions yet to be answered about this approach are whether local disease control and survival are improved. These can only be answered by randomized studies. A number of preliminary reports of randomized studies testing the value of neoadjuvant chemotherapy have been presented (Chauvergne *et al.* 1988; Souhami *et al.* 1988). On the basis of these limited reports survival does not appear to be improved. Unfortunately the regimens used in these studies were not the most active that have been reported and the number of patients included were inadequate to be certain of not missing a significant difference in outcome. Studies with the most active reported regimens are currently in progress but until these are completed this approach will remain of unproven value.

Adjuvant therapy

Carcinoma of the uterine cervix is a curable disease if it is detected and treated at an early stage. Survival in treated women with early stage (I/IIa) disease is high but despite the apparently favourable prognosis, in what is increasingly a young patient population, around 20–25% of women presenting with early stage disease relapse within 5 years of primary treatment. The prognosis for women with recurrent disease is poor with less than 15% alive 1 year after diagnosis (Disaia & Rich 1975).

Conventional therapy fails either because the disease extends beyond the treatment field by direct extension of the primary tumour and metastatic spread to regional and distant lymph nodes or because the disease is not sensitive to the treatment; radiobiological differences between tumours are unpredictable. These limitations suggest a potential role for highly active systemic adjuvant therapy. This approach can only be justified if patients at high risk of recurrence can be accurately identified prospectively.

In patients treated by radical surgery the presence of metastases in the pelvic and para-aortic lymph nodes represents a well recognized adverse prognostic factor. Around 50% of patients with positive pelvic lymph nodes are alive five years after conventional treatment (Piver & Chung 1975). This group of patients may benefit from systemic adjuvant therapy after radical surgery. A substantial proportion of patients with early disease are also treated primarily with radiotherapy. As yet there is no satisfactory means of identifying which patients in this group are at high risk of developing recurrence.

Recently there have been a number of phase II studies reported in the literature exploring the feasibility of giving adjuvant chemotherapy in patients who are found to have involved pelvic nodes after radical surgery for early stage disease (Hakes et al. 1987; Shirozimu et al. 1988). While this is a logical progression from the development of highly active cisplatin containing systemic chemotherapy regimens in recurrent disease, and studies of neoadjuvant chemotherapy in advanced disease, enthusiasm for this approach must be tempered with the knowledge that not all patients found to have positive nodes relapse after conventional treatment. Furthermore, around 10% of node negative patients also relapse (Piver & Chung 1975). There is therefore a need to more precisely define patients at high risk of relapse.

The group from the Memorial Sloan-Kettering Cancer Centre also included patients selected on the basis of other parameters associated with a high risk of relapse including tumour diameter >4 cm, invasion of the parametrium or involved excision margins, lymphatic and blood vessel invasion and poor differentiation (Hakes et al. 1987). Thirty-four of the 44 patients entered had multiple risk factors. The regimen comprised bleomycin 40 mg/m² divided between a 24-h infusion and an intravenous bolus dose repeated for 3 days followed by cisplatin at 75 mg/m². This was repeated after 21 days followed by external beam radiotherapy. After completion of the radiotherapy two further cycles were given omitting the bleomycin. Five-year relapse free survival was 71% in the 44 patients with no evidence of greater toxicity than in historic controls.

As in phase II studies of neoadjuvant chemotherapy in advanced disease, while the feasibility of this approach has been confirmed, the possibility that relapse rates could be reduced and survival improved can only be answered by randomized trials. Such studies are in progress but an answer is unlikely for some years.

Radiosensitizers

Failure to cure cervical cancer with radical radiotherapy may be a reflection of the fact that the disease is not radiosensitive. Radiobiological differences are unpredictable. One potential cause of radioresistance is the presence of hypoxic cell populations within a tumour, a phenomenon which is well recognized. A number of drugs are known to act as hypoxic cell radiosensitizers and clearly have potential to improve control of tumour within the radiation fields. A number of these drugs have been evaluated in clinical trials.

The Medical Research Council carried out a randomized trial of misonidazole (Dische et al. 1984). This study, however, was prematurely closed after an interim analysis of 153 of the planned total of 300 cases revealed that significant and occasionally severe neurotoxicity occurred in 36% of patients receiving misonidazole. There was no apparent benefit to this group either in disease free survival or local disease control. Subsequent studies from other groups have corroborated these findings (Liebel et al. 1987). The cytotoxic hydroxyurea also acts as a radiation potentiator. This is thought to occur through several distinct mechanisms. It prevents repair of sublethal radiation damage within cells and is preferentially cytotoxic in S phase of the cell cycle also preventing transition of cells from G0/G1 of the cycle, when they are most radiosensitive, to S phase. In a small randomized study of 40 patients Piver et al. demonstrated that patients in the arm receiving hydroxyurea had significantly longer survival (Piver et al. 1983). The caveats to these results are the small numbers in the trial and the highly selected population; only patients proven to have negative para-aortic nodes at pretreatment surgical staging were included. In a randomized study of radiotherapy with either hydroxyurea or misonidazole in 296 patients with stage IIb−IVa disease, Stehman et al. found greater short term toxicity in the hydroxyurea arm but a lower rate of recurrence (36.7% vs. 43.9%) with 57% of recurrences being pelvic (Stehman et al 1988). At the time of this preliminary analysis there was no statistically significant difference between the two treatments in terms of progression free interval, or survival.

Other cytotoxics may also interact with radiotherapy. Among these are cisplatin, 5-fluorouracil and mitomycin C. The results of phase II studies using these cytotoxics as concurrent radiation potentiators suggest that the approach is feasible with no apparent increase in acute or long term radiation toxicity (Thomas *et al*. 1984; Orielly *et al*. 1986).

Intra-arterial chemotherapy

The blood supply to pelvic tumours lends itself to the possibility of arterial infusion of cytotoxics, the potential advantage of this approach being the increased regional tissue concentrations that can be achieved. Additionally it may be possible to achieve these tissue levels with little or no increase in systemic toxicity or even reduced toxicity. The disadvantage of this approach is that it requires arterial cannulation and it may not be as efficient as systemic administration in dealing with micrometastases.

There have been a number of studies evaluating cytotoxic administration by this route but it remains to be demonstrated that this approach has any clear advantage over conventional routes of administration.

Endometrial adenocarcinoma

Adenocarcinoma of the endometrium has become the most common gynaecological malignancy in many countries. Although the majority (75%) of patients present with stage I disease somewhat surprisingly the overall 5-year survival is only around 68% (FIGO 1985). At present chemotherapy has no place in the management of the majority of patients presenting with primary disease amenable to surgery. In patients with inoperable, metastatic or recurrent disease chemotherapy may be appropriate but should only be considered in cases with disease that has failed to respond to hormonal manipulation either with progestogens or antioestrogens such as tamoxifen. Both of these groups of drugs will produce response in around one-third of patients and they are essentially nontoxic. Unfortunately many patients who present with advanced or recurrent disease are unsuitable for intensive chemotherapy because they are frail, often with intercurrent illness, and may have coexistent medical disorders such as diabetes, cardiovascular and renal disease.

There is some evidence that the tumours most likely to respond to chemotherapy with progestins and antioestrogens are those with a high progestogen or oestrogen receptor content (Kneale 1986). Whether receptor levels can be used to prospectively identify those patients most likely to benefit from treatment with hormones or cytotoxics is under investigation.

There have been comparatively few studies, with adequate patient numbers, of chemotherapy in this disease. Adriamycin is one of the agents that is active. Thigpen *et al*. reported the results of a GOG phase II study using this drug. They observed 16 responses in 43 patients treated with 60 mg/m^2 (Thigpen *et al*. 1979). In a later randomized phase II study conducted by the GOG responses were seen in 22/97 patients (22%), with seven complete responses (Thigpen *et al*.

1985). The other treatment arm in this study comprised adriamycin and cyclo-phosphamide which produced response in 34/105 patients (32%) with 15 complete responses. The median progression free intervals were 3.4 months and 4.0 months and median survivals 6.8 months and 7.6 months, respectively, for the two study arms. None of the differences were statistically significant. Some studies with adriamycin have produced lower response rates than the GOG studies possibly because of variations in the dose given.

Cisplatin also has activity in this disease. Response was seen in 11/26 patients (42%) reported by the MD Anderson group but as with adriamycin the duration of remission (median 5 months) and survival were short (Seski et al. 1981b). A third of the patients in this study stopped treatment because of toxicity (neuro- and nephrotoxicity). Although this study evaluated three different doses the patient numbers were too small to identify any dose response relationship with this drug. Deppe et al. reported a 31% response rate in 13 patients treated after failing therapy for advanced or recurrent disease (Deppe et al. 1980). In a GOG study of a similar group of patients only one response was seen in 25 patients treated with 50 mg/m^2 (Thigpen et al. 1984). Carboplatin also appears to be active with a reported response rate of 33% in a small study of 15 patients (Long et al. 1987).

There have been a number of reports of combination regimens in this disease. The Gynecologic Oncology Group reported on 257 evaluable patients with re-current or advanced disease entered into a randomized phase II study of either melphalan, 5-fluorouracil and medroxyprogesterone acetate or adriamycin, 5-fluorouracil, cyclophosphamide and medroxyprogesterone acetate (Cohen et al. 1984). A further 63 patients with cardiovascular disease were not randomized and received melphalan, 5-fluorouracil and medroxyprogesterone acetate. The objective response rates were identical in both arms of the study with 37% of patients in each group responding. The median response duration and survival were similar in both groups. Haematological toxicity with these regimens was considerable. Piver et al. reported a 48% response rate with 20% complete responses in 50 patients treated with melphalan, 5-fluorouracil and medroxy-progesterone acetate (Piver et al. 1986). The median progression free interval in this series was only 5 months and 14% of patients experienced severe haema-tological toxicity. Response rates of 27% and 31% have been demonstrated for cyclophosphamide and adriamycin with or without a progestin (Seski et al. 1981a; Horton et al. 1982).

Trope et al. treated 19 patients (18 recurrent and one stage IV disease) with adriamycin and cisplatin and observed an objective response rate of 60% (Trope et al. 1984). The regimen appeared to cause minimal toxicity apart from alopecia. The EORTC has reported response in 17/26 patients (60%) treated with combi-nation cyclophosphamide, adriamycin and cisplatin. There were eight complete responses and prior hormone therapy appeared to have no bearing on response rates (DeOliveira et al. 1986).

Uterine sarcomas

Sarcomas of the uterus are rare comprising between 3% to 5% of all uterine tumours. The prognosis for patients with this disease is poor with an overall 5-year survival of between 22% and 39% with around 54% of patients with stage I disease surviving 5 years (Salazar *et al.* 1978a). Although histologically these tumours are heterogeneous for the purposes of treatment they are usually grouped with tumours of other sites under the general heading of soft tissue sarcomas. The hallmark of treatment of uterine sarcomas has traditionally been surgery with or without adjuvant radiotherapy to the pelvis; however, the value of radiotherapy in this setting has been questioned (Salazar *et al.* 1978b). Salazar *et al.* reported on 73 patients of whom 47 had developed recurrence. Only 4% of patients had pelvic recurrence alone, 49% had both pelvic and distant metastases and the remainder presented with distant metastases alone (Salazar *et al.* 1978b).

Recurrent and advanced disease

The results of treatment for advanced and recurrent soft tissue sarcomas in adults are disappointing. Around half of patients with stage I disease and 90% of those with stage II/IV disease will relapse within 5 years of primary therapy. Patients with recurrence are unlikely to be cured with chemotherapy but useful palliation of disease related symptoms may be achieved. Adriamycin is one of the most important drugs in this disease. Omura *et al.* reported that adriamycin produced response in 13/80 patients (16%) with stage III/IV and recurrent disease (Omura *et al.* 1983). One of the problems with adriamycin is the occurrence of dose limiting cardiotoxicity. In soft tissue sarcomas in general, studies comparing other anthracyclines with adriamycin, in an effort to limit toxicity while maintaining response rates, show that none of the analogues evaluated has superiority or comparability to adriamycin (Santoro & Bonadona 1985).

Dacarbazine and cyclophosphamide also have activity in soft tissue sarcoma (Bersagel & Levin 1960; Korst *et al.* 1963; Luce *et al.* 1970; Gottleib *et al.* 1976). Cisplatin has also shown activity producing response in five of 28 patients (18%) with advanced or recurrent mixed mesodermal sarcoma (Thigpen *et al.* 1982). Ifosfamide has activity in soft tissue sarcoma with a reported response rate of up to 38% in some studies (Sutton 1988, personal communication; Stuart-Harris *et al.* 1983) and overall appears to have greater activity than cyclophosphamide (Bramwell *et al.* 1986). However, in the latter study the response rates in women were 23% for ifosfamide and 20% for cyclophosphamide, respectively.

Although there is experimental data to suggest an additive effect between adriamycin and dacarbazine this does not appear to be translated into either improved survival or response rates in the clinical situation. In a randomized study of 240 patients Omura *et al.* showed no difference in response rate in 146 evaluable patients (16.3% vs. 24.2%) and no difference in progression free interval in the whole group (10 months vs. 8 months) (Omura *et al.* 1983). Responses were more frequently seen in lung metastases in patients receiving the combination but this did not produce a survival advantage. There was, however, evidence of increased toxicity with the drugs combined. Similarly in a randomized study of 104 patients addition of cyclophosphamide to adriamycin produced no increase in response rates (19%) or survival (median 11.6 months single agent, 10.9 months combination) (Disaia & Creasman 1984). CYVADIC (cyclophosphamide, vincristine, adriamycin and DTIC) has been the most widely used combination chemotherapy in the treatment of advanced soft tissue sarcoma and response rates of 11–52% have been achieved with this regimen (Bonadona & Santoro 1984). This variation of reported response rates is probably a reflection of differences in patient selection and the composition of the study groups in terms of tumour type and site.

Neoadjuvant and adjuvant therapy

Because of the poor survival associated with conventional treatment and the obvious predeliction of this tumour for distant spread the possibility of giving adjuvant chemotherapy to patients with this disease is clearly attractive. There have been comparatively few studies reporting the results of neoadjuvant therapy and these have been in tumours of various sites rather than specifically uterine sarcomas. Generally the results of adjuvant studies in soft tissue sarcomas have been disappointing, although many studies have suffered from serious methodological flaws in both design but more importantly in the number of patients included. Buchsbaum *et al.* reported 17 patients with stage I/II uterine sarcoma treated with postoperative vincristine, actinomycin D and cyclophosphamide (VAC) (Buchsbaum *et al.* 1979). Only 10 of the 17 patients completed the planned six cycles of treatment. These authors suggested that survival benefit was seen in patients with more than 10 mitoses/hpf; however, this was not a randomized study and the claim was based on a comparison with historic controls. In a prospective randomized study conducted by the GOG adjuvant adriamycin was compared to no adjuvant therapy in 159 evaluable patients with stage I/II sarcomas in which all gross disease had been removed (Omura *et al.* 1985). In this study radiation therapy was allowed prior to randomization. There was no significant difference in progression free interval or survival in either group.

Sarcomas in other sites

Childhood rhabdomyosarcomas are an example of a tumour where chemotherapy has transformed management. These tumours frequently arise within the pelvis, a common site being the vagina in very young children although the cervix may be involved, particularly in the older child. The VAC schedule of vincristine, actinomycin D, cyclophosphamide with or without adriamycin can be effective even in advanced disease and in combination with surgery and radiotherapy produces high cure rates for early stage disease. The value of this combination as adjuvant and neoadjuvant therapy is being tested (Maurer 1980).

The most common mesenchymal tumours of the vulva are leiomyosarcomas. Primary management should consist of surgery if possible and/or radical radiotherapy with consideration being given to chemotherapy as in other sarcomas.

Vulval cancer

Vulval cancer comprises around 8% of gynaecological malignancies (Green 1978). It is a disease of older patients with the majority being over 60 years of age. Despite this between 85 and 95% are operable and surgery should be the treatment of choice. Because of their age and general condition many patients are not suitable for intensive chemotherapy but in selected cases chemotherapy may be useful for palliative therapy of inoperable advanced or recurrent disease and for neoadjuvant therapy. Preoperative cytoreductive chemotherapy may not only make surgery easier but also make surgery possible for what was initially unresectable disease.

Bleomycin is active in this disease and produces objective response rates of around 60% (Deppe et al. 1979). Other active agents include methotrexate, vincristine and mitomycin C. Unlike cervical carcinoma this tumour does not appear to be particularly sensitive to cisplatin (Thigpen et al. 1986b). There have been comparatively few studies of combination chemotherapy but combinations of bleomycin, methotrexate and mitomycin C appear to be the most active. Belinson reported tumour regression in five of six patients with primary advanced disease but few responses in recurrent disease with no enhancement of quality of life using the combination of bleomycin, vincristine, mitomycin C and cisplatin (Belinson et al. 1985).

Neoadjuvant chemotherapy

The possibility of neoadjuvant chemotherapy has been explored. Durrant reported the results of an EORTC study of low dose bleomycin, methotrexate, and CCNU as neoadjuvant therapy in inoperable vulvar cancer (Durrant 1988, personal communication). Although a 65% response rate was seen and in 28% disease was rendered resectable toxicity was considerable with some toxic deaths. Chemotherapeutic agents may also act as radiosensitizers when given in combination with radiotherapy. The danger of this approach is that normal tissues may also be rendered more radiosensitive so that both local and systemic toxicity become unacceptable (Iverson 1982; Arnott 1988, personal communication). Despite these problems significant tumour regression and improved resectability have been achieved in some series (Levin et al. 1986).

Other vulval tumours

Vulval melanoma is an uncommon tumour which may occur in this site. Treatment is usually surgical but in cases with deep penetration of the tumour chemotherapy may have a role. Frost *et al.* reported a partial response of 8 months duration in one patient treated with intra-arterial dacarbazine and cisplatin (Frost *et al.* 1985).

Carcinoma of the vagina

Vaginal cancer accounts for less than 2% of gynaecological cancers with over 90% of the tumours being squamous lesions. The principal treatments are surgery and/ or radiotherapy. There have been few reported studies evaluating chemotherapy in carcinoma of the vagina and many comprise anecdotal reports of one or two patients. The GOG found insignificant activity with cisplatin (50 mg/m^2) in 22 evaluable patients with carcinoma of the vagina (Thigpen *et al.* 1986a). They reported one response in 16 cases with squamous disease but no responses in the remaining six cases. Holleboom *et al.* reported a single case with a skin metastasis which responded to cisplatin (Holleboom *et al.* 1987) and Katib *et al.* reported a complete response in an advanced primary tumour to the combination of bleomycin, methotrexate and cisplatin (Katib *et al.* 1985). Vaginal melanoma is rare but active agents include DTIC, vindesine and nitrosoureas.

References

Alberts D.S., Kronmal R., Baker L.H. *et al.* (1987) Phase II randomized trial cisplatin chemotherapy regimens in the treatment of recurrent or metastatic squamous cell cancer of the cervix: A Southwest Oncology Group study. *J. Clin. Oncol.*, **5**, 1791–95.

Arnott (1988) Personal communication.

Belinson J.L., Stewart J.A., Richards A.L. & McClure M. (1985) Bleomycin, vincristine, mitomycin-C and cisplatin in the management of gynaecological squamous cell carcinomas. *Gynecol. Oncol.*, **20**, 387–93.

Benedetti Panici P., Scambia G., Greggi S., DiRoberto P., Baiocchi G. & Mancuso S. (1988) Neoadjuvant chemotherapy and radical surgery in locally advanced cervical carcinoma: a pilot study. *Obstet. Gynecol.*, **71**, 344–48.

Bersagel D.E. & Levin W.C. (1960) A preclusive clinical trial of cyclophosphamide. *Cancer Chem. Rep.*, **8**, 120.

Bezwoda W.R., Nissenbaum M. & Derman D.P. (1986) Treatment of metastatic and recurrent cervix cancer with chemotherapy: a randomized trial comparing hydroxyurea with cisdiamminedichloro-platinum plus methotrexate. *Med. Pediatr. Oncol.*, **14**, 17–19.

Bonadona G. & Santoro A. (1984) Bone and soft tissue sarcomas. *In*: Pinedo H.M. & Chebner B.A. (eds), *Cancer Chemotherapy/6*, Elsevier Science Publishers B.V., Amsterdam. pp. 436–49.

Bonomi P., Blessing J.A., Stehman F.B., Disaia P.J., Walton L. & Major F.N. (1985) Randomized trial of three cisplatin dose schedules in squamous cell carcinoma of the cervix: a Gynecologic Oncology Group study. *J. Clin. Oncol.*, **3**, 1079–85.

Bonomi P., Brady M., Blessing J., Stehman F., Disaia P., Walton L. & Major F. (1988) Prognostic factors related to response and to survival in women with advanced squamous cell carcinoma of the cervix treated with cisplatin. A Gynecologic Oncology Group (GOG) study. *Proc. Am. Assoc. Cancer Res.*, **29**, 207 (Abstract 822).

Bramwell V., Mouridsen H.T., Santoro A. *et al.* (1986) Cyclophosphamide vs ifosfamide: preliminary report of a randomised phase II trial in adult soft tissue sarcoma. *Cancer Chemother. Pharmacol.*, **18** (Suppl.), 13–16.

Buchsbaum H.J., Lifshitz S. & Blythe J.G. (1979) Prophylactic chemotherapy in stage I and II uterine sarcoma. *Gynecol. Oncol.*, **8**, 346.

Buxton E.J., Meanwell C.A., Hilton C., Mould J.J., Spooner D., Chetiyawardana A., Latief T., Paterson M., Redman C.W., Luesley D.M. & Blackledge G.R. (1989) Combination bleomycin, ifosfamide and cisplatin chemotherapy in cervix cancer. *J. Nat. Cancer Inst.* (*in press*).

Buxton E.J., Meanwell C.A., Mould J.J. *et al.* (1988) Phase II studies of bleomycin, ifosfamide and cisplatinum in cervix cancer. *Acta Oncologica*, **27**, 545–49.

Chan W.K., Aroney R.S., Levi J.A., Tattersall M.H.N., Fox R.M. & Woods R.L. (1982) Four-drug combination chemotherapy for advanced cervical carcinoma. *Cancer*, **49**, 2437–40.

Chauvergne J., Rohart J., Heron J.F., Fargeot P., Berlie J., David P. & George M. (1988) Randomised phase III trial of neoadjuvant chemotherapy plus radiotherapy versus radiotherapy in stage IIb, III carcinoma of the cervix: a cooperative study of the French oncology centers. *Proc. Am. Soc. Clin. Oncol.*, **7**, 136 (Abstract 524).

Cohen C.J., Bruchner H.W., Deppe G., Blessing J.A., Homesley H., Lee J.H. & Watring W. (1984) Multidrug treatment of advanced and recurrent endometrial carcinoma: a Gynecologic Oncology Group study. *Obstet. Gynecol.*, **63**, 719–26.

Coleman R.E., Harper P.G., Gallagher M.C. *et al.* (1986) A phase II study of ifosfamide in advanced and relapsed carcinoma of the cervix. *Cancer Chemother. Pharmacol.*, **18**, 280–83.

Day T.G. Jr., Wharton J.T., Gottleib J.A. & Rutledge F.N. (1978) Chemotherapy for squamous carcinoma of the cervix: doxorubicin-methyl CCNU. *Am. J. Obstet. Gynecol.*, **132**, 545–48.

De Murua E.O., George M., Pejovic M.H., Dewailly J. & Wolff J.P. (1987) Combination cyclophosphamide, adriamycin, and cis-platinum in recurrent and metastatic cervical carcinoma. *Gynecol. Oncol.*, **26**, 225–27.

DeOliveira C.F., Van Der Berg M.E.L., Namer M., Van Oosterom A.T., Osorio M.T., Neijt J.P., Veenhof C.H.N., Rotmensz N. & Vermorken J.B. (1986) Phase II study of cyclophosphamide (C), adriamycin (A), cisplatin (P) in recurrent or advanced endometrial cancer (EC). *Proc. Am. Soc. Clin. Oncol.*, **5**, 123 (Abstract 480).

De Palo G.M., Bajetta E., Luciani L., Musumeci R., Di Re F. & Bonadonna G. (1973) Methotrexate (NSC-740) and bleomycin (NSC-125066) in the treatment of advanced epidermoid carcinoma of the uterine cervix. *Cancer Chemother. Rep.*, **57**, 429–35.

Deppe G., Cohen C.J. & Bruckner H.W. (1979) Chemotherapy of squamous cell carcinoma of the vulva. *Gynecol. Oncol.*, 345–348.

Deppe G., Cohen C.J. & Bruckner H.W. (1980) Treatment of advanced endometrial adenocarcinoma with cis-dichlorodiammine platinum (II) after intensive prior therapy. *Gynecol. Oncol.*, **10**, 51–54.

Disaia P. & Creasman W.T. (1984) *In: Clinical Gynecologic Oncology*, 2nd edition, CV Mosby Company, Missouri.

Disaia P.J. & Rich W.M. (1975) Advanced and recurrent carcinoma of cervix, *In*: Coppleson M. (ed), *Gynecologic Oncology*. Churchill Livingstone, New York. pp. 517–27.

Dische S. *et al.* (1984) The Medical Research Council trial of misonidazole in carcinoma of the uterine cervix. A report from the MRC working party on misonidazole for cancer of the cervix. *Br. J. Radiol.*, **57**, 491–99.

Durrant K.R. (1988) Personal communication.

Edmonson J.H., Johnson P.S., Wieand H.S. *et al.* (1988) Phase II studies of bleomycin, cyclophosphamide, doxorubicin and cisplatin, and bleomycin and cisplatin in advanced cervical carcinoma. *Am. J. Clin. Oncol.*, **11**, 149–51.

FIGO (1985) *Annual Report on the Results of Treatment in Gynecologic Cancer*, 19.

Freidlander M.L., Kaye S.B., Sullivan A. *et al.* (1983) Cervical carcinoma: a drug-responsive tumour-experience with combined cisplatin, vinblastine and bleomycin therapy. *Gynecol. Oncol.*, **16**, 275–81.

Frost D.B., Patt Y.Z., Mavligit G., Chuang V.P. & Wallace S. (1985) Arterial infusion of dacarbazine for recurrent regionally confined melanoma. *Arch. Surg.*, **120**, 478–80.

Green T.H. (1978) Carcinoma of the vulva; a reassessment. *Obstet. Gynecol.*, **52**, 462–68.

Gottlieb J.A., Benjamin R.S., Baker L.H. *et al.* (1976) Role of DTIC (NSC-45388) in the chemotherapy of sarcomas. *Cancer Treat. Rep.*, **60**, 199.

Hakes T., Nikrui M., Magill G. & Ochoa M. (1979) Treatment with combination vincristine and high doses of methotrexate. *Cancer*, **43**, 459–64.

Hakes T., Nori D. & Lewis J.L. (1987) Adjuvant cisplatin/bleomycin (C/B) for high risk stage Ib/IIa cervix carcinoma patients—a pilot study. *Proc. Am. Soc. Clin. Oncol.*, **6**, 116 (Abstract 455).

Hoffman M.S., Roberts W.S., Bryson S.C.P., Kavanagh J.J. Jr., Cavanagh D. & Lyman G.H. (1988) Treatment of recurrent and metastatic cervical cancer with cis-platin, doxorubicin, and cyclophosphamide. *Gynecol. Oncol.*, **29**, 32–36.

Holleboom C.A.G., Kock H.C.L.V., Nijs A.M. & Leers W.H. (1987) Cis-diamminechloroplatinum in the treatment of advanced primary squamous cell carcinoma of the vaginal wall: a case report. *Gynecol. Oncol.*, **27**, 110–15.

Homesley H.D., Blessing J.A. & Berman M. (1986) ICRF-159 (Razoxane) in patients with advanced non-squamous cell carcinoma of the cervix. *Am. J. Clin. Oncol.*, **9**, 325–26.

Hording U., Rose C., Jakobsen K. & Dirksen H. (1986) Mitoxantrone in advanced cervical carcinoma: a phase II study in patients not previously treated with chemotherapy. *Cancer Treat. Rep.*, **70**, 1239–40.

Horton J.E., Eelson P., Gordon P., Hann R. & Creech R. (1982) Combination chemotherapy for advanced endometrial cancer. An evaluation of three regimens. *Cancer*, **49**, 2441–45.

Hreschchyshyn M. (1963) Vincristine treatment of patients with carcinoma of the uterine cervix. *Proc. Am. Assoc. Cancer Res.*, **4**, 29.

Iverson T. (1982) Irradiation and bleomycin in the treatment of inoperable vulval carcinoma. *Acta Obstet. Gynaecol. Scand.*, **61**, 195–97.

Katib S., Kuten A., Steiner R.M., Yudelev M. & Robinson E. (1985) The effectiveness of multidrug treatment by bleomycin, methotrexate and cis-platinum in advanced vaginal carcinomas. *Gynecol. Oncol.*, **21**, 101–2.

Kavanagh J., Copeland L., Gershenson D., Saul P.B., Wharton J.T. & Rutledge F.N. (1985) Continuous infusion vinblastine in refractory carcinoma of the cervix. *Gynecol. Oncol.*, **21**, 211–14.

Kavanagh J.J., Gershenson D., Copeland L. & Roberts W.S. (1987) Combination chemotherapy for metastatic or recurrent adenocarcinoma of the cervix. *J. Clin. Oncol.*, **5**, 1621–23.

Keeney E.D., Freedman R.S., Drewinko B., Rutledge F.N. & Atkinson E.N. (1985) Clinical evaluation of high dose cytarabine and cisplatin in recurrent cervical carcinoma. *Cancer Treat. Rep.*, **69**, 1023–25.

Kirsten F., Atkinson K.H., Coppleson J.V.M. *et al.* (1987) Combination chemotherapy followed by surgery or radiotherapy in patients with locally advanced cervical cancer. *Br. J. Obstet. Gynaecol.*, **94**, 583–88.

Kneale B.L.G. (1986) Adjunctive and therapeutic progestins in endometrial cancer. *Clin. Obstet. Gynaecol.*, **13**, 789–809.

Korst D.R., Johnson F.D., Frenkel E.P. & Challenger W.L. (1963) Preliminary evaluation of the effect of cyclophosphamide on the course of human neoplasms. *Cancer Chem. Rep.*, **30**, 13.

Krakoff I.H., Cvitkovic E., Currie V., Yeh S. & LaMonte C. (1977) Clinical pharmacologic and therapeutic studies of bleomycin given by continuous infusion. *Cancer*, **40**, 2027–37.

Lahousen M., Pickel H. & Tamunssino K. (1987) Chemotherapy for advanced and/or recurrent cervical cancer. *Arch. Gynecol.*, **240**, 247–52.

Leibel S., Bauer M., Wasserman T. *et al.* (1987) Radiotherapy with or without misonidazole for patients with stage IIIb or stage IVa squamous cell carcinoma of the uterine cervix: preliminary report of the Radiation Therapy Oncology Group randomized trial. *Int. J. Radiat. Oncol. Biol. Phys.*, **13**, 541–49.

Leichman L.P., Baker L.H., Stanhope C.R. *et al.* (1980) Mitomycin C and bleomycin in the treatment of far-advanced cervical cancer: a Southwest Oncology Group pilot study. *Cancer Treat. Rep.*, **64**, 1139–40.

Levin W., Goldberg G., Altaras M., Bloch B. & Shelton M.G. (1986) The use of concomitous chemotherapy and radiotherapy prior to surgery in advanced stage carcinoma of the vulva. *Gynecol. Oncol.*, **25**, 20–25.

Lipsztein R., Kredentser D., Dottino P. *et al.* (1987) Combined chemotherapy and radiation therapy for advanced carcinoma of the cervix. *Am. J. Clin. Oncol.*, **10**, 527–30.

Long H.J., Pfeifle D.M. & Wieand H.S. (1987) Phase II evaluation of carboplatin (CBDCA) in advanced endometrial cancer: a collaborative trial of the North Central Cancer Treatment Group and the Mayo clinic. *Proc. Am. Soc. Clin. Oncol.*, **6**, 114 (Abstract 448).

Luce J.K., Thurman W.G., Isaacs B.L. & Talley R.W. (1970) Clinical trials with the antitumour agent 5-(3,3-dimethyl-1-triazeno)imidazole-4-carboxamide (NSC-45388). *Cancer Chem. Rep.*, **54**, 119—24.

Malkasian G.D. Jr., Decker D.G. & Jorgensen E.O. (1977) Chemotherapy of carcinoma of the cervix. *Gynecol. Oncol.*, **5**, 109—20.

Maurer H.M. (1980) The intergroup rhabdomyosarcoma study II. *J. Paediat. Surg.*, **15**, 371—72.

McGuire W.P., Arseneau J.C., Blessing J.A. *et al.* (1988) Randomized comparison of carboplatin (CP) and iproplatin (IP) in advanced squamous carcinoma of the uterine cervix (SCUC): a Gynecologic Oncology Group (GOG) study. *Proc. Am. Soc. Clin. Oncol.*, **7**, 135 (Abstract 521).

Meanwell C.A., Mould J.J., Blackledge G. *et al.* (1986) Phase II study of ifosfamide in cervical cancer. *Cancer Treat. Rep.*, **70**, 727—30.

Miyamoto T., Takabe Y., Watanabe M. & Terasima T. (1978) Effectiveness of a sequential combination of bleomycin and mitomycin C on an advanced cervical cancer. *Cancer*, **41**, 403—14.

Morgan L.S. & Nelson J.H. (1982) Surgical treatment of early cervical cancer. *Semin. Oncol.*, **9**, 312—30.

Omura G.A., Blessing J.A., Major F. *et al.* (1985) A randomized clinical trial of adjuvant adriamycin in uterine sarcomas: a Gynecologic Oncology Group study. *J. Clin. Oncol.*, **3**, 1240—45.

Omura G.A., Major F.G., Blessing J.A. *et al.* (1983) A randomized study of adriamycin with or without dimethyl triazenoimidazole carboxamide in advanced uterine sarcomas. *Cancer*, **52**, 626—32.

Omura G.A., Shingleton H.M., Creasman W.T., Blessing J.A. & Boronow R.C. (1978) Chemotherapy of gynecologic cancer with nitrosoureas: a randomized trial of CCNU and methyl-CCNU in cancer of the cervix, corpus, vagina, and vulva. *Cancer Treat. Rep.*, **62**, 833—35.

Omura G.A., Velez-Garcia E. & Birch R. (1981) Phase II randomized study of doxorubicin, vincristine, and 5-FU versus cyclophosphamide in advanced squamous cell carcinoma of the cervix. *Cancer Treat. Rep.*, **65**, 901—3.

OPCS (1988) Cancer statistics and registrations. *Series MB1 No. 16*. HMSO, London. p. 26.

Oreilly S.E., Swenerton K.D., Manji M., Acker B., Benedet J.L. & Elit L. (1986) Concomitant cisplatin (DDP) and radiotherapy (RT) in advanced cervical squamous cell carcinoma (SCC). *Proc. Am. Soc. Clin. Oncol.*, **5**, 115 (Abstract 448).

Panettiere F.J. (1976) Porfiromycin therapy for disseminated cancer of the cervix and other organs. *Proc. Am. Assoc. Cancer Res.*, **17**, 246.

Papavasiliou C., Pappas J., Aravantinos D. & Kaskarelis D. (1978) Treatment of cervical carcinoma with adriamycin combined with methotrexate. *Cancer Treat. Rep.*, **62**, 1387—88.

Picozzi V.J. Jr., Sikic B.I., Carlson R.W., Koretz M. & Ballon S.C. (1985) Bleomycin, mitomycin, and cisplatin therapy for advanced squamous carcinoma of the uterine cervix: a phase II study of the Northern California Oncology Group. *Cancer Treat. Rep.*, **69**, 903—5.

Piver M.S. & Barlow J.J. (1977) High dose irradiation to biopsy confirmed aortic node metastases from carcinoma of the uterine cervix. *Cancer*, **39**, 1243—46.

Piver M.S., Barlow J.J., Vongtama V. & Blumenson L. (1983) Hydroxyurea: a radiation potentiator in carcinoma of the uterine cervix. A randomized double-blind study. *Am. J. Obstet. Gynecol.*, **147**, 803—8.

Piver M.S. & Chung W.S. (1975) Prognostic significance of cervical lesion size and pelvic node metastases in cervical carcinoma. *Obstet. Gynecol.*, **46**, 507—10.

Piver M.S., Lele S.B., Patsner B. & Emrich L.J. (1986) Melphelan, 5-Fluorouracil and medroxyprogesterone acetate in metastatic endometrial cancer. *Obstet. Gynecol.*, **67**, 261—64.

Rhomberg W.U. (1986) Vindesine for recurrent and metastatic cancer of the uterine cervix: a phase II study. *Cancer Treat. Rep.*, **70**, 1455—57.

Rotmensch J., Senekjian E.K., Javaheri G. & Herbst A.L. (1988) Evaluation of bolus cis-platinum and continuous 5-fluorouracil infusion for metastic and recurrent squamous cell carcinoma of the cervix. *Gynecol. Oncol.*, **29**, 76—81.

Salazar O.M., Bonfiglio T.A., Patten S.F. *et al.* (1978a) Uterine sarcomas: natural history, treatment and prognosis. *Cancer*, **42**, 1152—60.

Salazar O.M., Bonfiglio T.A., Patten S.F., Keller B.E., Feldstein M., Dunne M.E. & Rudolph J. (1978b) Uterine sarcomas; analysis of failures with special emphasis on the use of adjuvant radiation therapy. *Cancer*, **42**, 1161—70.

Santoro A. & Bonadona G. (1985) Soft tissue and bone sarcomas. In: Pinedo H.M. & Chabner B.A. (eds), Cancer Chemotherapy/7. Elselvier Science Publishers B.V., Amsterdam. pp. 426—38.

Seski J.C., Edwards C.L., Gershenson D.M. & Copeland L.J. (1981a) Doxorubicin and cyclophosphamide chemotherapy for disseminated endometrial cancer. Obstet. Gynecol., 58, 88—91.

Seski J.C., Edwards C.L., Herson J. & Rutledge F.N. (1981b) Cisplatin chemotherapy for disseminated endometrial cancer. Obstet. Gynecol., 59, 225—28.

Shirozimu K., Matsuzawa M., Takahashi M. & Ishihara O. (1988) Is postoperative radiotherapy and maintenance chemotherapy necessary for carcinoma of the uterine cervix. Br. J. Obstet. Gynaecol., 95, 503—06.

Slayton R.E., Blessing J.A. & Homesley H.D. (1984) Phase II trial of etoposide in the management of advanced or recurrent non-squamous cell carcinoma of the cervix: a Gynecologic Oncology Group study. Cancer Treat. Rep., 68, 1513—14.

Souhami L., Gil R.A. & Allan S.E. (1988) Randomized trial of neoadjuvant chemotherapy followed by pelvic radiotherapy versus radiotherapy alone in stage IIIb carcinoma of the cervix. Proc. Am. Soc. Clin. Oncol., 7, 137 (Abstract 538).

Stehman F.B., Bundy Y.B.N., Keys H., Currie J.L., Mortel R. & Creasman W.T. (1988) A randomized trial of hydroxyurea versus misonidazole adjunct to radiation therapy in carcinoma of the cervix. A preliminary report of the Gynecologic Oncology Group. Am. J. Obstet. Gynecol., 159, 87—94.

Stuart-Harris R.C., Harper P.G., Parson C.A., Kaye S.B., Mooney C.A., Gowin N.F. & Wiltshaw E. (1983) High dose alkylation therapy using ifosfamide infusion with mesna in the treatment of adult advanced soft tissue sarcoma. Cancer Chemother. Pharmacol., 11, 69—72.

Sutton G.P. (1988) Personal communication.

Symonds R.P., Watson E.R., Habeshaw T. & Kaye S.B. (1987) Chemotherapy prior to radical radiotherapy for stage III and IV carcinoma of the cervix. Clinical Radiology, 38, 273—74.

Thar T.L., Million R.R. & Daly J.W. (1982) Radiation treatment of carcinoma of the cervix. Semin. Oncol., 9, 299—311.

Thigpen J.T., Blessing J., Disaia P. & Ehrlich C. (1985) A randomised comparison of adriamycin with or without cyclophosphamide in the treatment of advanced or recurrent endometrial carcinoma. Proc. Am. Soc. Clin. Oncol., 4, 115 (Abstract C-448).

Thigpen J.T., Blessing J., Disaia P., Shingleton H. & Fowler W. (1986d) Cisplatin in the management of patients with advanced or recurrent squamous carcinoma of the cervix: effects of prolonged infusion. Proc. Am. Soc. Clin. Oncol., 5, 116 (Abstract 452).

Thigpen J.T., Blessing J.A., Fowler W.C. Jr. & Hatch K. (1986c) Phase II trials of cisplatin and piperazinedione as single agents in the treatment of advanced or recurrent non-squamous cell carcinoma of the cervix: a Gynecologic Oncology Group study. Cancer Treat. Rep., 70, 1097—1100.

Thigpen J.T., Blessing J.A., Homesley H.D., Berek J.S. & Creasman W.T. (1986a) Phase II trial of cisplatin in advanced or recurrent cancer of the vagina: a Gynecologic Oncology Group study. Gynecol. Oncol., 23, 101—4.

Thigpen J.T., Blessing J.A., Homesley H.D. & Lewis G.C. Jr. (1986b) Phase II trials of cisplatin and piperazinedione in advanced or recurrent carcinoma of the vulva: a Gynecologic Oncology Group study. Gynecol. Oncol., 23, 358—63.

Thigpen J.T., Blessing J.A., Lagasse L.D., Disaia P.J. & Homesley H.D. (1984) Phase II trial of cisplatin as second line chemotherapy in patients with advanced or recurrent endometrial carcinoma. A Gynecologic Oncology Group study. Am. J. Clin. Oncol., 7, 253—56.

Thigpen J.T., Buchsbaum H.J., Mangan C. & Blessing J.A. (1979) Phase II trial of adriamycin in treatment of advanced or recurrent endometrial carcinoma. A Gynecologic Oncology Group study. Cancer Treat. Rep., 63, 21—27.

Thigpen J.T., Shingleton H., Homesley H. & Blessing J. (1982) A phase II trial of cis-diammine dichloroplatinum (DDP) in treatment of advanced or recurrent mixed mesodermal sarcoma of the uterus. Proc. Am. Soc. Clin. Oncol., 1, 110 (Abstract C 127).

Thigpen J.T., Vance R., Lambuth B., Balducci L., Khansur T., Blessing J. & McGehee R. (1987) Chemotherapy for advanced or recurrent gynecological cancer. Cancer, 60, 2104—16.

Thomas G., Denbo A., Beale F. et al. (1984) Concurrent radiation, mitomycin C and 5 fluorouracil in poor prognosis carcinoma of the cervix: preliminary results of a phase I—II study. Int. J. Radiat. Oncol. Biol. Phys., 10, 1785—90.

Trope C., Johnsson J.E., Grundsell H. & Mattsson W. (1980) Adriamycin-methotrexate combination chemotherapy of advanced carcinoma of the cervix: a third look. *Obstet. Gynecol.*, **55**, 488−92.

Trope C., Johnsson J.E., Simonsen E., Christiansen A., Cavallin-Stahl E. & Horvath G. (1984) Treatment of recurrent endometrial adenocarcinoma with a combination of doxorubicin and cisplatin. *Am. J. Obstet. Gynecol.*, **149**, 379−81.

Trope C., Johnsson J.E., Simonsen E., Sigurdsson K.J., Stendahl U., Mattsson W. & Gullberg B. (1983) Bleomycin-mitomycin C in advanced carcinoma of the cervix. *Cancer*, **51**, 591−93.

Van Der Burg M.E.L., Subandono A.J., Mangioni C. *et al.* (1984) Vincristine, bleomycin, mitomycin C, cisplatin chemotherapy as additive treatment to radiotherapy in poor risk patients with squamous cell carcinoma of the uterine cervix. *Proc. Am. Soc. Clin. Oncol.*, **165** (Abstract 644).

Vermorken J.B., Pecorelli S., Mangioni C., Van Der Burg M.E.L., Kenis Y. & Rotmensz N. (1984) Phase II study of vindesine (DVA) in disseminated squamous cell carcinoma of the uterine cervix (SCCUC). *Proc. Am. Soc. Clin. Oncol.*, **165** (Abstract 645).

Vermorken J.B., Van Der Burg M.E.L., George M., Mangioni C., Pecorelli S., Rotmensz N. & Dalesio O. (1987) Phase II study of bleomycin (B), vindesine (E), mitomycin C (M) and cisplatin (P) in recurrent and or metastatic squamous cell cancer of the uterine cervix (SCCUC). *Proc. Am. Soc. Clin. Oncol.*, **6**, 120 (Abstract 470).

Wallace H.J., Hreschchyshyn M.M., Willbanks G.D., Boronow R.C., Fowler W.C. Jr. & Blessing J.A. (1978) Comparison of the therapeutic effects of adriamycin alone versus adriamycin plus vincristine versus adriamycin plus cyclophosphamide in the treatment of advanced carcinoma of the cervix. *Cancer Treat. Rep.*, **62**, 1435−41.

Weiner S.A., Aristizabal S., Alberts D.S., Surwit E.A. & Deatherage-Deuser K. (1988) A phase II trial of mitomycin C, vincristine, bleomycin, and cisplatin (MOBP) as neoadjuvant therapy in high risk cervical carcinoma. *Gynecol. Oncol.*, **30**, 1−6.

14

Trophoblastic Disease

RICHARD H.J. BEGENT

The trophoblast is a unique tissue, being among the first to differentiate from developing foetus and comprising foetal tissue which forms an interface with the maternal circulation. Not surprisingly, gestational trophoblastic disease presents unique biological and clinical features. Gestational trophoblastic diseases comprise neoplasms of trophoblast and conditions which predispose to neoplasia. They include hydatidiform mole which comprises complete and partial hydatidiform mole, invasive mole, gestational choriocarcinoma and placental site trophoblastic tumour. Choriocarcinoma arising in germ cell tumours is excluded because it is not gestational in origin. This classification is defined by a WHO Scientific Group (Gestational Trophoblastic Diseases 1983) and acknowledges the Histological Classification of Tumours (Poulsen 1975) but modifies it because of the subsequent discovery (Vassilakos *et al.* 1977) that complete and partial hydatidiform mole are separate entities of different aetiology.

Pathology and origin

Complete hydatidiform mole

Hydatidiform mole was recognized as a cause of abortion by Hippocrates and his pupil, Diocles. Its origin from the chorion was recognized in Paris in the nineteenth century (for review see Ober 1987). The macroscopic structure of multiple hydropic vesicles probably led the attendants of Margaret, Countess of Henneberg, in 1276 to believe that each vesicle was a separate conception and christen half John and half Mary.

The universal hydropically dilated trophoblastic villi connected by narrow bridges bear hyperplastic syncytio- and cytotrophoblast on their surface with varying degrees of exuberance. The villi initially contain oedematous mesenchyme. Cisterns form within the mesenchyme which involutes with increasing gestational age. Any blood vessels in the mesenchyme also tend to die out leaving the fluid filled cistern as the feature causing hydropic villous dilatation. There being no foetus, no nucleated foetal erythrocytes are seen in any vessels present.

Complete hydatidiform mole originates from fertilization of an ovum from

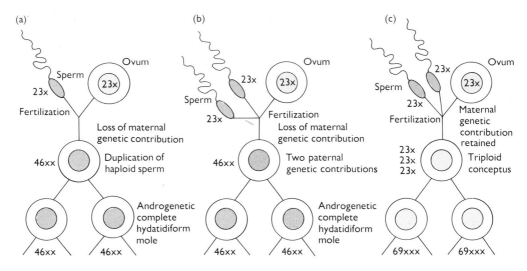

Fig. 14.1. Genetic origin of (a) complete hydatidiform mole, single sperm >90% of moles; (b) complete hydatidiform mole, dispermy 4–8% of moles; (c) partial hydatidiform mole.

which the maternal genetic material is lost or inactivated (Fig. 14.1). A single sperm bearing a 23X set of chromosomes produces the fertilization and then duplicates to 46XX in about 90% of cases (Kajii & Ohama 1977; Vassilakos *et al.* 1977; Lawler *et al.* 1979, 1982a; Davis *et al.* 1984; Lawler & Fisher 1987). Occasionally fertilization takes place with two spermatozoa, resulting in the XY configuration (Ohama *et al.* 1981). The 46XX constitution can probably also originate in this way. A 46YY conceptus would be theoretically possible by this mechanism but is not described and is presumably non-viable. The most frequent variants are shown in Fig. 14.1a, b. While the nuclear genetic material is paternal, the mitochondrial DNA is of maternal origin (Edwards *et al.* 1984). The conceptus in complete hydatidiform mole is thus entirely paternally derived and a total allograft in the mother. Twin pregnancies with a complete hydatidiform mole and normal fetus have been reported (Fisher *et al.* 1982; Berrebi *et al.* 1988). The latter paper reviewed this literature and found birth of a viable fetus in 27%, fetal death *in utero* in 46% and birth of a non-viable fetus in 23%.

Partial hydatidiform mole

This condition is now recognized as of different cytogenetic origin from complete hydatidiform mole although discrimination by morphology is not always straightforward. There is evidence of a fetus as part of the same conception in which the placenta contains some normal and some abnormal villi. These villi are swollen, showing trophoblastic hyperplasia and cistern formation. In older examples (more than 18–20 weeks) a maze-like outline is sometimes seen in the cisterns. If the fetus is alive the vessels in the villi contain nucleated fetal red blood cells. There is a characteristic scalloping of the outline of the villi and stromal trophoblastic inclusions are common. The affected villi are mixed in the form of a mosaic with normal trophoblastic villi within the placenta. The trophoblastic hyperplasia is often less marked than in complete hydatidiform mole and is usually confined to the syncytiotrophoblast. The fetus usually dies at 8–9 weeks of menstrual age. This is followed by fibrosis of the villous mesenchyme in unaffected and affected villi.

Cytogenetic and biochemical studies show that partial moles are triploid, differing from complete hydatidiform mole by retaining a maternal genetic contribution. They most often arise by diandry with two paternal and one maternal set of chromosomes (Jacobs et al. 1982; Lawler et al. 1982b, 1987) (Fig. 14.1c). Triploidy occurs in 1–3% of all recognized conceptions and in about 20% of spontaneous abortions with abnormal karyotype. Not all of these become partial hydatidiform mole. Exceptionally, partial mole can be tetraploid with three paternal contributions (Sheppard et al. 1982). Flow cytometry can now be used to determine whether trophoblastic disease is triploid or diploid. This offers a practical solution to the problem of discriminating complete and partial mole because it can be done on formalin fixed, paraffin embedded tissue (Fisher et al. 1987; Lage et al. 1988). It is not certain whether partial hydatidiform mole can give rise to choriocarcinoma. However, after evacuation human chorionic gonadotrophin (HCG) levels have failed to fall to normal in some patients, indicating persistent growth of trophoblast which could be explained by the development of choriocarcinoma or invasive mole.

Invasive mole

Invasive mole occurs when complete or partial hydatidiform mole invades deep into the myometrium. This extension is well beyond the usual decidual site of implantation and has been likened to placenta accreta or percreta in the non-molar placenta (Szulman 1987). Invasive mole is distinguished from choriocarcinoma by the presence of chorionic villae. However, the diagnosis is often obscure because uterine curettage cannot gain access to the tumour deep in the myometrium and the absence of chorionic villae in fragments of trophoblast does not exclude the presence of villae deep in the myometrium. Similarly it is not possible to determine whether a pulmonary metastasis after hydatidiform mole is choriocarcinoma or hydatidiform mole without resecting it. This is hardly ever done.

The principal risk is of uterine perforation or severe uterine bleeding. Invasive mole may metastasize to the lungs, cervix, vulva and vagina. It may regress spontaneously and although it can occasionally progress to choriocarcinoma it does not usually exhibit the progression of true malignancy. There is some evidence that heterozygosity is more common in moles subsequently requiring chemotherapy because of invasive mole or choriocarcinoma (Davis et al. 1984; Sheppard et al. 1985; Lawler & Fisher 1986).

Choriocarcinoma

Choriocarcinoma is a malignant tumour comprising, principally, villous trophoblast. It has the essential features of the rapidly dividing and invasive trophoblast
of the implanting blastocyst but maintains these features, instead of differentiating to a more stable form as occurs in the progress of a normal pregnancy.
Chorionic villi are absent. The characteristic morphology is of pleomorphic cytotrophoblast surrounded by some syncytium with extensive areas of haemorrhage
and necrosis. The syncytiotrophoblast is largely responsible for production of
hCG and other hormones of pregnancy. Because of the similarity to early trophoblast in normal pregnancy, caution is needed in making the diagnosis on scanty
uterine curettings when an early pregnancy is possible. Viable choriocarcinoma
cells may comprise only a rim on a mass of necrotic and haemorrhagic tissue. The
tumour has no stroma or vasculature of its own and relies on vessels of the tissue
which it invades. Choriocarcinoma may follow normal pregnancy, non-molar
abortion, ectopic pregnancy or hydatidiform mole. It is not practical to make
the diagnosis on uterine curettings after hydatidiform mole since it is necessary
to obtain more comprehensive material in order to practically exclude the presence of chorionic villi. For this reason doubt often exists at the time the patient
comes to treatment whether she has invasive mole or choriocarcinoma. Gestational choriocarcinoma must also be distinguished from choriocarcinoma arising
in an ovarian germ cell tumour or trophoblastic differentiation in a common epithelial carcinoma. Gestational choriocarcinoma metastasizes widely, particularly
to the lungs, pelvic organs and brain.

Placental site trophoblastic tumour

These tumours are composed principally of placental site (intermediate) trophoblast. This is normally separate from villous trophoblast and infiltrates the
deciduum, myometrium and spiral arteries of the placental site. The cells are
mostly mononuclear, though multinucleate forms occur. Their appearance in the
normal placenta and placental site tumour has been reviewed by Mazur &
Kurman (1987). Serum hCG levels are low in relation to the volume of tumour
but produce abundant human placental lactogen which can be valuable in discriminating from carcinomas or sarcomas by immunohistochemistry. At first
they were thought to behave in a benign fashion leading to the name 'trophoblastic pseudotumour' which was ascribed to them by Kurman et al. (1976). Later
experience shows that these tumours may metastasize and usually prove resistant
to cytotoxic chemotherapy (Scully & Young 1981; Eckstein et al. 1982). The term
placental site trophoblastic tumour is therefore preferred. They probably constitute
about 1% of trophoblastic tumours, have a slow growth rate and may present
years after term delivery, non-molar abortion or complete hydatidiform mole.

Only about 50 cases are reported and they are best treated by hysterectomy if still localized to the uterus.

Hydropic degeneration

This is characterized by dilatation with increased fluid content or liquefaction of placental villi. It has also previously been known as molar degeneration and hydropic change. The trophoblastic proliferation and other characteristic features of complete or partial hydatidiform mole are absent and there is no increased risk of neoplastic sequelae compared with a natural pregnancy. It is mentioned here in order to exclude it from the definition of trophoblastic disease.

Incidence of trophoblastic disease

Complete hydatidiform mole

The incidence of hydatidiform mole has been reviewed by a WHO Scientific Group (Gestational Trophoblastic Diseases 1983) and Bracken *et al.* (1984). Epidemiological studies have not in general taken into account the fact that complete and partial hydatidiform mole have a different pathological basis. The situation is further complicated by variation in the classification of hydropic degeneration, a harmless condition, which is sometimes included in studies of hydatidiform mole. There is probably a tendency for hospital based studies to exaggerate the incidence of hydatidiform mole, particularly in the developing countries where the hospital population will reflect a selected group of patients with a greater incidence of complications of pregnancy. Reports are also difficult to compare because some relate the incidence of hydatidiform mole to the number of pregnancies, others to normal deliveries and others to the number of live births.

Overall incidence

The incidence from hospital based studies varies between 0.7 and 10 cases of hydatidiform mole per 1000 pregnancies. The highest values have been from South-East Asia and western Africa where the effect of the selection of hospital is likely to be high. Population based studies do not reflect the same differences, with the exception of Japan where higher incidences have been reported than in other parts of the world. There are not sufficient studies to establish with certainty that incidence does vary substantially in different parts of the world and the incidence of the order of 1 per 1000 pregnancies appears representative.

Information on temporal trends of hydatidiform mole is more conflicting and again tends to suffer from the problems of hospital based studies. No clear trend emerges from them.

Ethnic origin

Large differences in the incidence of hydatidiform mole do seem to be established in various ethnic groups. In the USA, for 1970–77, hydatidiform mole was only half as frequent in black women as in others (Hayashi 1982) and in Singapore from 1963–65 Eurasian women had a rate of hydatidiform mole twice as high as that of Chinese, Indian or Malaysian (Teoh et al. 1971). A higher incidence was also seen in Jewish women over 45 years old who lived in Israel and came from Europe than those of the same age who were born in Africa, Asia or Israel (Matalon & Moden 1972). A study by Jacobs et al. (1982), showed that Filipinos seem to maintain the high risk of hydatidiform mole which prevails in their own country whereas Japanese and other East Asians seem to lose the high incidence of their own countries when they live in Hawaii. This suggests that cultural factors affect the immigrants when they move to a new environment.

Age

In the UK the lowest incidence appears to be between 25 and 29 years with a 6-fold increase in relative risk in pregnancies in girls under 15 years. There is also an increased risk above the age of 40 years with a relative risk of 3-fold between 40 and 45 years, 26-fold between 45 and 49 and more than 400-fold over 50 years of age (Bagshawe et al. 1986). The effect of paternal age is difficult to separate from that of maternal age and conflicting studies of the independent effect of paternal age have been reported (Yen & McMahon 1968; La Vecchia et al. 1984). No clear effect from gravidity seems to apply but women who have had a previous hydatidiform mole have a substantially increased risk of having another. For instance in the UK, the incidence rises from 1 in 1000 pregnancies for the first mole to 1 in 74 in women who have already had one mole (Bagshawe et al. 1986).

Incidence of partial mole

Partial mole was found to be less frequent than complete hydatidiform mole (24% of the total) in a series in which cases were selected because of suspicion of hydatidiform mole (Lawler & Fisher 1986). Similarly, Berkowitz & Goldstein (1981) found 3% of partial hydatidiform moles in their series. However, in patients presenting as spontaneous abortion the frequency of partial hydatidiform mole was 69% relative to complete hydatidiform mole (Jacobs et al. 1982).

Incidence and epidemiology of choriocarcinoma

This is influenced by the incidence of hydatidiform mole and about 3% of patients with hydatidiform mole finally develop choriocarcinoma. Problems with definition arise in this group where the histology is not always available and discrimination between invasive mole and choriocarcinoma is not possible. Hydatidiform mole is probably the commonest antecedent to choriocarcinoma, comprising 29−83% in studies from various parts of the world, abortion or ectopic pregnancy being the next most common (11−42%), followed by live births (5−34%) (Gestational Trophoblastic Diseases 1983). The incidence following term delivery without hydatidiform mole is of the order of 1 in 50000. No very clear trends emerge for greater frequency in particular parts of the world (Bracken *et al.* 1984) but more extensive population based studies are needed.

Genetic factors

Cytogenetic studies show 4.6% of balanced translocations in women with complete hydatidiform mole compared with 0.6% of normal populations. The ABO blood groups of women with hydatidiform mole and their spouses do not appear to differ from normal populations. However, choriocarcinoma after term delivery is about twice as common when patient and partner have different A and O blood groups as when they are the same (for review see Gestational Trophoblastic Diseases 1983).

Clinical features

Presentation of hydatidiform mole

Hydatidiform mole including complete and partial hydatidiform mole presents in the first trimester most commonly with vaginal bleeding which may be fresh or altered, light or heavy enough to require transfusion and is frequently asso ciated with anaemia. The uterus may be enlarged or small for gestational age. Hyperemesis and toxaemia occur with greater frequency than in normal pregnancy. Passage of vesicles is not infrequent and occasionally the entire mole is evacuated spontaneously. Theca lutein cysts are frequently found when hCG levels are high. Pulmonary, vaginal and cervical metastases may occur but do not necessarily imply development of invasive mole or choriocarcinoma since they may resolve after evacuation of the mole. Hyperthyroidism (Fradken *et al.* 1989) and pulmonary emboli of trophoblast occur occasionally. The clinical features of hydatidiform mole have been reviewed by Goldstein *et al.* (1981). Pregnancy terminated for medical or social reasons may be a mole and escape detection when no histological examination is done.

Invasive mole

This is usually diagnosed in the weeks following evacuation of hydatidiform mole because invasion of the myometrium produces heavy bleeding, lower abdominal pain or intraperitoneal haemorrhage. These life threatening presentations of invasive mole should not be awaited before treatment is started since they can be predicted in most cases by monitoring hCG levels in urine or serum. Occasionally the bladder or rectum is infiltrated producing haematuria or rectal bleeding. Enlarging pulmonary, vulval or vaginal metastases may occur.

Choriocarcinoma

Choriocarcinoma is 1500 times more common after a molar pregnancy than after a term delivery. In the former case it should be suspected if hCG levels are not normal 6 months after evacuation. It may occur sooner than this after a mole but then is often difficult to distinguish from invasive mole without performing a hysterectomy to determine the diagnosis histologically. Hysterectomy is only rarely justified or necessary at this stage so there remain many cases in which it is never known whether the patient had invasive mole or choriocarcinoma even after treatment. Choriocarcinoma and placental site tumour are the only possible gestational trophoblastic tumours originating from a term delivery or a non-molar abortion.

Presentation of choriocarcinoma

The majority of patients with choriocarcinoma present within a year of an apparently normal pregnancy or non-molar abortion. The presentation may be delayed for several years, however, the longest interval in the Charing Cross Hospital series being 17 years. Vaginal bleeding or bloodstained discharge, sometimes with abdominal pain and mass, are most common. Extra uterine masses and ovarian involvement are frequent. In about one-third of cases, however, the presenting features are not gynaecological but originate from distant metastases (McGrath *et al.* 1971). Pulmonary, cerebral and hepatic deposits are most frequent (see Table 14.1) (Begent & Bagshawe 1982). Pulmonary deposits (Fig. 14.5) may cause dyspnoea or haemoptysis and when widespread can be associated with pneumonia. Choriocarcinoma can grow within the pulmonary artery and cause pulmonary hypertension (Bagshawe & Begent 1981). Cerebral metastases may present with focal neurological signs, convulsions, evidence of raised intracranial pressure or of haemorrhage intracerebrally or into the sub-arachnoid space (Athanassiou *et al.* 1983). These features are not specific for choriocarcinoma and it may be many years since the causative pregnancy. It is important, therefore, to remember to measure hCG levels (see below) when they occur in women who have had a pregnancy. Metastases in viscera such as the liver, kidney, spleen or bowel may also present with haemorrhage intraperitoneally or into the lumen of the bowel. Skin metastases are usually purple and most frequently occur late in the course of the disease. Lymph node and bone metastases are so rare that their presence should lead to review of the evidence for the diagnosis.

Occasionally thyrotoxicosis is present in patients with very high hCG levels because of cross reaction between the alpha subunit of hCG and thyroid stimulating hormone (Fradken *et al.* 1989).

Table 14.1. Sites of metastases outside the pelvis detected at presentation in 72 patients with high risk gestational choriocarcinoma

Site	No. of patients
Lungs	57
Brain	11
Liver	9
Breast	1
Spleen	1
Cauda equina	1
None detected	8

Investigation

Human chorionic gonadotrophin (HCG)

This hormone is only one of a range produced by normal and neoplastic trophoblast. It is a polypeptide composed of two subunits with a combined molecular weight of 37 000 daltons. It is excreted in the urine with a half-life of approximately 24–36 h and has so far proved the most sensitive and specific marker for trophoblastic tumours when compared with other placental proteins (PP) such as PP5 and beta 1 SP1. Pregnancy tests employing haemagglutination inhibition or complement fixation methods have a lower limit of sensitivity of about 2000 i.u./l whereas the best radioimmunoassays are sensitive to 1 i.u./l in serum and 20 i.u./l in urine (Kardana & Bagshawe 1976). Immunoenzymatic, immuno-chemiluminescent and fluoroimmunoassays also have the potential to match this sensitivity. It is important to be aware that simple pregnancy tests can also give false negative results when hCG values are very high.

When it is wished to exclude a trophoblastic tumour, one of the more sensitive assays must be used. HCG assays do not discriminate between trophoblastic tumours and normal pregnancy though very high values outside the range for twin pregnancy may lead to suspicion of a trophoblastic tumour. HCG levels are frequently within the pregnancy range. Considering that pregnancy is much the commoner cause of a raised hCG this possibility must always be considered before embarking on investigation or treatment of a suspected trophoblastic tumour. Germ cell tumours containing trophoblastic elements can produce hCG levels as high as gestational trophoblastic tumours (GTT) (for review see Bagshawe & Begent 1983). About 15% of common epithelial malignancies produce measurable amounts of hCG (Vaitukaitis 1979) and exceptionally levels can exceed 20 000 i.u./l.

In gestational trophoblastic disease, hCG values give an indication of the volume of tumour. It has been estimated from tissue culture experiments that serum values of hCG of the order of 5 i.u./l correspond to 10^4 to 10^5 viable tumour cells making these assays orders of magnitude more sensitive than the most sensitive imaging methods. Total tumour volume can be estimated from hCG measurements and used to determine prognosis (Bagshawe 1976). Serial measurements allow progress of the disease or response to therapy to be monitored (Fig. 14.2). Development of drug resistance can be detected at an early stage. Estimates may be made of the time for which chemotherapy should be continued after hCG is undetectable in serum in order theoretically to eradicate all tumour cells. In these respects it is the best tumour marker known and is of wider interest as a model for the way in which tumour markers may eventually be used in other diseases.

Ultrasound

This investigation has transformed the investigation of the uterus and pelvic organs in trophoblastic tumours. It has largely displaced arteriography which was used previously to show the distinctive circulation of hydatidiform mole and choriocarcinoma. Ultrasound is used to discriminate between normal pregnancy

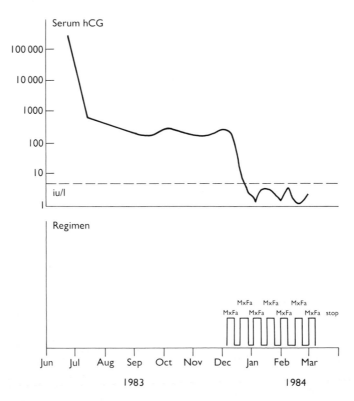

Fig. 14.2. Serum hCG values after evacuation of hydatidiform mole. Levels fell after evacuation of the uterus but remained raised 6 months later. Chemotherapy with methotrexate and folinic acid (MxFa) (Table 14.5) was given because the patient fell into the low risk group. HCG fell to undetectable levels and chemotherapy was continued for a further 8 weeks.

and hydatidiform mole, not solely by the pattern of echogenicity (Fig. 14.3) which is not entirely specific but by the presence of this pattern when there is a history consistent with hydatidiform mole or normal pregnancy and when hCG levels are raised. An example of the appearance of choriocarcinoma is shown in Fig. 14.4. An indication of uterine volume can be obtained which is more accurate than estimations obtained by palpation and is useful as a prognostic indicator (Halpin *et al.* unpublished). It is helpful in showing extension of the tumour through the uterine wall and separate extra uterine masses. Theca lutein cysts of the ovary and other ovarian masses are also well seen. Hepatic and renal deposits can be shown. Ultrasound is convenient to use for monitoring the progress of the disease (Requard & Mettler 1980) although it does not match the sensitivity of hCG measurements and should not be used as a substitute. When uterine or ovarian masses are present at the start of treatment it is worth repeating the ultrasound examination at the end of treatment to ensure that the changes were not due to some other pathology.

Arteriography

Arteriography still has a limited place. It shows the great vascularity of trophoblastic tumours and the arteriovenous malformations which exist within them. This vascular pattern sometimes persists after eradication of the mole and can cause severe haemorrhage. Arteriography is also useful in determining the extent and vascular supply of deposits of choriocarcinoma in the liver if resection is planned for drug resistant disease.

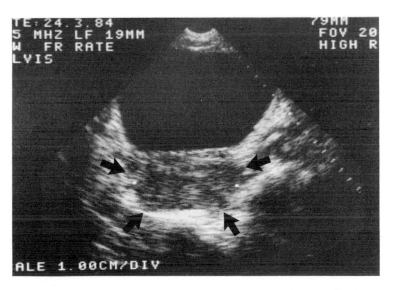

Fig. 14.3. Ultrasound of the uterus (arrowed) in transverse section showing the characteristic pattern of hydatidiform mole.

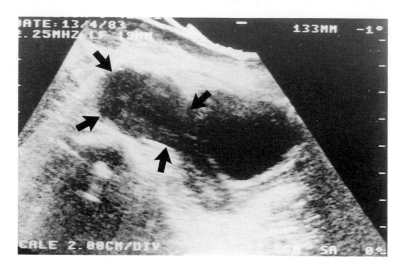

Fig. 14.4.   Ultrasound of the uterus (arrowed) in sagittal section showing choriocarcinoma after term delivery of a normal fetus.

Plain radiography of the chest

This demonstrates the diverse patterns of metastases of GTT. The most common appearance (Fig. 14.5) is of multiple discrete rounded lesions but large solitary lesions or a miliary pattern can occur (Bagshawe & Begent 1981). Pleural effusions are rare but dilatation of the pulmonary arteries occurs in patients with pulmonary hypertension.

X-ray computerized tomography (CT)

CT is more sensitive than plain radiography being able to detect metastases of 3—4 mm in the lungs (Fig. 14.6). It is not necessary to perform the investigation routinely but it is invaluable in determining the extent of disease if resection of drug resistant deposits of choriocarcinoma is being considered. CT is also valuable along with ultrasound in assessing intraabdominal disease, particularly in the liver and pelvis. In the brain, CT is better than isotope scanning (Athanassiou *et al*. 1983) and is now the standard method for imaging cerebral metastases.

Magnetic resonance imaging (MRI)

MR imaging (for review see Steiner & Radda 1983) can also be used to give images of choriocarcinoma in the pelvis and liver. It is not yet clear whether it will be superior to CT in these areas but it does have advantages in the brain where better images of the posterior fossa are obtained. In imaging of choriocarcinoma in the cerebral hemispheres it is able to locate deposits of choriocarcinoma

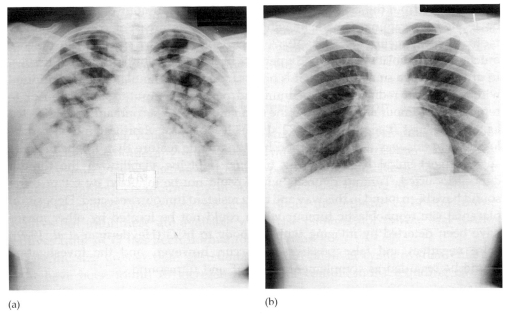

(a)   (b)

Fig. 14.5. Multiple pulmonary metastases of choriocarcinoma, (a) before and (b) after treatment.

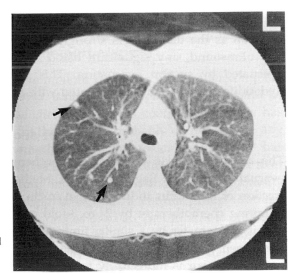

Fig. 14.6. CT of the lungs showing small metastases which were not detectable by plain radiography.

close to the bone of the skull which have been undetectable by CT. These have been resected eradicating drug resistant disease.

Radioimmunolocalization

In this method, radiolabelled antibody directed against hCG (anti-hCG) is given intravenously. Anti-hCG is retained in hCG-producing tumours but is cleared

lower incidence of those subsequently requiring chemotherapy than in untreated patients (Fasoli *et al.* 1982). Actinomycin D probably provides a more satisfactory agent. In one study it reduced the proportions subsequently requiring chemotherapy (Goldstein *et al.* 1981). Xia *et al.* (1988) and Kashimura *et al.* (1986) have defined groups of patients more likely to require chemotherapy than others after evacuation of hydatidiform mole and given prophylactic chemotherapy only to them. However, mortality was lower in the series of Bagshawe *et al.* (1986) in which prophylactic chemotherapy was not given (see below).

The administration of cytotoxic drugs to a group of patients of whom 90% do not need them is unattractive but it may be a reasonable approach in areas where a follow up of hCG levels (see below) is not practical. It seems clear that some patients relapse with all the regimens so that prophylactic chemotherapy does not remove the need for follow up of hCG values. It is recommended that prophylactic chemotherapy should not be given in the UK or other countries where adequate hCG follow up is possible. This is because survival is very close to 100% if such follow up is undertaken (Bagshawe *et al.* 1986) as described below without prophylactic chemotherapy.

Follow up of HCG levels

An alternative approach to prophylactic chemotherapy is to follow up patients with hCG estimations after evacuation of hydatidiform mole and only treat those in whom there is evidence of invasive mole or choriocarcinoma. Such a scheme has existed in the UK since 1972 under the auspices of the Royal College of Obstetricians and Gynaecologists. Patients are registered by their gynaecologist at one of three centres where an hCG is assayed (Charing Cross Hospital in London, Sheffield and Dundee). Urine samples are then sent by post every 2 weeks until hCG levels are normal. In a study of 4205 patients hCG levels fell to undetectable levels within 56 days of uterine evacuation in 42% of patients none of whom required chemotherapy (Bagshawe *et al.* 1986). Follow up is continued for 6 months in these patients and for 2 years after the levels have been normal in the remainder.

A number of indications for treatment have evolved which are designed to pick out those patients who have developed choriocarcinoma or are at risk of dangerous sequelae of invasive mole. They depend heavily on the results of assays for hCG but other clinical factors are important and clinical follow up of these patients is also necessary by the referring gynaecologist. The indications for treatment are shown in Table 14.3. A very high hCG, of the order of 20 000 i.u./l, 4 weeks after evacuation of a mole or rising values in this range at an earlier stage indicate that the patient is at risk of severe haemorrhage or uterine perforation with intraperitoneal bleeding. These complications can be life threatening and the ability to predict them to some extent with hCG values usually enables treatment to be started before complications develop. Chemotherapy is

Table 14.3. Indications for chemotherapy of gestational trophoblastic tumours

---

Rising hCG after evacuation
Very high hCG after evacuation (e.g. 25 000 i.u./l after 4 weeks)
HCG not falling 4 months after evacuation
Raised hCG 6 months after evacuation even if still falling slowly
Pulmonary, vulval or vaginal metastases unless hCG falling
Metastases at any other site
Heavy vaginal bleeding or evidence of gastrointestinal or intraperitoneal bleeding
Histological evidence of choriocarcinoma
Raised hCG with a clinical picture strongly suggestive of choriocarcinoma if the patient is too ill for a
  suitable biopsy

---

in general the best way of dealing with heavy bleeding. Repeated dilatation and curettage have not been shown to be beneficial provided that the uterus was thoroughly evacuated on the first occasion.

Metastases in the lungs, vulva or vagina are not necessarily indications for treatment provided that hCG levels are falling. However, chemotherapy should be started if metastases are present and hCG levels are not dropping. Metastases at other sites are an indication of the development of choriocarcinoma and chemotherapy is required. Although choriocarcinoma cannot be diagnosed on uterine curettings (see above) histological evidence of choriocarcinoma from other specimens is an indication for chemotherapy since it is known that this tumour will not die out spontaneously. The development of choriocarcinoma can also be predicted if hCG levels are rising 4 months after evacuation of a mole or if hCG is detectable at all 6 months after evacuation. Mortality from the sequelae of hydatidiform mole was 0.1% in patients followed up according to this scheme.

Patients requiring chemotherapy

Staging

Anatomical staging systems such as that of FIGO would be relevant if surgical treatment was appropriate after the diagnostic evacuation. Since surgery is virtually never indicated at this time, these systems play no part in treatment planning.

Prognostic factors

The indications for chemotherapy given above define a group of patients with a spectrum of trophoblastic tumours which vary from invasive mole with a tendency to die out spontaneously but which is causing local complications to choriocarcinoma with a tendency to grow and metastasize, progressing rapidly to death. The responsiveness of these different conditions to cytotoxic drugs is also varied, invasive mole usually being very sensitive to methotrexate whereas some choriocarcinomas require intensive combination chemotherapy for there to be any chance of tumour eradication. A number of prognostic factors have been recognized and are used to divide patients into risk groups in terms of the prospects for eradication of the tumour by cytotoxic drugs. It was noted in the 1960s that the proportion of patients achieving long term complete remission was lower if hCG concentrations were markedly raised and if there was a long interval after the antecedent pregnancy. It subsequently became clear that there are several factors influencing prognosis in this context and a scoring system incorporating them and giving due weight to each was described by Bagshawe (1976). A system applicable to patients with metastases was also described by Hammond *et al.* (1973). Since that time attempts have been made to simplify the system in the light of further experience of chemotherapy. Azab *et al.* (1988) have used multivariate analysis to try and improve on the univariate methods of other authors but their patients were already treated differently according to previously identified risk factors. This makes their system less satisfactory than that adopted by the World Health Organization (Table 14.4) (Gestational Trophoblastic Diseases 1983). Patients are divided on the basis of these scores into three risk groups.

General principles of management

Examination of the criteria for treatment and prognostic factors identifies a group of patients with life-threatening complications of a trophoblastic tumour. The most common of these are heavy vaginal or intraperitoneal bleeding or pulmonary metastases producing respiratory impairment. Before considering chemotherapy regimens it is necessary to consider the immediate management of these complications.

It is usually possible to control vaginal bleeding with chemotherapy. It may, however, be necessary to transfuse many units of blood while waiting for the chemotherapy to be effective. Control is usually achieved within a few days. It is important to be ready to do a hysterectomy if bleeding cannot be controlled, but fortunately this can usually be avoided.

Intraperitoneal bleeding may come from invasive mole or choriocarcinoma which has invaded through the myometrium, from tubal choriocarcinoma or from metastases of choriocarcinoma in the liver or kidneys. Patients sometimes present in this way, the diagnosis being made at laparotomy. As with vaginal bleeding it is usually possible to control intraperitoneal haemorrhage with chemotherapy and blood transfusion. These patients are sometimes considered too unwell for intensive chemotherapy on presentation, particularly if there is hepatic or renal impairment. Actinomycin D has a reputation for producing early cessation of bleeding and can be used as a single agent for the first course in the most seriously ill patients. Usually, however, it is possible to use the chemotherapy regimen dictated by the risk group in which the patient is classified. Particular attention must be paid here to hepatic and renal function. Seriously ill patients, especially if they have lost a lot of blood, are prone to have significant renal

Table 14.4. Scoring system based on prognostic factors

Prognostic factors	Score[b]			
	0	1	2	4
Age (years)	<39	>39		
Antecedent pregnancy	HM*	abortion	term	
Interval[a]	4	4–6	7–12	>12
hCG (i.u./l)	10^3	10^3–10^4	10^4–10^5	>10^5
ABO groups (female × male)		OXA	B	
		AXO	AB	
Largest tumour, including uterine tumour		3–5 cm	>5 cm	
Site of metastases		spleen	GI tract	brain
		kidney	liver	
No. of metastases identified		1–4	4–8	>8
Prior chemotherapy			single drug	2 or more drugs

[a] Interval time (months) between end of antecedent pregnancy and start of chemotherapy.
[b] The total score for a patient is obtained by adding the individual scores for each prognostic factor.
Total score: <4: low risk; 5–7: middle risk; >8: high risk.
* HM = hydatidiform mole.

impairment. The excretion of drugs such as methotrexate by the kidney will be delayed and this can easily produce fatal toxicity. Similarly hepatic impairment delays metabolism of methotrexate and vincristine with augmentation of toxicity. It is essential, therefore, that the metabolism of the drugs to be used is well understood and that reversible conditions such as pre-renal uraemia are detected and treated at the earliest possible stage.

Pulmonary metastases producing significant respiratory impairment at the start of treatment should also be handled with caution. When the disease is diffuse it is often accompanied by fever with or without purulent sputum. In many of these cases the patients have superadded infection in the lungs and if there is any doubt about this, antibiotic therapy should be given after taking cultures of blood and sputum. Respiratory function often seems to deteriorate after beginning cytotoxic chemotherapy and it is thought that this is because of oedema and inflammation around tumour deposits which are becoming necrotic. Serial measurements of arterial blood gases provide the best means of monitoring such patients. Dyspnoea can often be relieved by administration of oxygen but if this is not sufficient, artificial ventilation has to be considered but is rarely successful. It is thought that vigorous combination chemotherapy at the outset of treatment often precipitates a more severe initial deterioration than if treatment is started in a less aggressive fashion. This is very difficult to submit to a randomized study but it does appear that nearly all patients will respond at first to a simple therapy with one or two drugs. After the initial crisis is over intensive therapy can be instituted.

Central nervous system metastases also present special problems during the first few weeks of treatment. This topic will be dealt with separately (see below).

Strategy for eradication of disease and prevention of drug resistance

After dealing with immediate life-threatening problems it is necessary to develop a strategy which gives the best chance of tumour eradication in the shortest time with the minimum of toxicity. Placing the patient in an appropriate risk group is the basis of this approach. However, the duration of treatment will need to be different for each patient and some will develop drug resistance and then require to change to other therapy. Twice weekly measurement of serum hCG provides a basis for making these decisions in any individual. The rate of fall of hCG is monitored and when it becomes normal an estimate is made of the duration for which chemotherapy should be continued in order to reduce the tumour mass theoretically to zero cells. This is done on the assumption that an hCG value at the limit of detectability of the most sensitive assays corresponds to 10^4 to 10^5 tumour cells. For the average patient in the low risk group who has responded reasonably rapidly to therapy, about 8 weeks further treatment is required (Fig. 14.2). With a slow fall patients in the high risk group may require treatment for as much as 12 or 16 weeks after hCG levels become normal (Fig. 14.9). If drug resistance develops during treatment then this can be seen by a failure of hCG to fall. Normally hCG should fall by about half a log with each course of chemotherapy, rates of fall below this are suggestive of a degree of drug resistance. Very slow rates of fall or a sustained rise in values are an indication to change chemotherapy (see Fig. 14.7). In this context it is important that patients are treated where results of hCG assays can be obtained rapidly otherwise significant delays tend to occur between development of resistance and an appropriate change of treatment.

In order to be sure that the patient is responding in the initial weeks of therapy and to minimize risks associated with haemorrhage or respiratory deterioration which may occur after the start of treatment, patients are kept in hospital for the first 3−5 weeks of their treatment. Later they are admitted only as necessary for the administration of chemotherapy. In parts of the world where it is difficult for patients to come back repeatedly to hospital they may receive the entire course of therapy as an inpatient.

Low risk therapy

The regimen used for this group for the last 10 years at Charing Cross Hospital and widely followed in other centres is shown in Table 14.5. It is simple to

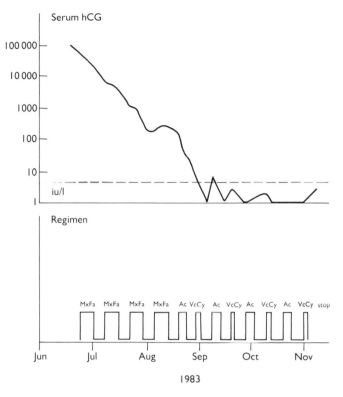

Fig. 14.7. Serum hCG values during chemotherapy after hydatidiform mole in a patient in the low risk group. After four courses of methotrexate and folinic acid (MxFa) hCG failed to maintain a satisfactory rate of fall but the tumour then responded to alternating courses of actinomycin D (Ac) and vincristine and cyclophosphamide (VcCy) (Table 14.6).

Table 14.5. Regimen for low risk patients

MX/FA	
Methotrexate	50 mg (or 1 mg/kg with maximum 70 mg) by i.m. injection repeated every 48 h ×4
Calcium folinate	6 mg, 30 h after each injection of methotrexate by i.m. injection

Courses repeated after a 1-week interval without treatment, i.e. days 1, 14, 28, etc.

administer and in the later stages can sometimes be given by the district nurse in the patient's own home. Toxicity is either absent or modest. There is no alopecia but oral ulceration may occur in patients with fluid intake below 2–3 l per day and in some others presumably due to individual variations in the rate of methotrexate metabolism. If this is a problem then folinic acid can be given earlier than 30 h after methotrexate administration but not usually less than 24 h after methotrexate. Some patients experience pleuritic chest pains and vaginal or, rarely, perianal ulceration. Allergic reactions occur in a small proportion of patients. Methotrexate induces photosensitivity and patients are advised to avoid sunbathing. Myelosuppression is infrequent but it is essential to measure haemoglobin, white cell and platelet counts before each course of chemotherapy. Renal and hepatic function should be measured at least every week during treatment. An example of a patient successfully treated in this way is shown in Fig. 14.2.

In about 75% of 'low risk' patients the tumour will be eradicated by this treatment alone, 20% need to change to combination, the medium risk regimen because of drug resistance and about 5% do so because of intolerance to methotrexate (Bagshawe *et al.* 1989).

Medium risk

This regimen is shown in Table 14.6, the alternating courses comprising etoposide and actinomycin D, being the second and third most important agents after methotrexate. This strategy of including several effective agents reduces the chances of development of drug resistance. Etoposide is an important recent addition to the drugs with high response rates in trophoblastic tumours (Newlands & Bagshawe 1982; Newlands *et al.* 1986; Hitchins *et al.* 1988). As well as being used for patients falling into the medium risk group from the outset the 'medium

Table 14.6. Regimens for medium risk patients

EHMMAC	
Regimen 1	(*Etoposide [VP16−213]*) Day 1−5 etoposide 100 mg/m^2 in 200 ml saline by i.v. infusion over 30 min daily
Regimen 2	(*HU, MX/FA, MP*) Day 1 hydroxyurea, 0.5 g repeated after 12 h (2 doses) orally Day 2−8 methotrexate 50 mg i.m. (or 1 mg/kg max 70 mg) repeated every 48 h ×4 calcium folinate (folinic acid), 6 mg i.m. 30 h after each dose of methotrexate mercaptopurine, 75 mg orally on alternate days ×4 (on calcium folinate days only)
Regimen 3	(*Actinomycin D*) Day 1−5 actinomycin D 0.5 mg i.v. daily
Regimen 4	(*VC, CY*) Day 1 and 3 vincristine, 1 mg/m^2 i.v. Day 1 and 3 cyclophosphamide, 400 mg/m^2 i.v.

The sequence of regimens in EHMMAC is 1, 2, 3, 4, 1, 2, etc.
Alternatively, regimen 4 may be held in reserve, to be used if one of the other regimens proves ineffective or toxic. The preferred sequence then is 1, 2, 3, 2, 1, 2, 3, etc.
The interval between the end of one course and the start of the next should not be less than 7 days or more than 10 days, but some extension is sometimes necessary.

risk' regimen is also used for those showing evidence of drug resistance on the low risk regimen. In those patients, if it is clear that hCG levels are rising during methotrexate therapy, then the methotrexate containing component is omitted. The medium risk regimen produces alopecia and is occasionally associated with myelosuppression. Oral ulceration with etoposide is rare but actinomycin D sometimes produces this and nausea or vomiting. An example of the use of this regimen is shown in Fig. 14.8. 86% of patients had complete response with no modification of the regimen and the remainder.did so with some modification. 4% of patients relapsed but all achieved sustained complete remission with EMA/CO therapy (see high risk, below). No deaths occurred in 76 patients treated in this way (Newlands *et al.* 1986).

High risk disease

These patients require intensive combination chemotherapy because deaths from drug resistance are still a significant problem. The aim is to give chemotherapy with the highest practical dosages as rapidly and consistently as possible. The

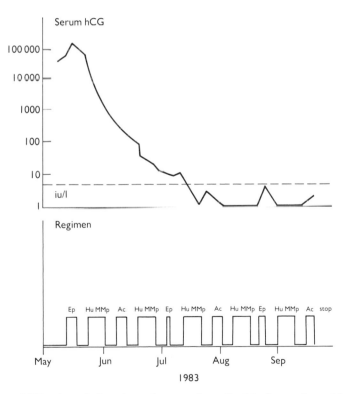

Fig. 14.8. Serum hCG values during chemotherapy of a patient in the medium risk group. Ep = etoposide; Hu MMP = hydroxyurea, methotrexate, folinic acid and mercaptopurine; Ac = actinomycin D (Table 14.6).

CHAMOCA regimen (Bagshawe & Begent 1981) was developed for this purpose containing the best drugs available in the early and mid-1970s. It has now been superseded by EMA/CO (Newlands *et al.* 1986) as shown in Table 14.7. An example of the response achieved with this therapy is shown in Fig. 14.9. Complete remission has been achieved in 67% of patients receiving this regimen whereas only approximately 50% of patients treated with CHAMOCA achieved sustained complete remission (Bagshawe & Begent 1981). Relapse after treatment occurred in 3% who had no prior chemotherapy and in 19% who had. Sustained complete remission was eventually achieved in 93% of patients who had no prior chemotherapy and 74% who had prior chemotherapy (Newlands *et al.* 1986). Similar results have also been reported with EMA/CO by Bolis *et al.* (1988). Most patients are able to have this therapy with only one night in hospital every 2 weeks. With a weekly chemotherapy regimen it is sometimes necessary to maintain treatment despite a low white cell and platelet count. Chemotherapy is continued unless total white count falls below $1.5 \times 10^9/l$ or platelets below $60 \times 10^9/l$ or unless mucosal ulceration develops. The combination of neutropaenia and mucosal ulceration seems to be particularly associated with development of febrile episodes presumably because there is already a portal for entry of bacteria into the circulation via the ulcerated mucosa. Other therapy regimens used have been reviewed by Rustin & Bagshawe (1984).

Table 14.7. Regimen for high risk patients

EMA/CO		
Course 1 (EMA)		
Day 1	etoposide	100 mg/m^2, by i.v. infusion in 200 ml 0.9% saline over 30 min
	actinomycin D	0.5 mg, i.v. *stat.*
	methotrexate	300 mg/m^2, in 1 l 0.9% saline by i.v. infusion over 12 h
Day 2	etoposide	100 mg/m^2, by i.v. infusion in 200 ml 0.9% saline over 30 min
	actinomycin D	0.5 mg, i.v. *stat.*
	calcium folinate	(folinic acid), 15 mg, i.m. or orally every 12 h for 4 doses beginning 24 h after starting methotrexate
Course 2 (CO)		
Day 8	vincristine	1.0 mg/m^2, i.v. *stat.*
	cyclophosphamide	600 mg/m^2, i.v. in saline

This regimen consists of two courses. Course 1 is given on days 1 and 2. Course 2 is given on day 8. Course 1 may require overnight admission, course 2 does not.
These courses can usually be given on days 1 and 2, 8, 15 and 16, 22, etc and the intervals should not be extended without cause.

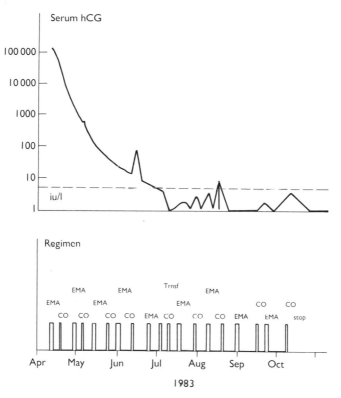

Fig. 14.9. Serum hCG values during chemotherapy of a patient in the high risk group receiving the EMA/CO regimen (Table 14.7). Chemotherapy was continued for 12 weeks after levels fell to within the normal range (<5 i.u./l).

Drug resistant disease

The development of drug resistance in any of the three risk groups is shown by failure of hCG fall at a satisfactory rate and is an indication to move on to a regimen of the next highest group. Occasionally patients in a low risk group will require high risk therapy having failed to respond to the medium risk regimen. This is very unusual, however, if etoposide is used in the medium risk group. Patients in the high risk group have only one remaining major drug, that is cisplatinum (Newlands & Bagshawe 1979; Begent & Bagshawe 1983). Those who fail on the EMA/CO regimen receive cisplatinum in combination with vincristine and methotrexate. If cisplatinum fails there are few promising options for therapy.

Surgery for drug resistant disease

When chemotherapy fails to eradicate the tumour, surgical resection of truly localized disease can sometimes lead to sustained complete response (Begent & Bagshawe 1982). This depends, of course, on the residual tumour being localized and it being technically possible to resect it. Sensitive and specific imaging methods become of great importance in this context. First, the major sites of the tumour must be defined and secondly, the imaging methods must be sufficiently sensitive to exclude metastases at other sites within reason.

Hammond *et al.* (1980) have advocated surgery at the start of treatment for high risk patients. In our experience this is sometimes dangerous due to the profuse vasculature around an infiltrating choriocarcinoma and also because some patients are left unnecessarily infertile.

CT is important in this context, being able to detect lesions of a few millimetres in the lungs and being a sensitive indicator of brain metastases.

Outside the pelvis these are the two sites most likely to contain metastases which can be resected. The uterus is the most common site in which drug resistant disease can be resected by hysterectomy (Begent & Bagshawe 1982). CT or ultrasound may show the uterus to be enlarged. If both investigations are negative and no other sites of disease can be found a hysterectomy should be performed. It is unusual for it to be possible to resect disease at sites other than the pelvis, lung and brain but exceptions do exist in other intraabdominal sites, particularly the bowel. Radioimmunolocalization is an imaging method with particular attraction in this context (see above) since it shows the site at which hCG is being produced. Choriocarcinoma frequently leaves mass lesions visible by conventional radiology after tumour has been eradicated from the site concerned. Histological examination of these lesions shows them to contain only necrotic disease. Here radioimmunolocalization could discriminate between viable and necrotic deposits of tumour giving important information for selection for surgery. Study of radioimmunolocalization using radiolabelled antibody directed against hCG in this context at Charing Cross Hospital has shown that it is sometimes possible to locate tumour when CT scanning or ultrasound are negative (Begent *et al.* 1980, 1987; Begent 1989). A positive result is evidence of hCG production in the site. Unfortunately, some false negative and false positive results do occur. This investigation should be seen as complementary to the other imaging methods and if both are positive in one site then the probability of there being viable tumour present in that location is very high. An example of the fall in serum hCG levels in such a patient after surgery is shown in Fig. 14.10. It has been the experience at Charing Cross Hospital that multiple metastases may appear within a few weeks of such surgery suggesting that there has been a spread of tumour at the time of the operation. For this reason it is our practice to give methotrexate 50 mg intravenously at the time of operation.

Central nervous system metastases

The central nervous system (CNS) is the second commonest site of metastases in the high risk group (Begent & Bagshawe 1982). In the study of patients treated at Charing Cross Hospital over a period of 23 years (Athanassiou *et al.* 1983) nearly

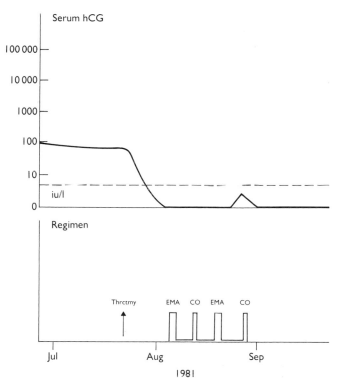

Fig. 14.10. Serum hCG values in a patient with drug resistant choriocarcinoma. CT and radioimmunolocalization suggested the presence of tumour in the right lung. When this was resected (arrow) hCG levels fell to normal and the patient remains in complete remission 3 years later. It is the policy of Charing Cross Hospital to give chemotherapy postoperatively as shown.

all patients with brain metastases also had lung deposits. Also, if lung metastases developed during chemotherapy the chance of their eradication was very small, whereas if they were diagnosed at the start of treatment prospects of cure were good. For these reasons prophylactic intrathecal methotrexate is now given to all patients at risk of cerebral metastases, namely those with pulmonary metastases in any risk group and those in the high risk group regardless of whether lung metastases are detected. Since this policy has been in use, development of brain metastases without evidence of drug resistance elsewhere, has been much less frequent (Athanassiou *et al.* 1983). In order to increase the chance of detection of CNS metastases, hCG concentrations are measured in the CSF at the start of treatment. A level of greater than 1/60 the serum value suggests the presence of CNS metastases. The poor penetration of most cytotoxic drugs into the central nervous system means that conventional chemotherapy is not effective against brain metastases. In the regimen for central nervous system prophylaxis 12.5 mg of methotrexate is given intrathecally with each course of chemotherapy until hCG becomes normal. In the case of the EMA/CO regimen, this is given with the CO part of each course.

Established CNS metastases

Patients with CNS metastases on presentation sometimes already have serious neurological signs. This accounts for the fact that approximately 25% of these patients die within 2 weeks of starting treatment (Athanassiou *et al.* 1983). Some patients present with extremely severe neurological damage whilst others develop this soon after starting treatment often as a result of haemorrhage into the area or tumour. Early resection of solitary deposits in patients presenting with serious neurological signs can sometimes be life saving (Ishizuka 1983; Song & Wu 1988; Rustin *et al.* 1989). Earlier consideration of a diagnosis of choriocarcinoma could probably also improve this situation.

Dexamethasone is given at the start of treatment to reduce oedema. If there is no evidence of raised intracranial pressure, chemotherapy comprises intrathecal methotrexate 12.5 mg once with each course and high dose intravenous methotrexate (1 g/m^2) given in the EMA/CO regimen in place of the medium dose methotrexate previously used. Folinic acid is increased to 30 mg 8-hourly over 3 days starting 32 hours after the beginning of the methotrexate intravenously on 1 week and intrathecal methotrexate on alternate weeks (given with CO). Patients surviving the first 3 weeks of treatment have a good prognosis, the chance of tumour eradication then being 89% (Athanassiou *et al.* 1983; Rustin *et al.* 1989). This therapy is continued until the end of treatment.

Cerebral metastases developing during chemotherapy

Prospects of tumour eradication for this group are poor since the development of cerebral tumour during chemotherapy implies that it is already drug resistant. The patients who have been cured in these circumstances in our series have had the tumour deposit resected as soon as it was diagnosed (Athanassiou *et al.* 1983; Rustin *et al.* 1989). While CT is usually sufficient for location of brain deposits, MRI has located deposits of choriocarcinoma in the cerebral hemispheres close to the skull which were not detected by CT and which have been successfully removed. A raised CSF: serum ratio of hCG often gives a guide to the presence of a CNS deposit.

Radiation therapy

Radiation therapy has some activity against cerebral deposits of choriocarcinoma but has not been shown to eradicate tumour without chemotherapy in addition. Regimens which include radiation (Weed *et al.* 1982; Ishizuka 1983) with cytotoxic chemotherapy have been less successful than those depending on chemotherapy alone (Athanassiou *et al.* 1983).

Survival

One hundred percent of patients in the low risk group can be expected to survive long term. In the medium risk group, an analysis in 1981 showed 98% long term survival. However, there have been no fatalities since etoposide has been introduced into the regimen (Newlands *et al*. 1986). In the high risk group, survival has progressively improved since the introduction of methotrexate in the 1950s when 30–50% survival could be expected. This figure has risen progressively and with the EMA/CO regimen it is currently 93% for patients who have not had prior chemotherapy and 74% for those who have (Newlands *et al*. 1986). This figure is only achieved, however, by the use of the additional drugs such as cisplatinum and appropriate use of surgery in those showing evidence of drug resistance. Relapse after apparently successful initial therapy does not necessarily imply a fatal outcome even in the high risk group. Complete responses can often be achieved by chemotherapy with or without surgery.

Many of the deaths occur in patients who present to a specialized unit with disease so advanced that they are close to death and there is no time for chemotherapy to be effective. The number of such patients can be diminished by a greater awareness of the possibility of the diagnosis of choriocarcinoma and by measurement of hCG on one of the most sensitive immunoassays if there is any suspicion of the diagnosis. The other major problem is drug resistant disease months or years after the initial treatment. Patients still die for this reason and it is probable that new drugs are necessary before the problem can be completely overcome.

Follow up and sequelae of the therapy

Because of the potential of choriocarcinoma to recur after a period of several years it is necessary to continue hCG follow up. It is our policy to do this for the rest of the patient's life. Samples can be posted into the central laboratory. Patients are advised against subsequent pregnancy for a year after completion of chemotherapy in order to avoid confusion between relapse and pregnancy and adverse effects on the ovum induced by chemotherapy. When a patient becomes pregnant it is important to confirm by ultrasound and other appropriate means that the pregnancy is normal. Follow up is then discontinued until the end of the pregnancy, being resumed in the normal way 3 weeks after delivery. Patients who have not received chemotherapy should have hCG measured 3 weeks and 3 months after the end of any further pregnancy because of the increased risk of trophoblastic tumours in this group.

Effects on fertility

The study of patients receiving chemotherapy for gestational trophoblastic tumours has shown that with the regimens described here 86% of patients wishing to have a further pregnancy have succeeded in having at least one live birth. The patients all receive methotrexate and it seems that, given in the way described here, this drug and etoposide have little effect on subsequent fertility (Rustin *et al.* 1984; Adewole *et al.* 1987). Song *et al.* (1988) have reported similar findings from China. Neither study showed an increased incidence of fetal abnormalities.

The incidence of second malignancies in the Charing Cross series is also of the order that would be expected in the normal population, there having been one case of breast cancer and one of acute myeloid leukaemia (Rustin *et al.* 1983). Here the expected figure would be 3.5 cases.

Contraceptive advice

Studies in the UK have found that patients given oral contraceptives before hCG falls to normal after evacuation of hydatidiform mole have an increased incidence of sequelae requiring chemotherapy (Stone *et al.* 1976). For this reason patients are advised to avoid oral contraceptives until hCG has been normal for 3 months if they have had a hydatidiform mole not requiring chemotherapy, or for 6 months after completion of chemotherapy. The mechanisms by which oestrogens and progestogens may influence trophoblastic tumours is unclear.

Conclusions

The 33 years since cytotoxic chemotherapy came into use for treatment of gestational trophoblastic tumours have seen great advances in our understanding of these diseases. About 90% of patients with hydatidiform mole do not need chemotherapy and can be followed up by their gynaecologist in conjunction with a central laboratory which monitors hCG levels in samples sent by post. Long term disease free survival is now expected for the great majority of patients requiring chemotherapy but this is only achieved with careful attention to detail by experienced staff. Even though it may mean spending time away from their homes and families, there can be little doubt that the chances of long term survival are greater if the small proportion of patients who need chemotherapy are managed in special centres.

Acknowledgements

The author wishes to thank Professor K.D. Bagshawe, Dr E.S. Newlands and Dr G.J.S. Rustin and his other colleagues at Charing Cross Hospital, without whom this review would not have been possible. He is also indebted to the gynaecologists who have referred patients contributing to the unique experience of trophoblastic disease at Charing Cross Hospital. The author is supported by the Cancer Research Campaign.

References

Adewole I.F., Rustin G.J.S., Newlands E.S., Dent J. & Bagshawe K.D. (1987) Fertility in patients with gestational trophoblastic tumours treated with etoposide. Eur. J. Cancer Clin. Oncol., 22, 1479.

Athanassiou A., Begent R.H.J., Newlands E.S., Parker D., Rustin G.J.S. & Bagshawe K.D. (1983) Central nervous system metastases of choriocarcinoma: 23 years experience at Charing Cross Hospital. Cancer, 52, 1728−35.

Azab M.B., Pejovic M-H., Theodore C. et al. (1988) Prognostic factors in gestational trophoblastic tumours. A multivariate analysis. Cancer, 62, 585−92.

Bagshawe K.D. (1976) Risk and prognostic factors in trophoblastic neoplasia. Cancer, 38, 1373−85.

Bagshawe K.D. & Begent R.H.J. (1981) Trophoblastic tumours: clinical features and management. In: Coppleson M. (ed), Gynaecologic Oncology. Vol 2. Churchill Livingstone, Edinburgh. pp. 757−72.

Bagshawe K.D. & Begent R.H.J. (1983) Staging markers and prognostic factors in germ cell tumours. In: Bagshawe K.D., Newlands E.S. & Begent R.H.J. (eds), Clinics in Oncology 2, Germ Cell Tumours. Ch. 8, No. 1. W.B. Saunders, London. pp. 159−81.

Bagshawe K.D., Dent J., Newlands E.S., Begent R.H.J. & Rustin G.J.S. (1989) The role of low-dose methotrexate and folinic acid in gestational trophoblastic tumours (GTT). Br. J. Obstet. Gynaecol., 96, 795−802.

Bagshawe K.D., Dent J. & Webb J. (1986) Hydatidiform mole in the United Kingdom 1973−1983. Lancet, ii, 673.

Begent R.H.J. (1989) Immunoscintigraphy with radiolabelled antibody directed against hCG. In: Chatal J.-F. (ed), Monoclonal Antibodies in Immunoscintigraphy. CRC press, pp. 299−309.

Begent R.H.J. & Bagshawe K.D. (1982) The management of high risk choriocarcinoma. Sem. Oncol., 9, 198−203.

Begent R.H.J. & Bagshawe K.D. (1983) Treatment of advanced trophoblastic disease. In: Griffiths C.T. & Fuller A.F. (eds), Gynecologic Oncology. Martinus Nijhoff, Boston. pp. 155−86.

Begent R.H.J., Bagshawe K.D., Green A.J. & Searle F. (1987) The clinical value of imaging with antibody to human chorionic gonadotrophin in the detection of residual choriocarcinoma. Br. J. Cancer, 55, 657−60.

Begent R.H.J., Keep P.A., Green A.J. et al. (1982) Liposomally entrapped antibody improves imaging with radiolabelled (first) antitumour antibody. Lancet, ii, 739−42.

Begent R.H.J., Searle F., Stanway G., Jewkes R.F., Jones B.E., Vernon P. & Bagshawe K.D. (1980) Radioimmunolocalization of tumours by external scintigraphy after administration of 131I antibody to human chorionic gonadotrophin. J. Roy. Soc. Med., 73, 624−30.

Berkowitz R.S. & Goldstein D.P. (1981) Pathogenesis of gestational trophoblastic neoplasms. In: Ioachim H.L. (ed), Pathobiology Annual. Raven Press, New York. pp. 391−411.

Berrebi A., Mercier B., Sarramon M.F. et al. (1988) A new case of hydatidiform mole occurring on one of the ova of a twin pregnancy. Rev. Fr. Gynecol. Obstet., 83, 439−41.

Bolis C., Bonazzi C., Landoni F., Mangili G., Vergadoro F., Zanaboni F. & Mangioni C. (1988) EMA/CO regimen in high-risk gestational trophoblastic tumor (GTT). Gynecol. Oncol., 31, 439−44.

Bracken M.B., Brinton L.A. & Hayashi K. (1984) Epidemiology of hydatidiform mole and choriocarcinoma. Epidemiol. Rev., 6, 52−74.

Brandes J.M., Grunstein S. & Peretz A. (1966) Suction evacuation of the uterine cavity in hydatidiform mole. Obstet. Gynecol., 28, 689−91.

Curry S.L., Hammond C.B., Tyrey L., Creasman W.T. & Parker R.T. (1975) Hydatidiform mole: diagnosis, management and long term follow up of 347 patients. Obstet. Gynecol., 45, 1−8.

Davis J.R., Surwit E.A., Garay J.P. & Fortier K.J. (1984) Sex assignment in gestational trophoblastic neoplasia. Am. J. Obstet. Gynecol., 148, 722−25.

Eckstein R.P., Paradinas F.J. & Bagshawe K.D. (1982) Placental site trophoblastic tumour: a study of four cases requiring hysterectomy, including one fatal case. Histopathology, 6, 211−26.

Edwards Y.H., Jeremiah S.J., McMillan S.L., Povey S., Fisher R.A. & Lawler S.D. (1984) Complete hydatidiform moles combine maternal mitochondria with a paternal nuclear genome. Ann. Hum. Genet., 48, 119−27.

Fasoli M., Ratti E., Franceschi S., La Vecchia C., Pecorelli S. & Mangioni C. (1982) Management of gestational trophoblastic disease: results of a cooperative study. Obstet. Gynecol., 60, 205−9.

Fisher R.A., Lawler S.D., Ormerod M.G., Imrie P.R. & Povey S. (1987) Flow cytometry used to distinguish between complete and partial hydatidiform moles. *Placenta*, **8**, 249—56.

Fisher R.A., Sheppard D.M. & Lawler S.D. (1982) Twin pregnancy with complete hydatidiform mole (46, XX) and fetus (46, XY): genetic origin proved by analysis of chromosome polymorphisms. *Br. Med. J.*, **1**, 1218—20.

Fradken J.E., Eastman R.C., Lesniak M.A. & Roth J. (1989) Specificity spillover at the hormone receptor — exploring its role in human disease. *N. Engl. J. Med.*, **320**, 640—45.

Gestational Trophoblastic Diseases (1983) *Technical Report Series 692*. World Health Organization, Geneva.

Goldenberg D.M., Kim E.E., DeLand F.M., Van Nagell J.R. & Javadapour N. (1980) Clinical radio-immunodetection of cancer with radiolabelled antibodies to human chorionic gonadotrophin. *Science*, **208**, 1284—86.

Goldstein D.P. (1971) Prophylactic chemotherapy with molar pregnancy. *Obstet. Gynecol.*, **38**, 817—22.

Goldstein D.P., Berkowitz R.S. & Bernstein M.R. (1981) Management of molar pregnancy. *J. Repro. Med.*, **26**, 208—12.

Hammond C.B., Borchert L.G., Tyrey L., Creasman W.T. & Parker R.T. (1973) Treatment of metastatic trophoblastic disease: good and poor prognosis. *Am. J. Obstet. Gynecol.*, **115**, 451—57.

Hammond C.B., Weed J.C. & Currie J.L. (1980) The role of operation in the current therapy of gestational trophoblastic disease. *Am. J. Obstet. Gynecol.*, **136**, 844—58.

Hayashi H. (1982) Hydatidiform mole in the United States (1970—1977): a statistical and theoretical analysis. *Am. J. Epidemiol.*, **115**, 67—77.

Heyderman R.S., Begent R.H.J., Buckley R.G., Searle F., Southall P. & Bagshawe K.D. (1989) Antibody imaging to locate a placental site trophoblastic tumour following a complete hydatidiform mole. *J. Roy. Soc. Med.*, **82**, 299—300.

Hitchins R.N., Holden L., Newlands E.S., Begent R.H.J., Rustin G.J.S. & Bagshawe K.D. (1988) Single agent etoposide in gestational trophoblastic tumours. Experience at Charing Cross Hospital 1978—1987. *Eur. J. Cancer Clin. Oncol.*, **24**, 1041—46.

Ishizuka T. (1983) Intracranial metastases of choriocarcinoma. A clinicopathologic study. *Cancer*, **52**, 1896—903.

Jacobs P.A., Hunt P.A., Matsuuro J.S. & Wilson C.C. (1982) Complete and partial hydatidiform mole in Hawaii: cytogenetics, morphology and epidemiology, *Br. J. Obstet. Gynaecol.*, **89**, 258—66.

Kajii T. & Ohama K. (1977) Androgenetic origin of hydatidiform mole. *Nature*, **268**, 633—34.

Kardana A. & Bagshawe K.D. (1976) A rapid, sensitive and specific radioimmunoassay of human chorionic gonadotrophin. *J. Immunol. Methods*, **9**, 297—305.

Kashimura Y., Kashiimura M., Sugimori H. *et al.* (1986) Prophylactic chemotherapy of hydatidiform mole. *Cancer*, **58**, 624—29.

Kurman R.J., Scully R.E. & Norris H.J. (1976) Trophoblastic pseudotumour of the uterus. *Cancer*, **38**, 1214—26.

Lage J.M., Driscoll S.G., Yavner D.L., Olivier A.P., Mark S.D. & Weinberg D.S. (1988) Hydatidiform moles. Application of flow cytometry in diagnosis. *Am. J. Clin. Pathol.*, **89**, 596—600.

La Vecchia C., Parrazini F., Decarli A. *et al.* (1984) Age of parents and risk of gestational trophoblastic disease. *J. Natl. Cancer Inst.*, **73**, 639—42.

Lawler S.D. & Fisher R.A. (1986) Genetic aspects of gestational trophoblastic tumors. *In*: Ichinoe K. (ed), *Trophoblastic Diseases*. Igaku-Shoin Tokyo, New York. pp. 23—33.

Lawler S.D. & Fisher R.A. (1987) Genetic studies in hydatidiform mole with clinical correlations. *Placenta*, **8**, 77—88.

Lawler S.D., Fisher R.A., Pickthall V.G., Povey S. & Wyn Evans M. (1982a) Genetic studies on hydatidiform moles I: the origin of partial moles. *Cancer Gen. Cytogen.*, **4**, 309—20.

Lawler S.D., Pickthall V.G., Fisher R.A., Povey S., Wyn Evans M. & Szulman A.E. (1979) Genetic studies of complete and partial hydatidiform mole (letter). *Lancet*, **ii**, 580.

Lawler S.D., Povey S., Fisher R.A. & Pickthall V.G. (1982b) Genetic studies on hydatidiform moles II: the origin of complete moles. *Ann. Human Gen.*, **46**, 209—22.

Matalon M. & Modan B. (1972) Epidemiologic aspects of hydatidiform mole in Israel. *Am. J. Obstet. Gynecol.*, **112**, 107—12.

Mazur M.T. & Kurman R.J. (1987) Choriocarcinoma and placental site trophoblastic tumour. *In*: Szulman A.E. & Buchsbaum H.J. (eds), *Gestational Trophoblastic Disease*. Springer Verlag, New York.

McGrath I.T., Golding P.R. & Bagshawe K.D. (1971) Medical presentations of choriocarcinoma. *Br. Med. J.*, **2**, 633–37.

Newlands E.S. & Bagshawe K.D. (1979) Activity of high dose platinum (NC1 119875) in combination with vincristine and methotrexate in drug resistant choriocarcinoma. A report of 17 cases. *Br. J. Cancer*, **40**, 943–45.

Newlands E.S. & Bagshawe K.D. (1982) Role of VP16–213 (Etoposide; NSC 141540) in gestational choriocarcinoma. *Cancer Chemother. Pharmacol.*, **7**, 211–14.

Newlands E.S., Bagshawe K.D., Begent R.H.J., Rustin G.J.S., Holden L. & Dent J. (1986) Developments in chemotherapy for medium- and high-risk patients with gestational trophoblastic tumours (1979–1984). *Br. J. Obstet. Gynaecol.*, **93**, 63–69.

Ober W.B. (1987) Choriocarcinoma: historical notes. In: Szulman A.E. & Buchsbaum H.J. (eds), *Gestational Trophoblastic Tumours.* Springer Verlag, New York. p. 1.

Ohama K., Kajii T., Okamoto E., Fukuda Y., Imaizumi K., Tsukahara M., Kobayashi K. & Hagiwara K. (1981) Dispermic origin of XY hydatidiform mole. *Nature*, **292**, 551–52.

Poulsen H.E. (1975) Histological typing of female genital tract tumours. *International Histological Classification of Tumours*, No. 13. World Health Organization, Geneva. pp. 70–73.

Ratnam S.S., Teoh E.S. & Dawood M.Y. (1968) Methotrexate for prophylaxis of choriocarcinoma. *Am. J. Obstet. Gynecol.*, **111**, 1021–27.

Requard C.K. & Mettler F.A. (1980) The use of ultrasound in the evaluation of trophoblastic disease and its response to therapy. *Radiology*, **135**, 419–22.

Rustin G.J.S. & Bagshawe K.D. (1984) Gestational trophoblastic tumours. *Crit. Rev. Oncol.* CRC Press Inc., USA.

Rustin G.J.S., Booth M., Dent J., Salt S., Rustin F. & Bagshawe K.D. (1984) Pregnancy after cytotoxic chemotherapy for gestational trophoblastic tumours. *Br. Med. J.*, **288**, 103–6.

Rustin G.J.S., Newlands E.S., Begent R.H.J., Dent J. & Bagshawe K.D. (1989) Weekly alternating chemotherapy (EMA/CO) for treatment of central nervous systems of choriocarcinoma. *J. Clin. Oncol.*, **7**, 900–3.

Rustin G.J.S., Rustin F., Dent J., Booth M., Salt J. & Bagshawe K.D. (1983) No increase in second tumors after chemotherapy for gestational trophoblastic tumors. *New Engl. J. Med.*, **308**, 473–76.

Scully R.E. & Young R.H. (1981) Trophoblastic pseudotumour: a reappraisal. *Am. J. Surg. Pathol.*, **5**, 75–76.

Sheppard D.M., Fisher R.A. & Lawler S.D. (1985) Karyotypic analysis and chromosome polymorphisms in four choriocarcinoma cell lines. *Cancer Gen. Cytogen.*, **16**, 251–58.

Sheppard D.M., Fisher R.A., Lawler S.D. & Povey S. (1982) Tetraploid conceptus with three paternal contributions. *Hum. Genet.*, **62**, 371–74.

Song H-Z. & Wu B-Z. (1988) Treatment of brain metastases in choriocarcinoma and invasive mole. In: Song H-Z. & Wu P-C. (eds), *Studies in Trophoblastic Diseases in China*. Pergamon Press, Oxford. Ch. 22, pp. 231–37.

Song H-Z., Wu P-C., Wang Y-E., Yang X-Y. & Dong S-Y. (1988) Pregnancy outcomes after successful chemotherapy for choriocarcinoma and invasive mole: long term follow-up. *Am. J. Obstet. Gynecol.*, **158**, 538–45.

Steiner R.E. & Radda G. (eds) (1983) Nuclear magnetic resonance and its clinical applications. *Br. Med. Bull.*, Churchill Livingstone, Edinburgh, **40**, (2).

Stone M. & Bagshawe K.D. (1979) An analysis of the influence of maternal age, gestational age, contraceptive method, and the mode of primary treatment of patients with hydatidiform moles on the incidence of subsequent chemotherapy. *Br. J. Obstet. Gynaecol.*, **86**, 782–92.

Stone M., Dent J., Kardana A. & Bagshawe K.D. (1976) Relationship of oral contraception to development of trophoblastic tumour after evacuation of a hydatidiform mole. *Br. J. Obstet. Gynaecol.*, **83**, 913–16.

Szulman A.E. (1987) Complete hydatidiform mole: clinicopathologic features. In: Szulman A.E. & Buchsbaum H J. (eds), *Gestational Trophoblastic Disease*. Springer Verlag, New York.

Teoh E.S., Dawood M.Y. & Ratnam S.S. (1971) Epidemiology of hydatidiform mole in Singapore. *Am. J. Obstet. Gynecol.*, **110**, 415–20.

Vaitukaitis J.L. (1979) Human chorionic gonadotrophin—a hormone secreted for many reasons. *New Engl. J. Med.* (Editorial), **301**, 324–26.

Vassilakos P., Riotton G. & Kajii T. (1977) Hydatidiform mole: two entities. A morphologic and cytogenetic study with some clinical considerations. *Am. J. Obstet. Gynecol.*, **127**, 167–70.

Weed J.C., Kent T.W. & Hammond C.B. (1982) Choriocarcinoma metastatic to the brain: therapy and prognosis. *Sem. Oncol.*, **9**, 208–12.

Xia Z-F., Song H-Z. & Tang M-Y. (1988) Risk of malignancy and prognosis using a provisional scoring system in hydatidiform mole. *In*: Song H-Z. & Wu P-C. (eds), *Studies in Trophoblastic Diseases in China*. Pergamon Press, Oxford. pp. 175–85.

Yen S. & MacMahon B. (1968) Epidemiological features of trophoblastic disease. *Am. J. Obstet. Gynecol.*, **101**, 126–32.

Zongfu X., Hongzhao S. & Minyi T. (1979) Risk of malignancy and prognosis using a provisional scoring system in hydatidiform mole. *Chin. Med. J.*, **93**, 605–12.

15

Malignant Disease of the Genital Organs in Childhood

SIR JOHN DEWHURST

Malignant disease of the genital organs is, happily, rare in children. However, when it does occur it can be of a highly malignant nature and, unless recognized early and treated efficiently, results may be poor.

The organs most commonly affected — accepting that the word 'commonly' is used in a relative sense — are the vagina, cervix and ovary. Malignant disease of the vulva and body of the uterus is extremely rare and of the fallopian tube unknown at this period of life.

Lesions of the vagina and cervix

Malignant lesions of the vagina and cervix are first considered together since both organs may be affected by the same disease at the time the patient is seen, making it difficult, in some instances, to determine where the tumour actually originated.

The lesions to be considered in this section are the embryonal rhabdomyosarcoma, the clear cell adenocarcinoma and, more rarely, the endodermal sinus tumour.

Embryonal rhabdomyosarcoma

Clinical features

This disease known for many years by gynaecologists as the botryoid sarcoma on account of the grape-like appearance it sometimes shows is a highly malignant lesion which is most commonly seen in the very young 2 years of age or less although also occurring in older children.

The site of the tumour varies. A loose, general rule, to which there are, however, many exceptions, is that in the youngest children the tumour will originate in the lower vagina and in the older ones in the upper vagina and cervix.

The gross appearance of the lesion, although sometimes grape-like, as shown in Fig. 15.1, may be a haemorrhagic mass or an apparently simple polyp (Fig.

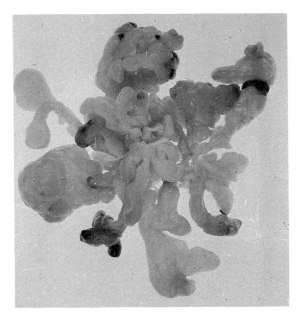

Fig. 15.1. Embryonal rhabdomyosarcoma showing a markedly grape-like appearance. (By courtesy of Marcel Dekker & Co.)

15.2). It is worthy of emphasis at this stage, that simple polypi of the vagina and cervix in childhood are extremely rare; a gynaecologist should always have a strong suspicion that an apparently innocent cervical polyp in a child will, in fact, turn out to be malignant.

Only in the earliest cases will the tumour affect a limited area of the vagina. Spread is rapid beneath the epithelium of the vagina (Fig. 15.3) which is lifted up into the polypoid, grape-like shapes already discussed. These appear soft and translucent because of the myxomatous nature of the underlying tumour tissue. In more advanced cases the vagina will be filled with tumour and will probably constitute a sizeable mass in the pelvis which is likely to be palpable *per abdomen*. A tumour spreads locally in the early stages and before long may be found extending forwards into the bladder, upwards into the pelvis and backwards to involve the rectum. Blood and lymph spread are late, but will certainly occur in advanced cases.

The presenting clinical feature is almost invariably bleeding which may be slight and intermittent at first, but will be heavier and more continuous later. There will be no constitutional upset until the late stages of the disease although if bleeding is profuse a considerable degree of anaemia may develop.

Pathology

The histological appearance, like the gross appearance in some instances, may also suggest a benign lesion in early cases since sections may not show obvious malignant features. There is a loose, myxomatous stroma beneath an intact

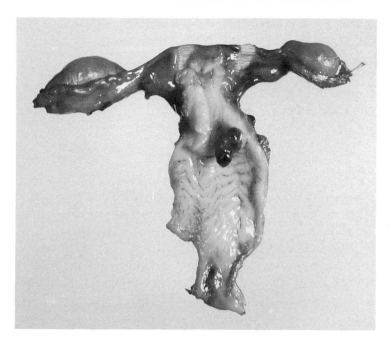

Fig. 15.2. A small cervical polyp which appears innocent, but is, in fact, a malignant embryonal rhabdomyosarcoma in a 5-month-old child. (By courtesy of Marcel Dekker & Co.)

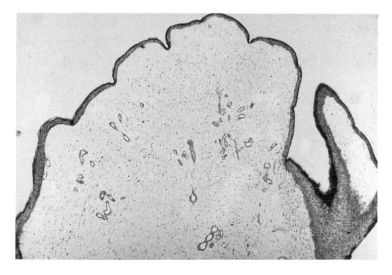

Fig. 15.3. Histological appearance of an embryonal rhabdomyosarcoma showing typical myxomatous stroma containing fusiform cells beneath an intact epithelium.

epithelium (Fig. 15.3). Fusiform cells are scattered throughout the tumour substance and these may be collected into groups. Pleomorphism is invariable and is usually evident even in early cases. Two characteristic features are the presence of rhabdomyoblasts—large cells with a vacuolated eosinophilic cytoplasm and cross striated muscle fibres (Fig. 15.4); the search for the latter may need to be prolonged, however, since striations may not be well defined and the cells are sparse. Examination beneath the electron microscope will disclose their presence more readily. This technique allows the lesion to be distinguished from the so-called pseudosarcoma botryoides which has been described in young women, sometimes in association with pregnancy (Mitchell *et al*. 1987).

Management

The immediate management of a child with vaginal bleeding who is suspected of having a malignant vaginal tumour involves examination under anaesthesia. At this examination it will often be possible to see the lesions within the introitus as soon as the labia are withdrawn laterally thus permitting a view of the lower part of the organ. If this is not possible, one or two small Langenbeck's retractors can be gently inserted allowing posterolateral retraction on each side of the perineum and permitting visualization to a higher level.

Vaginoscopy must always be performed to establish the possible presence of an upper vaginal lesion if none is seen near the introitus and to assess upward spread if the lesion did exist at a lower level. The vagina of the child may be inspected with a variety of instruments but the best view is undoubtedly obtained if a 30° adult cystoscope is introduced into the vagina; continuously running bladder irrigation fluid then permits distension of the vagina, gives excellent visibility and allows direct biopsies to be taken. Failing this an infant McGill laryngoscope can be helpful in a somewhat older child, the narrow blade allow-

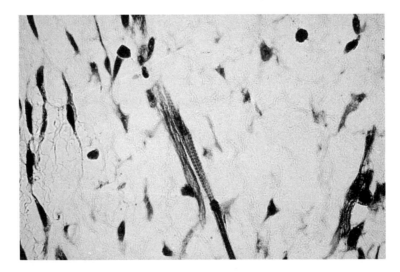

Fig. 15.4. High power view of the tumour seen in Fig. 15.3 to illustrate the striated muscle fibre which indicates the true nature of the tumour.

ing its insertion through the hymen without damage with illumination being satisfactory.

A representative biopsy must be obtained from any lesion that is seen. This must be sent off for histological study both with the light and electron microscope.

The examination under anaesthesia must also include cystoscopy, to detect the possibility of anterior spread into the bladder, and rectal examination with the little finger to establish the possible spread posteriorly. Other investigations which are generally appropriate are a chest X-ray, a body scan, an ultrasonic scan of the lower abdomen and an intravenous pyelogram and, in older children, lymphangiography, although there is doubt as to its value.

Treatment

The treatment of the embryonal rhabdomyosarcoma has undergone a change in recent years since it has been realized that the tumour is sensitive to modern chemotherapy (Hilgers *et al.* 1970; Grosfeld *et al.* 1972; Tank *et al.* 1972; Ghavimi *et al.* 1973; Hilgers *et al.* 1973). The most satisfactory regimen is yet to be determined, but the most popular and successful is with triple chemotherapy using vincristine, actinomycin D and cyclophosphamide. These agents have been given at 2–3 weekly intervals for 1 year or even more and repeat examination and repeat biopsy has been undertaken at 3-monthly intervals to determine progress. The further examinations under anaesthesia will probably show shrinkage of the gross mass of the tumour perhaps to a considerable extent, and even total disappearance may be seen. The histological study will allow some assessment to be made of the viability of the tumour cells as treatment continues although this is an unusually difficult assessment to make. On the basis of this response, it must be determined whether additional treatment should be used or whether chemotherapy alone will be satisfactory. A more recent regimen employs bleomycin, etoposide and cis-platinum; the same careful supervision is essential. Surgery and radiotherapy are available and each may have a place.

If regression during chemotherapy is less than complete, surgery will generally be indicated. It is seldom necessary nowadays to consider exenteration procedures. The standard operation is an extended hysterectomy of the Wertheim type with the addition of total vaginectomy. Pelvic lymphadenectomy should also be undertaken since it is a comparatively simple step if limited, as it should be, to the removal of the glands on the side wall of the pelvis. This type of surgery is simpler than it sounds since the uterus and cervix are much more abdominal than pelvic organs in the child and come readily into the wound to facilitate removal. The performance of the procedure should follow conventional lines and can be accomplished *per abdomen* until the upper three-quarters of the vagina have been freed. At that point it is necessary to approach the lower quarter of the vagina from below to separate the posterolateral parts from the rectum in the manner of the performance of a perineorrhaphy although sharp dissection is usually required to free the anterior wall of the vagina from beneath the urethra. The ovaries may be preserved without in any way detracting from the efficacy of the procedure.

If the tumour extends so far down the vagina as to reach the introitus even total vaginectomy will mean that the line of excision is immediately adjacent to the tumour. In this circumstance radiotherapy may be required (Grosfeld *et al.* 1972; Ghavimi *et al.* 1973). The disadvantage of radiotherapy is the effect it has upon the growing pelvic bones of the child and although this treatment formed a part of a former protocol (Dewhurst 1980), it is best avoided if possible. Nonetheless, if surgery cannot completely excise the lesion with a satisfactory margin and complete regression has not occurred with chemotherapy, radiotherapy is indicated. It may be applied conventionally as external beam therapy or it may be possible to build a small obturator carrying a radium source from which intravaginal radiation takes place.

Some authorities still use pelvic radiotherapy and claim improved results. Reynolds (1984), reporting on a group of patients with either vaginal, vesical or prostate tumours, quoted survival rates with VAC alone as 50%, with VAC and radiotherapy 68%, VAC and surgery 67% but when all three were employed 88%.

The likely ill effect of any radiotherapy on the ovaries may be avoided by oophoropexy. It is possible to elevate the gonads high into the paracolic gutters close to the level of the lower pole of the kidneys where they can be fixed in position by a few Prolene sutures and a metal clip attached for radiological location (Shepherd 1989).

Prognosis

It is usually difficult to give a firm prognosis to a rare lesion and this one is no exception. There can be no doubt that the results of treatment are far better now than they were 10–20 years ago. Initially, only 12 cases with long term survival had been reported (Dewhurst 1963). The author had eight patients under his care who had been treated between 22 years and 7 years ago and all are apparently well and tumour free; one other patient has been lost to follow up, one developed a recurrence and one died. This gives an estimate of the degree of improvement in treatment which has occurred and compares favourably with the figures mentioned by Reynolds (1984) above. It is worthy of emphasis that the fatal case mentioned above was initially diagnosed incorrectly at the first biopsy which was reported to be benign. The tumour recurred very quickly with fatal consequences.

Clear cell adenocarcinoma

This malignant lesion, although known as a rare genital tract tumour for many years, came to prominence in 1970 when six cases of it and one of the closely related endometrioid carcinoma were reported in women between the ages of 15 and 22 (Herbst & Scully 1970). At about the same time an eighth case was recorded (Herbst 1981), and a case-controlled epidemiological study of all eight revealed, in seven, a history of treatment of the mothers of these patients with diethylstilboestrol (DES). No history of DES medication was found in 32 control mothers whose babies were born in the same hospital within 5 days of the birth of the index patients (Herbst et al. 1971). Since that time numerous excellent papers have appeared (Gunning 1976; Mattingly & Staft 1976; Noller et al. 1976a, b; Ulfelder 1976; Bibbo et al. 1977; Herbst et al. 1977; Robboy et al. 1977; Poskanzer & Herbst 1977; Herbst 1978) and many other cases have been reported in young women. Not all show a positive history of maternal DES exposure, but most do. Out of 429 cases referred to by Herbst (1981) 243 were positive for exposure to DES, dinoestrol or hexoestrol, nine for exposure to a steroidal oestrogen or progestogen or both, two for treatment with thyroid hormone and 36 for an unknown medication for high risk pregnancy; in 99 no positive maternal history of this therapy was obtained and in 40 the maternal history was unknown. Thus of 353 cases of clear cell adenocarcinoma where a reliable history was available, 243 (69%) were associated with prior DES therapy. Since, in addition, 36 other patients received unknown treatment for a high risk pregnancy, the true association is probably higher still.

The amount of DES prescribed to the mothers of affected patients has varied considerably. Many received large doses for weeks or months, but very low doses have also been recorded; as little as 1.5 mg per day of DES throughout pregnancy having been associated with the development of a clear cell adenocarcinoma in the offspring. An association with treatment of short duration — perhaps only 1–2 weeks — is also established. In all cases where a precise treatment regimen has been determined, the DES therapy has always been started prior to the 18th week of pregnancy.

Attempts to compute the risk of a female exposed to DES in utero developing clear cell adenocarcinoma in later life have led to the estimated incidence of 0.14 to 1.4 per 1000 up to and including age 24 (Herbst et al. 1977). The risk is, therefore, a low one, but it should be mentioned that the risk of the exposed girl developing benign adenosis of the vagina is very high — perhaps as high as 90%. Other deformities of the vagina and cervix have been recognized such as the coxcomb appearance of the cervix and transverse vaginal septum formation.

Clinical features

The youngest DES exposed patient to develop a clear cell adenocarcinoma to date was 7 years old and the oldest 31. Examination of incidence figures reveals a sharp rise at about age 14 followed by a plateau of increased risk until age 21.

Beyond that age there is a fall, but the incidence is uncertain since few exposed females had reached that age at the time the calculations for the curve of incidence were completed. Ninety-five percent of cases of clear cell adenocarcinoma in DES exposed individuals have occurred at or after 14 years of age, so comparatively few fall within the childhood period. This section should therefore be read in conjunction with Chapter 8.

The presenting symptom has almost always been vaginal bleeding or the occurrence of a bloodstained discharge except in those patients in whom an early lesion has been detected at routine screening before any symptoms become evident.

Either the vagina or the cervix or both may be the site of a tumour. In approximately two-thirds of the patients the vagina alone has been affected. In the remaining third the cervix alone has been affected in some, and both vagina and cervix in others; in this latter group the tumours are classified as cervical, although in a number an origin from the vagina appears likely. Patients in the Registry for Research on Hormonal Transplacental Carcinogens in the USA have been classified according to the staging recommended by the International Federation of Gynaecology and Obstetrics (FIGO) (Herbst & Anderson 1981).

There has been great variation in size and extent of the tumours. Some have been very tiny, perhaps only a millimetre or two across and others very extensive. Spread is usually local at first, but lymph and blood spread may occur later and, as with other tumours, the earliest treatment has given the best results.

Growths tend to be nodular and polypoid in appearance and are usually firm, indurated or granular on palpation. Ulceration of the tumour may be evident. Some tumours are predominantly flat in appearance, projecting little above the vaginal wall and, on rare occasions, the tumour may even be covered by intact squamous epithelium.

Herbst & Anderson (1981) recorded tumour size and depth of invasion and correlated this with the presence of positive lymph node metastases in 200 cases as follows:

Tumour size	*Positive nodes*
Less than 1 cm^2	6%
1.1−6.0 cm^2	12%
More than 6.0 cm^2	24%

Depth of invasion	*Positive nodes*
Less than 3 mm	11%
3.1−6.0 mm	10%
More than 6.0 mm	23%

Pathology

The gross tumour may affect the vagina alone, the cervix alone or both. It has already been indicated that some two-thirds of the tumours are classified as vaginal and one-third as cervical, although the cervix and vagina may be affected together in some of these. Scully & Welch (1981) report that if tumours are classified on a basis of predominant location, the ratio of vagina to cervix is 7:3. In the vagina the anterior wall in the upper third is the usual site of the growth, although any part may be affected. On the cervix the ectocervix is generally the site of the tumour, although the endocervix may be involved by spread in some instances. Scully & Welch (1981) report a variation in size from 0.2 cm to more than 10.0 cm.

The histology of the tumour shows two main patterns — the tubulocystic with tubules and cysts being evident without papillae, and a papillary form in which numerous papilliferous projections are seen within the cyst spaces of the growth. Two main cell types are encountered; the most common is the clear cell type due to the presence of large quantities of glycogen in the cytoplasm and the less common, the hob-nailed cell (Fig. 15.5) which appears as tiny protrusions into the cystic spaces. Other features include mucin production and the presence of psammoma bodies. A diagnostic feature which may give rise to confusion between an innocent or malign lesion is the presence of microglandular hyperplasia, sometimes evident in benign adenosis (Robboy et al. 1977).

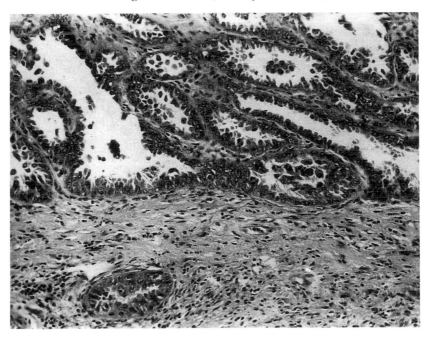

Fig. 15.5. Adenocarcinoma showing markedly hob-nailed features in the cervix and vagina of a child.

Management

Biopsy of suspicious lesions either in the presence of symptoms or if carrying out a routine screening examination on an exposed patient, is mandatory. Exfoliative cytology may be used in addition but cannot be relied upon alone, even though four-fifths of the cases have been reported as positive or suspicious (Taft *et al.* 1974). Colposcopy may be of great assistance in identifying the areas from which biopsies should be taken; Noller *et al.* (1981) considered this procedure mandatory for follow-up of a patient from whom a positive cytological smear has been obtained. Staining with Lugol's iodine can be a helpful step also, with failure to take up the stain indicating, in some instances, the suspicious area.

Treatment has generally been radical and has involved an extended hysterectomy of the Wertheim type with the removal of part of all of the vagina and pelvic lymph node dissection in the manner described for embryonal rhabdomyosarcoma. If radiotherapy is not used, which will generally be the case, one or both ovaries may be preserved without significant risk since ovarian metastases appear to be rare. Exenteration procedures have only infrequently been carried out and all have been in extensive tumours. Local excision has sometimes been tried, with or without extraperitoneal lymph node excision, but the rate of recurrence has been high (Herbst *et al.* 1979) and such conservative measures are seldom now employed. Their aim has been to preserve reproductive function by the performance of an excision of some or all of the vagina which may be grafted at once or soon afterwards (Hudson *et al.* 1983).

Radiation therapy is sometimes employed for various reasons. It was used in a conventional fashion in the manner employed for the management of carcinoma of the cervix in one of the author's patients because of an extensive anterior area of growth beneath the bladder base in the upper half of the vagina which would have involved a primary exenteration procedure (Dewhurst *et al.* 1980). Occasionally, radiation therapy has been employed after surgery where extensive lymph node involvement has been detected. In general, radiation therapy has not given as good results as surgery. Herbst *et al.* (1979) report a recurrence rate of only 8% in stage I cervical or vaginal cases treated with radical surgery compared with one of 37% where radiotherapy had been used.

The results of treatment of clear cell adenocarcinoma of the vagina and cervix have, in general, been comparatively good. Herbst & Anderson (1981) comment that of 400 patients with this disease, of whom details are available in the Registry, 297 are living and well, 12 have had a recurrence treated and are living and well, 12 are living with the disease and 79 have died. Senekjian & Herbst (1985) report for stage I lesions a 5-year survival figure of 90%, for stage IIA cervix and stage II vagina 82%, for stage IIB cervical lesions 60% and for stage III cases only 37%; for all patients the survival figure was 80%.

The good results for early cases has tempted some to attempt less than radical treatment in order to preserve fertility. Of 27 Registry patients with early lesions receiving such management however only five conceived, while there were six recurrences and two deaths among the remainder. Recurrences have occurred at a variety of sites, metastases in the lungs and supraclavicular lymph nodes being somewhat more frequent than in patients with squamous cell carcinoma of the cervix and the vagina.

DES exposed patients

Brief mention must be made of the screening procedures which may be appropriate in DES exposed patients. It is generally thought to be unrewarding to carry out routine examination of the vagina and cervix in very young patients. It is Herbst's (1983) view that routine screening should begin after the age of 14 or after the menarche, whichever is earlier. If the procedure is to be carried out in the young, general anaesthesia will be necessary, but as the girl grows older this may be dispensed with in many instances. Careful visualization of the whole vagina is necessary; smears for exfoliative cytology should be taken from the cervix and from other lesions within the vagina; a careful plan should be drawn of the extent and appearance of any benign vaginal adenosis lesions that are seen and biopsies should be taken from any suspicious areas. Colposcopy or iodine staining techniques may be employed as an aid to diagnosis. How frequent examination should be is a matter of opinion, but it appears that yearly examinations are appropriate and perhaps, in certain cases, more frequent examinations should be carried out if unusually extensive adenosis is present.

Vaginal endodermal sinus tumours

A rare vaginal tumour requiring brief mention is the endodermal sinus tumour. Allyn *et al.* (1971) reviewing the literature on vaginal carcinoma of childhood considered that two types could be discerned:

1 The clear cell adenocarcinoma which affected patients aged 7 years of age and above.

2 The endodermal sinus tumour which affected patients two years of age or less.

The histology of the latter tumour shows glomeruloid formations, hobnail patterns and the presence of PAS positive hyaline globules permitting a distinction histologically between it and the clear cell adenocarcinoma. Alphafetoprotein levels in the blood will also be raised.

Radical surgery has been the treatment most often employed in the past but the better results now being observed in modern chemotherapy in this lesion of the ovary suggest that this approach should be tried as well or even as an alternative. Results in earlier times were poor. Only three of 13 patients reported by Allyn *et al.* (1971) were alive, two after 2 years and a third after 7 years. Dewhurst & Ferreira (1981) reported a second alive and well 7 years later (Fig.

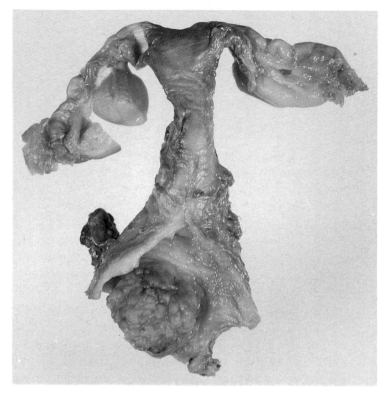

Fig. 15.6. An endodermal sinus tumour of the vagina in a 5-month-old child. The lesion was initially mistaken for a clear cell adenocarcinoma. (By courtesy of Marcel Dekker & Co.)

15.6) and this interval has now extended to 13 years. Goerzen *et al.* (1986) have reviewed the world literature for this condition.

Ovarian tumours

These lesions are uncommon in childhood and considerable clinical difficulty is often experienced in dealing with them. It should be stressed that most ovarian swellings encountered in children will not be malignant. In a series reported by Breen & Maxson (1977), 36% of ovarian swellings were non-neoplastic and, of the remainder which were new growths, two-thirds were benign and one-third malignant. Huffman (1968) reported a malignancy rate of 30% in 999 new growths encountered in children. Malignancy rates varying from 15 to 32% have been quoted by Carlson (1985).

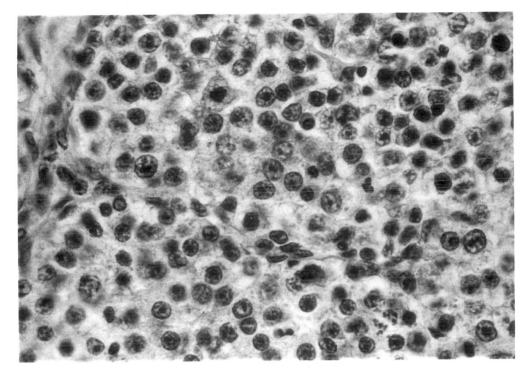

Fig. 15.7. Typical histological appearance of an ovarian dysgerminoma.

Pathology

The pattern of malignant ovarian tumours seen in children differs significantly from that seen in later life. The predominant ovarian tumours of the child are germ cell tumours and sex cord stromal tumours which clearly predominate over epithelial and other growths. In the malignant ovarian tumours in children reviewed by Breen & Maxson (1977), the commonest tumour was the dysgerminoma (11%) (Fig. 15.7) followed by the teratoma (7.4%), the endodermal sinus tumour (5.7%) and the granulosa cell tumour (4.3%).

Clinical features

It is characteristic of ovarian tumours in children that they present clinically in a somewhat different fashion from those in the adult. Pain is a common feature which was present in 54% of patients reviewed by Linfors (1971). It was not always possible to explain the pain although torsion was evident in a considerable proportion. Abdominal distension was a relatively uncommon feature, so it is easy to see why the ovarian tumours in the child escape detection for a period of time until some accident brings them to notice. It is always difficult to recognize a small tumour in the rather protuberant abdomen of a little girl, although if the tumour is large there should be no problem in detecting it.

X-rays have been used in the past in the hope of detecting the presence of a tooth in a benign teratoma, but nowadays an ultrasound scan of the lower abdomen and pelvis may be more rewarding and further experience with this method of investigation is proving of value.

Treatment

The management of a plainly malignant ovarian tumour in the child should, in the majority of instances, be radical with total hysterectomy, bilateral salpingo-oophorectomy and probably lymph node dissection as well as removal of the omentum. To carry out this treatment on a child, however, means the malignant nature of the lesion must be absolutely certain. Frozen section may provide this information although the assessment of unequivocal signs of malignancy in a frozen section of an ovarian tumour is not always easy. If there is doubt, it will probably be wisest in the first instance to carry out a conservative procedure such as a unilateral salpingo-oophorectomy and then consider what, if anything, should be performed later. It is wise practice to take blood from children with a suspected ovarian tumour for tumour marker studies, such as alphafetoprotein and human chorionic gonadotrophin, and if this has not already been done it should be done whilst the operation is in progress. Results will not of course be instantly available but they may be useful later to monitor follow up.

Since certain tumours such as the dysgerminoma are unusually radiosensitive and respond well to chemotherapy, a less than radical surgical procedure may be attempted and other treatment resorted to later should there be a recurrence. If the tumour in question is a granulosa cell tumour, the degree of malignancy is usually low and unilateral oophorectomy or salpingo-oophorectomy in a child presenting, for example, with precocious sexual development (Fig. 15.8a,b), would be entirely appropriate treatment in the first instance unless there was clear evidence of extension of the tumour.

Special gonadal tumours

Brief mention should be made of certain special gonadal tumours which arise in phenotypic females with a Y chromosome in their karyotype (Dewhurst 1981). In the circumstances where there is a displaced, but macroscopically normal testis, as in patients with androgen insensitivity or with a biosynthetic defect of testosterone production, there is probably a risk of testicular malignancy of the order of 5% at some time in the patient's life. Where the clinical features are predominantly those of gonadal dysgenesis and a Y chromosome is present the risk may be higher around 30% (Dewhurst et al. 1971). Manuel et al. (1976) attempted to relate the incidence of malignancy to age. In their view the percentage of

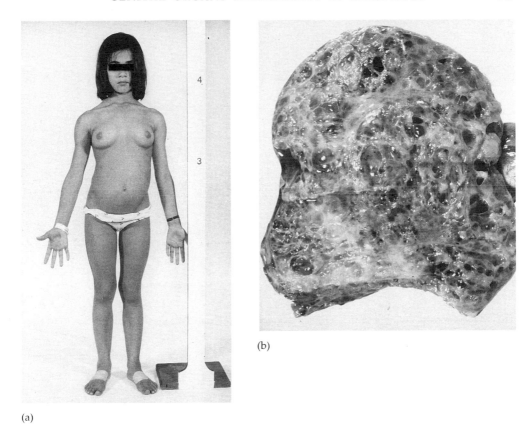

(a)

(b)

Fig. 15.8. (a) A child with precocious sexual development caused by an oestrogen secreting granulosa cell tumour seen in (b).

malignant tumours rose appreciably after puberty and they recommended gonadectomy before that time. The importance of these facts for the gynaecologist is that if a patient whose phenotype is predominantly female is found to have a 46XY karyotype or to have a Y chromosome in an abnormal karyotype, removal of the dysgenetic gonad is appropriate (Fig. 15.9) either before or soon after puberty depending upon the clinical features of the case.

Other tumours

Other genital tract malignant tumours are so rare as to be the greatest curiosities. Cases of carcinoma of the cervix have been described regularly over the years, but it is probable that these fall within the general pattern of clear cell adenocarcinoma of the cervix and vagina already mentioned, although the term mesonephroma has often been applied to them. Lister & Akinla (1972) reported a case of carcinoma of the vulva in a 13-year-old child which is the only case of this kind known to the author.

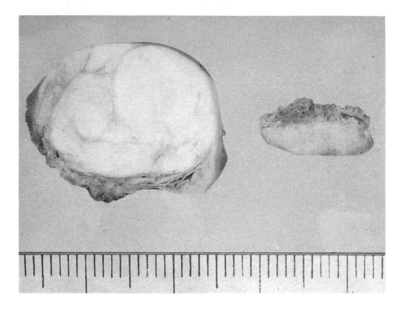

Fig. 15.9. Ovarian tumours of mixed dysgerminoma gonadoblastoma type in a child with gonadal dysgenesis and a Y chromosome.

References

Allyn D.L., Silverberg S.G. & Sakzberg A.M. (1971) Endodermal sinus tumour of the vagina; report of a case with 7-year survival and literature review of so-called 'mesonephromas'. *Cancer*, **27**, 1231−38.

Bibbo M., Gill W.B., Azizi F. *et al.* (1977) Follow-up study of male and female offspring of DES-exposed mothers. *Obstet. Gynecol.*, **49**, 1−8.

Breen J.L. & Maxson W.S. (1977) Ovarian tumours in children and adolescents. *Clin. Obstet. Gynaecol.*, **20**, 607−23.

Carlson J.A. (1985) *In*: Lavery J.P. & Sanfilippo J.S. (eds), *Gynecological Neoplasms in Pediatric and Adolescent Obstetrics and Gynecology*. Springer Verlag, New York. pp. 124−48.

Dewhurst C.J. (1963) *Gynaecological Disorders of Infants and Children*. Cassell, London.

Dewhurst Sir J. (1980) *Practical Pediatric and Adolescent Gynecology*. Marcel Dekker Inc., New York.

Dewhurst Sir J. (1981) Genital tract malignancy in the prepubertal child. *In*: Coppleson M. (ed.), *Gynecologic Oncology*. Churchill Livingstone, New York. p. 782.

Dewhurst Sir J. & Ferreira H.P. (1981) An endodermal sinus tumour of the vagina in an infant with seven year survival. *Br. J. Obstet. Gynaecol.*, **88**, 859−62.

Dewhurst Sir J., Ferreira H.P., Dalley V.M. & Staffurth J.F. (1980) Stilboestrol-associated vaginal carcinoma treated by radiotherapy. *J. Obstet. Gynaecol.*, **1**, 63−64.

Dewhurst C.J. Ferreira H.P. & Gillett P.G. (1971) Gonadal malignancy in XY females. *J. Obstet. Gynaecol. Br. Commonwealth*, **78**, 1077−83.

Ghavimi F., Exelby P.R., D'Angio G.J. *et al.* (1973) Combination therapy of urogenital embryonal rhabdomyosarcoma in children. *Cancer*, **32**, 1178−85.

Goerzen J.L., Grant R.M., Arthur K. & Stuart G.C.E. (1986) Primary endodermal sinus tumour of the vagina in childhood. *Pediatr. Adolesc. Gynecol.*, **3**, 131−56.

Grosfeld J.L., Smith J.P. & Clatworthy H.W. (1972) Pelvic rhabdomyosarcoma in infants and children. *J. Urol.*, **107**, 673−75.

Gunning J.E. (1976) The DES story. *Obstet. Gynaecol. Surv.*, **31**, 827−33.

Herbst A.L. (1978) Monograph. Intrauterine exposure to diethylstilbestrol in the human. *Am. Coll. Obstet. Gynaecol.*

Herbst A.L. (1981) The epidemiology of vaginal and cervical clear cell adenocarcinoma. *In*: Herbst A.L. & Bern H.A. (eds), *Developmental Effects of Diethylstilbestrol (DES) in Pregnancy*. Thieme-Stratton Inc., New York. pp. 63−800.

Herbst A.L. (1983) Personal communication.

Herbst A.L. & Anderson D. (1981) Clinical correlations and management of vaginal and cervical clear cell adenocarcinoma. *In*: Herbst A.L. & Bern H.A. (eds), *Developmental Effects of Diethylstilbestrol (DES) in Pregnancy*. Thieme-Stratton Inc., New York. pp. 71−80.

Herbst A.L., Cole P., Colton T. *et al.* (1977) Age-incidence and risk of diethylstilbestrol-related clear cell adenocarcinoma of the vagina and cervix. *Am. J. Obstet. Gynecol.*, **128**, 43−50.

Herbst A.L., Kurman R.J., Scully R.E. *et al.* (1979) Clear cell adenocarcinoma of the genital tract in young females: Registrar Report. *New Engl. J. Med.*, **287**, 1259−64.

Herbst A.L. & Scully R.E. (1970) Adenocarcinoma of the vagina in adolescence: a report of 7 cases including 6 clear-cell carcinomas (so-called mesonephromas). *Cancer*, **25**, 745−57.

Herbst A.L., Ulfelder H. & Poskanzer D.C. (1971) Adenocarcinoma of the vagina: association of maternal stilbestrol therapy with tumor appearance in young women. *New Engl. J. Med.*, **284**, 878−81.

Hilgers R.D., Ghavimi F., D'Angio G.J. *et al.* (1973) Memorial Hospital experience with pelvic exenteration and embryonal rhabdomyosarcoma of the vagina. *Gynecol. Oncol.*, **1**, 262−70.

Hilgers R.D., Malkasian G.D. & Soule E.H. (1970) Embryonal rhabdomyosarcoma (botryoid type) of the vagina. *Am. J. Obstet. Gynecol.*, **107**, 484−502.

Hudson C.N., Crandon A.J., Baird P.J. & Willcocks D. (1983) Preservation of reproductive potential in diethylstilbestrol-related vaginal adenocarcinoma. *Am. J. Obstet. Gynecol.*, **145**, 375−77.

Huffman J.W. (1968) *The Gynecology of Childhood and Adolescence*. W.B. Saunders, Philadelphia.

Linfors O. (1971) Primary ovarian neoplasms in infants and children: study of 81 cases diagnosed in Finland and Sweden. *Ann. Chir. Gynaecol.*, **60**, suppl. 177, 7.

Lister U.M. & Akinla O. (1972) Carcinoma of the vulva in childhood. *J. Obstet. Gynaecol. Br. Commonwealth*, **79**, 470−73.

Manuel M., Katayama K.P. & Jones H.W. (1976) The age of occurrence of gonadal tumours in intersex patients with a Y chromosome. *Am. J. Obstet. Gynecol.*, **124**, 293−300.

Mattingly R.F. & Stafl A. (1976) Cancer risk in diethylstilbestrol-exposed offspring. *Am. J. Obstet. Gynecol.*, **126**, 543−48.

Mitchell M., Talerman A., Sholl J.S., Okagaki T. & Cibils L.A. (1987) Pseudosarcoma botryoides in pregnancy. *Obstet. Gynecol.*, **70** (2), 522−26.

Noller K.L., Decker D.G., Fish C.R. & Gaffey T.A. (1976a) Identification, examination and management of diethylstilbestrol-exposed offspring. *Clin. Obstet. Gynaecol.*, **19**, 699−705.

Noller K.L., Decker D.G., Symmonds R.E. *et al.* (1976b) Clear cell adenocarcinoma of the vagina and cervix: survival data. *Am. J. Obstet. Gynecol.*, **124**, 285−88.

Noller K.L., Townsend D.E. & Kaufman R.H. (1981) Genital findings, colposcopic evaluation, and current management of the diethylstilbestrol-exposed female. *In*: Herbst A.L. & Bern H.A. (eds), *Developmental Effects of Diethylstilbestrol (DES) in Pregnancy*. Thieme-Stratton Inc., New York. pp. 81−102.

Poskanzer D.C. & Herbst A.L. (1977) Epidemiology of vaginal adenosis and adenocarcinoma associated with exposure to stilbestrol *in utero*. *Cancer*, **39**, 1892−95.

Reynolds V.H. (1984) (in discussion of Fleming I.D., Etcubanas E., Patterson R., Rao B., Pratt C., Hutsu O. & Kumar M.) The role of surgical resection when combined with chemotherapy and radiation in the management of pelvic rhabdomyosarcoma. *Ann. Surg.*, **199**, 509−14.

Robboy S.J., Scully R.E., Welch W.R. & Herbst A.L. (1977) Intrauterine diethylstilbestrol exposure and
    its consequences. *Arch. Pathol. Lab. Med.*, **101**, 1–5.
Scully R.E. & Welch W.R. (1981) Pathology of the female genital tract after prenatal exposure to
    diethylstilbestrol. *In*: Herbst A.L. & Bern H.A. (eds), *Developmental Effects of Diethylstilbestrol
    (DES) in Pregnancy*, Thieme-Stratton Inc., New York. pp. 26–45.
Senekjian E.L. & Herbst A.L. (1985) Diethylstilbestrol exposure *in utero*. *In*: Lavery J.P. & Sanfilippo
    J.S. (eds), *Pediatric and Adolescent Obstetrics and Gynecology*. Springer Verlag, New York. pp.
    149–60.
Shepherd J.H. (1989) Personal communication.
Taft P.D., Robboy S.J., Herbst A.L. & Scully R.E. (1974) Cytology of clear cell adenocarcinoma of the
    genital tract in young females: review of 95 cases from the Registry. *Acta Cytol.*, **18**, 279–90.
Tank E.S., Fellman S.L., Wheeler E.S. *et al.* (1972) Treatment of urogenital tract rhabdomyosarcoma in
    infants and children. *J. Urol.*, **107**, 324.
Ulfelder H. (1976) The stilbestrol-adenosis-carcinoma syndrome. *Cancer*, **38**, 426–31.

16

Cancer Complicating Pregnancy

JOHN H. SHEPHERD

Pregnancy and cancer evoke directly opposite responses in young women. The first results in pleasure and excitement with optimism for a new future to plan ahead, the other in pessimism, fear and horror. When occurring together, the patient is inevitably distraught, confused and terrified whilst her obstetrician is faced with a therapeutic dilemma. Many other opinions will be sought to help answer surgical, perinatal, obstetric, oncological and psychological as well as moral and religious questions.

This situation is thankfully uncommon but occurs 2–3 times a year in the average obstetric unit. An incidence of one case in every thousand pregnancies has been reported (Potter & Schoeneman 1970). Two basic principles must be obeyed in order to follow a coherent plan of treatment. First, the patient should be treated as though she were not pregnant although the timing and details of therapy vary according to the individual case. Nevertheless, the fact that a potentially lethal condition has been detected must not be forgotten in an ideological attempt to please all. The primary concern must not be to save the pregnancy at the expense of curing the malignancy. The cancer may well be at an early and curative stage when presenting, but will progress if left to await fetal maturity. Secondly, in no condition is it more important to discuss fully and frankly the situation with the patient and her partner so that they may be part of the final decision and understand the doctor's quandary. Absolute honesty, even if there is no categorical answer, is vital to obtain the confidence of the patient. This is even more important when the cancer is advanced with the patient perhaps deciding to sacrifice all for the sake of the unborn child.

Five questions are generally raised requiring careful consideration.

1 *Is the natural history of the cancer affected by the pregnancy?* This is usually not the case, with the exception of malignant melanomas. However, the great physiological and anatomical changes of various organs that inevitably occur, especially the breast and cervix, may affect the management. The increase in vascularity and lymphatic drainage as a result of hypertrophy as well as the expansion in tissue planes, should be remembered. A vaginal delivery in the presence of a cervical carcinoma with lymphatic or vascular space permeation could lead to widespread dissemination of malignant cells.

2 *Is the fetus affected by the cancer?* Not in any developmental way but rarely transplacental transfer of metastases has been reported.

3 *Does termination offer any therapeutic value?* Not necessarily, but this may be inevitable and advisable as part of the treatment plan decided upon.

4 *Is the fetus affected by the treatment?* This depends on which modality of treatment is selected for a particular tumour. Systemic chemotherapy, especially antimetabolites may have teratogenic effects and cause abortion. Radiotherapy to the pelvis in curative doses inevitably leads to fetal death and usually abortion.

5 *Are future pregnancies possible?* Under some circumstances, this may be possible, after allowing some time for follow up.

Malignancy during the reproductive years

Cancer as a rule is a disease of an elderly population. However, the age groups who become pregnant have different primaries to consider. Up to the age of 14 years leukaemias account for 35% of all cancer registrations. The central nervous system (CNS) including the brain accounts for 19% and other organs, such as bone (9%), soft tissue sarcomas (6%) and renal tumours (5%), a small proportion. From the age of 15–34 years, CNS lesions, cervical tumours and Hodgkin's disease occur more often. Between the ages of 35 and 50, breast (22%), colon and rectum (13%), skin (11%), lung (9%), uterus, including cervix and corpus (8%) and ovarian tumours (5%) peak in their incidence (Cancer Statistics 1983).

Emancipation and modern society has resulted in many women, for personal and career reasons, delaying their decision to bring up a family. As a result, a large number of women embark upon their first pregnancy in their 30s and 40s. At the other end of the reproductive age group, pregnancy may be the first time that many women are actually fully examined medically. Not only are the breasts carefully palpated, but abdominal and pelvic examinations are performed and a Papanicolaou cervical smear is taken. At this time, the importance of regular medical screening should be stressed to this captive and hopefully attentive audience. If one includes breast cancer, 37 000 gynaecological cancers occur each year. Education will make women and doctors more aware of this. Earlier detection is probably the most important factor for improving cure rates in general.

Cancer complicating pregnancy may be divided into pelvic and extrapelvic malignancies. As a rule, the pelvic cancers complicating this condition are best treated surgically. This is because cancer is still basically a surgical disease and the ideal treatment is to excise it widely if this is possible with an acceptably low mortality and morbidity. This predominantly applies to early stage disease. Radiotherapy on the other hand is most beneficial in well vascularized and oxygenized tissues. Once the pregnancy is destroyed by radiation, an anoxic environment results which is not ideal for maximum effect. Secondly, surgical treatment aims for a decisive cure in a short and limited time. Even with a coexisting pregnancy, extirpation of the malignant tissue is an important principle.

With the generally improving results of cancer therapy, more women will conceive during or shortly after treatment. This is an important consideration. At the same time, with expanding screening programmes, more women will present during pregnancy with their cancer. Guidelines may be applied for the treatment of various primary tumours according to the trimester of presentation, or the postpartum period. These principles will be flexible, however, according to the cancer and organ involved, as well as the needs of the patient herself.

Pelvic cancers complicating pregnancy

These may arise from gynaecological genital organs, either the lower or upper genital tracts, or from the bladder or rectum. Gynaecological tumours include those of the vulva, vagina, and cervix, from the lower tract, and from the endometrium, ovary and fallopian tube from the upper genital tract. The breast is an extrapelvic, but still gynaecological, organ.

Carcinoma of the cervix

There have been approximately 2000 cases of invasive carcinoma of the cervix complicating pregnancy reported in the world literature, although many others remain unreported. Most authors accept patients either diagnosed during pregnancy or within 12 months of delivery as being eligible for inclusion in these figures. An incidence of between 1 and 13 per 10 000 is quoted. The average incidence in larger centres is 1:2000—2500 pregnancies (Kistner et al. 1957). The incidence of carcinoma in situ during pregnancy is 1:750 (Hacker et al. 1982). With increasing screening programmes and widespread availability of cervical smears at antenatal clinics, it is reasonable to assume that the incidence of the latter will increase. At the same time, the number of invasive cancers will hopefully decrease as they are detected earlier.

Of the 20 cases dealt with over the last 7 years by the author, five had microinvasive lesions. Three patients had adenocarcinoma and the rest (12) were squamous cell tumours. One patient was stage IIB at presentation and the remainder stage IB. Five of these patients had caesarean Wertheim radical hysterectomies and the remainder were treated stage for stage either by surgery or radiotherapy regardless of the pregnancy. The ratio of carcinoma in situ to invasive cancer at this time was 4:1 during pregnancy.

Diagnosis

Approximately 10—15 abnormal smears are reported per thousand pregnancies from the average antenatal clinic. Management is shown in the flow chart, see Fig. 16.1. Colposcopic assessment may be readily performed and although tedious during pregnancy because of the hypertrophy and increased vascularity, a satisfactory view of the lower endocervical canal and ectocervix can be obtained. It is most important to exclude invasive carcinoma. This may usually be achieved by colposcopy and cytology alone in the hands of an experienced colposcopist (Benedet *et al.* 1977). Pregnancy with its consequent anatomical and physiological changes results in an exaggerated and altered colposcopic appearance of intra-epithelial neoplasia. If invasive disease cannot be excluded then an adequate biopsy is essential. Although this may be colposcopic, on occasions a larger wedge biopsy or cone biopsy may be necessary, especially if the limits of the lesions within the canal may not be visualized. However small the biopsy, the increased vascularity may lead to excessive bleeding. As a result, packing or a suture may be necessary, performed as an inpatient procedure. A colposcopic diagnosis of microinvasion necessitates conization to exclude invasive disease, although this procedure is required less as colposcopy becomes more generally

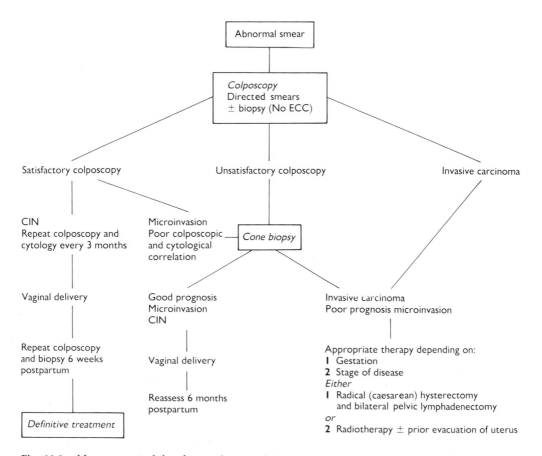

Fig. 16.1.   Management of the abnormal smear during pregnancy.

available and accepted. However, cone biopsy during pregnancy carries an almost 50% morbidity including immediate or delayed haemorrhage, subsequent cervical laceration, abortion and perinatal mortality (Hannigan *et al*. 1982). The procedure does not significantly increase first trimester abortions, but fetal wastage from mid-trimester cone biopsy is substantial. Therapeutic cervical encirclage is advisable if the pregnancy is to continue.

Many patients, especially those with cervical intraepithelial neoplasia, are asymptomatic. The commonest presenting symptom in invasive carcinoma is vaginal bleeding. These points emphasize the need for examination and the taking of a cytological smear of the cervix in all patients at their initial antenatal visit. Any vaginal bleeding, threatened abortion or antepartum haemorrhage warrants another careful speculum examination of the cervix with a further smear. Regrettably, a delay in diagnosis often results because of a reluctance on behalf of the obstetrician to follow these guidelines (Stander & Lein 1960).

Management of pregnant patients found to have cervical cancer

This depends entirely on whether invasion is present or not. Cervical intraepithelial neoplasia may be observed through the pregnancy by repeated colposcopic and cytological examination 3 monthly with a check at 36 weeks to confirm the absence of invasive disease (see Fig. 16.1). A vaginal delivery is then permitted unless obstetric contraindications supervene. Definitive treatment may then be decided upon at the postnatal visit after a suitable colposcopic biopsy. An alternative approach is to consider caesarean hysterectomy. This procedure in experienced hands has a definite place, with a negligible increase in morbidity (Plauché *et al*. 1981). For many patients it would avoid a further hospital admission and subsequent time away from home, the family and work. This obviously only applies if childbearing is complete and sterilization is being seriously considered. Under these circumstances, hysterectomy is therefore a realistic option for treatment regardless of the pregnancy.

Microinvasive disease requires very careful assessment and a cone biopsy to exclude invasion (see Chapter 4). Although the definition by FIGO staging is less than 5 mm of invasion through the basement membrane, most gynaecologic oncologists accept 5 mm as a practical depth of invasion. For those cases with a single bud of invasion stage IaI and a well differentiated tumour with a low number of malignant cells invading through the basement membrane, conization would be sufficient therapy and a vaginal delivery at a suitable time anticipated. However, with multiple foci of invasion involving lymphatic or vascular spaces and a high morphological tumour load, especially with moderate or poor histological differentiation, then it would be wise to treat this as invasive disease and not allow a vaginal delivery.

Vaginal delivery in such cases or with deeper invasion risks dissemination of malignant cells into the lymphatic or vascular channels as well as into interstitial spaces, as progressive cervical dilatation and vaginal delivery occur. Haemorrhage, sepsis and cervical laceration may result. Transport of malignant cells down the vagina with subsequent growth in an episiotomy site may herald recurrent disease unexpectedly some time later. Interestingly, there is little difference in maternal survival if the pregnancy is terminated by caesarean section or vaginal delivery. This, however, is not an endorsement of vaginal delivery because considerable difficulties may be experienced, especially if the lesions are large. The majority of patients delivering in this way have their diagnosis made postpartum.

The choice between radiotherapy and surgery

The treatment of invasive cervical cancer remains an individual decision depending on the patient and the stage of disease as well as the facilities available. Full and early assessment for staging is clearly essential under anaesthesia with a thorough review of all available histopathology specimens.

Surgical treatment is indicated in most young patients with early invasive disease (stage IB and IIA). This would involve radical abdominal hysterectomy, bilateral salpingectomy, with conservation of both ovaries if possible, in conjunction with a bilateral pelvic lymphadenectomy. Excision of a 3–4 cm cuff of vagina with the specimen is necessary. This procedure may be performed during the first and second trimester with the fetus *in utero* (Fig. 16.2). In the late second trimester fetal viability may be awaited and corticosteroids administered to accelerate fetal lung maturity prior to caesarean section with transfer of the fetus to a suitable neonatal unit. The lower segment should be avoided in view of the increased vascularity and relation of the tumour: hence this is an indication for

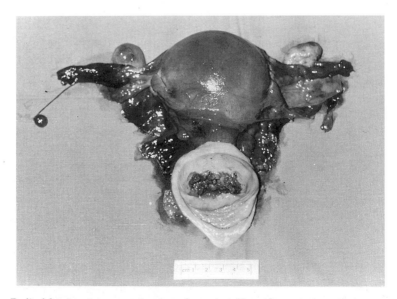

Fig. 16.2.   Radical hysterectomy specimen performed at 12 weeks gestation.

the classical caesarean incision (Fig. 16.3). A radical hysterectomy and pelvic node dissection may then be proceeded with. This would also apply to the third trimester and postpartum when surgery may proceed without undue delay. If possible, the fetus should not be exposed to unnecessary X-rays, so intravenous urography is limited during pregnancy to a single view whenever possible (Fig. 16.4). Improving ultrasound techniques and equipment with better resolution should indicate para-aortic node involvement or ureteric dilatation and obstructive uropathy. A chest X-ray should always be performed preoperatively with suitable shielding of the abdomen.

Radiotherapy is the preferred treatment in more advanced lesions (stage IIB and beyond) and for some earlier lesions not deemed suitable for surgery. During the second and third trimesters when a non-viable fetus is present, external irradiation with at least 3000 centigrays (cGy) to the uterus is administered. Spontaneous abortion is preferable to induced abortion as the latter reduces the 5-year survival. An afterloading intrauterine tandem and colpostat may then be inserted. Following this, the whole pelvis is further irradiated with a booster to the pelvic side walls and nodal areas, increasing the dosage to 5000 to 6000 cGy.

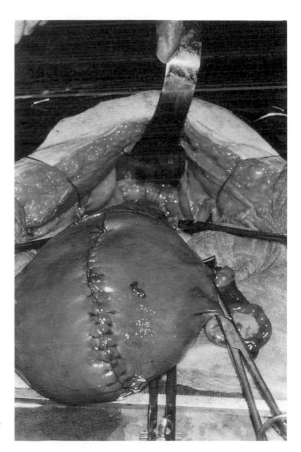

Fig. 16.3. Classical caesarean section preceding radical abdominal hysterectomy at 32 weeks gestation.

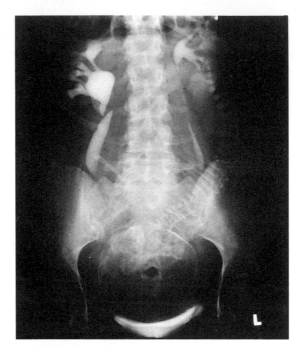

Fig. 16.4. Intravenous urogram performed prior to surgery at 32 weeks gestation: stage IB carcinoma of the cervix. Note the physiological dilatation of the right ureter.

When a viable fetus is present in the third trimester, then delivery by classical caesarean section is performed first, followed by external therapy and later caesium insertions. Postpartum radiation is carried out as in the non-pregnant patient. Because of the danger of infection, intracavitary caesium is usually divided into several applications.

Prognosis

Cervical intraepithelial neoplasia behaves as in a non-pregnant state with the same propensity for persistence, progression to invasive disease and recurrence. Definitive therapy postpartum should be followed up for life.

Five-year survival and prognosis for those with invasive disease is similar stage for stage to those patients with cervical cancer in the non-pregnant state. The overall 5-year survival is approximately 50% for all stages in both conditions. However, advanced stage disease may lead to dosimetry problems with radiotherapy due to repeated interruptions in treatment if sepsis occurs. On the other hand, a higher proportion of patients will present at an earlier stage than in the overall non-pregnant group.

Clinical staging is the most important factor for prognosis. The reason that patients with disease diagnosed and treated in the third trimester and postpartum fare significantly worse than those with disease diagnosed at an early time of pregnancy is because they have more advanced disease. The popular misconception that cervical cancer during pregnancy spreads more rapidly and aggressively than in the non-gravid state is unfounded. Most authorities favour abdominal delivery by classical caesarean section (Barber & Brunschwig 1963). However, this is questioned by others who show no difference in the survival rates (Lee *et al.* 1981). This emphasizes the necessity of assessing and individualizing each case; joint consultation between gynaecologist, radiotherapist, pathologist, neonatologist and the patient herself is of great importance.

Cancer of the vulva

This is rare during pregnancy, approximately 40 cases being reported with less than half of these being treated during the pregnancy itself (Barclay 1970). Although a disease of predominantly the seventh and eighth decades, when it does occur in pregnancy the patients are surprisingly young, between 25 and 35 years. The majority are well differentiated invasive epidermoid tumours with a small number of melanomas, sarcomas and adenocarcinomas. The pregnancy has no adverse effect on the prognosis and termination is not indicated in such patients (Kempers & Symonds 1965).

Vulvar intraepithelial neoplasia may be treated conservatively and watched closely until the puerperium. A wide excision may then be carried out. Initial biopsy under a local anaesthetic is advisable at the outset.

More established and advanced disease should be treated regardless of the pregnancy by the accepted procedure of radical vulvectomy and bilateral groin lymphadenectomy. During the first half of the pregnancy, this is quite feasible, but later in the second trimester due to uterine and therefore abdominal enlargement, this may become technically more difficult.

During the third trimester, if the lesion is small and will not interfere with vaginal delivery, then this should be allowed. Radical surgery may then be carried out 2–4 weeks later. If the lesion is very large, abdominal delivery would be necessary in order to avoid laceration, haemorrhage, and sepsis. Postpartum surgery may be proceeded with as in the non-pregnant state. Operative haemorrhage may be profuse due to increased vascularity but this may be controlled and treated in the standard way (Rahman *et al.* 1982).

Following a previous radical vulvectomy vaginal delivery may be allowed with suitable care of the introitus, and a timely episiotomy to avoid scar tissue tearing. If there is significant vaginal stenosis or fibrosis, abdominal delivery would be advisable. Should labour occur before the wound has healed or if there has been a degree of dehiscence, then elective caesarean section would be advisable.

Cancer of the vagina

Much rarer than cervical or vulval neoplasia, only 11 cases of vaginal cancer complicating pregnancy have been reported (Collins & Barclay 1973; Lutz *et al*. 1977). Follow up of these has been difficult but the prognosis would appear to be poor. It is often difficult to tell with advanced disease whether the tumour arises from the cervix or vagina, but if both are involved, then the primary is regarded as being cervical in origin.

As a rule the disease should be treated as though the patient were not pregnant. If the fetus is viable, classical caesarean section followed by radio-therapy is generally accepted. However, an early stage I localized tumour within the upper third of the vagina could be treated by radical hysterectomy, colpectomy and pelvic node clearance.

Following the reports of diethylstilboestrol (DES) exposure *in utero* and sub-sequent development of a vaginal clear cell carcinoma (Herbst *et al*. 1971), careful surveillance of such women is required. However, there is no evidence to suggest that adenosis progresses to carcinoma during a pregnancy. To date, 400 cases have been reported of such carcinoma arising in DES exposed infants and only two have arisen following progression from adenosis to carcinoma whilst under surveillance. Neither of these progressed during a pregnancy, but another case did present during a pregnancy initially. Treatment should obviously be as in the non-pregnant state.

Carcinoma of the endometrium

Endometrial carcinoma occurring with a pregnancy is extremely rare; eight cases have been reported, two of which were incidental findings in conjunction with abortions, one being spontaneous, the other therapeutic. Of the other six cases, four were over the age of 35 years (Karlen *et al*. 1972). Treatment is by total abdominal hysterectomy and bilateral salpingo-oophorectomy with supplemen-tary radiotherapy in high risk patients with poor prognostic features.

Ovarian cancer

Ovarian tumours are said to occur once in every 1000 pregnancies: one in 10 of these are normal physiological corpora lutea. Malignant ovarian tumours are quoted as complicating one in every 8–20000 pregnancies. Although overall one in five cysts are malignant, in the pregnant state this figure drops to one in 20. Of the 164 ovarian tumours detected during pregnancy reported by Beischer, half were either adult cystic teratomas or mucinous cyst adenomas (Beischer *et al*. 1971). The varied and favourable pathological type reflects an overall 5-year survival rate for ovarian neoplasia in pregnancy of 76% as compared to a general figure for all age groups of 25%. In Novak's series of 100 cases, 45 were common epithelial tumours, 14 gonadal stromal tumours, 33 germ cell tumours, two sarcomas, two Krukenberg tumours and four metastatic of which two were unclassifiable (Novak 1975).

The adnexal mass during pregnancy has a similar differential diagnosis as in the non-pregnant patients in a similar age group. The management depends on the gestation of pregnancy: as a rule surgery should be avoided during the first trimester to reduce the risk of abortion. Most ovarian cysts during this time are corpora lutea and some of these may actually increase in size during the second month of pregnancy as a result of the luteinization associated with high levels of chorionic gonadotrophin. Although a successful continuation and outcome of the pregnancy is of great concern, the tumour must be treated as if occurring in the non-pregnant state. Ultrasonic scanning is of great value to detect solid or semi-solid areas, septa or even osteoid tissue. Serial scans will confirm regression in the size of such a cyst which may become more difficult to palpate as the uterus enlarges. If it does not, however, exploration is mandatory. Peritoneal washings, ovarian cystectomy or oophorectomy if appropriate and biopsy of the other ovary and any suspicious lesions are the minimal acceptable procedures. Frozen section reporting of histopathology is very helpful if available. Interruption of the pregnancy has no beneficial effects on the outcome of this disease. Re-exploration may always be undertaken later if necessary, but if advanced disease is found then appropriate bulk-reducing surgery, followed by aggressive chemotherapy is essential if the patient is to survive. Approximately one-third of cases are stage III or IV at operation, therefore appropriate surgery must be undertaken for this degree of spread.

Fortunately, most malignancies in pregnancy are diagnosed at an early stage because the patient seeks medical advice at the booking clinic prior to symptoms related to the tumour occurring. The survival rate is much the same as in the non-pregnant state and is determined by the type of tumour and its staging. If the tumour is diagnosed in the third trimester, surgery may be delayed until the fetus is viable, but delay beyond that is not justifiable. Needless to say, inspection of fallopian tubes and ovaries is mandatory in any caesarean section.

In conclusion, it is important to have a high index of suspicion, to make an early diagnosis and treat promptly. Problems will occur when both obstetrician and patient delay or resist surgical exploration because of the fear of inducing an abortion. The risk of this may be reduced by using tocolytic agents such as salbutamol or ritodrine at the time. The dangers of delay to the mother far exceed the theoretical danger to the fetus. The possibility of ovarian cancer, let alone complications of torsion, haemorrhage or rupture must obviously be remembered whenever an ovarian cyst is detected or suspected during pregnancy.

Cancer of the rectum

Although not a gynaecological tumour, rectal and colonic cancers are for the most part pelvic in origin. More than 200 cases have been reported occurring in pregnancy (Barber & Brunschwig 1968) with a low incidence quoted as one case for every 50 000 pregnancies (McLean *et al.* 1955).

Rectal bleeding, abdominal pain, weight loss, a change in the bowel habit, persistent nausea and vomiting in late pregnancy and a palpable abdominal or pelvic mass may be the result of a colonic neoplasm and should certainly warrant thorough investigation to exclude the possibility. This is especially so in patients with a predisposing disease such as familial adenomatous polyposis coli, or ulcerative colitis. More advanced disease may present as a rectovaginal fistula at delivery. Occult blood studies followed by sigmoidoscopy, colonoscopy and biopsy as necessary should be carried out. Once the diagnosis is established, surgery is proceeded with. During the first and second trimester, this would involve an abdomino−perineal or anterior resection depending on the exact position of the rectal tumour or partial colectomy for a colonic lesion. Delivery later by the vaginal route may be anticipated unless obstetric complications arise.

In the late second and third trimester, surgical intervention should be delayed if possible until the fetus is viable. Then, caesarean section is usually required because of technical difficulties with the operation that would occur otherwise. Again, abdomino−pelvic or anterior resection is performed thereafter. If there is pelvic extension of disease, then hysterectomy and bilateral salpingo-oophorectomy may be necessary. However, if the surgery is delayed to allow fetal viability, haemorrhage, obstruction and perforation may complicate the situation.

Extrapelvic malignancies

Cancer of the breast

Over 22 000 new cases of breast cancer are reported each year in the UK. One in six occur in women aged less than 45 years and of these, 1−2% are pregnant at the time of diagnosis. There is a familial incidence of breast cancer, so that the risk of developing the disease increases by 5 to 10 times if a first degree relative has it. It is the leading site of mortality from cancer in the 25−74-year age group in women and in those 39−44 years of age, it is the leading cause of death. When women delay their first pregnancy until the age of 35 years or more, the risk of breast cancer increases by 3 times compared to those women who initially conceive prior to the age of 20. With changing contraceptive practices and this delay in starting a family, the incidence of this problem complicating pregnancy will increase. The dilemma for treatment is quite acute. Therapeutic abortion does not appear to improve the chance of a cure, even though this potentially lethal disease is hormone sensitive (Ribeiro & Palmer 1977). Hormone receptor studies to resolve these questions are not yet available, but may in the future give an indication as to which pregnancies should be terminated in view of a positive receptor status. Physiological changes continue throughout the pregnancy with alterations in vascularity, lymphatic permeation and the hormonal milieu. Widely differing views are held by those specializing in this disease, but the trend is away from radical surgery and mastectomy to localized excision of the primary tumour with lymph node sampling. This is followed by adjunctive therapy, either in the form of chemotherapy or radiotherapy. Numerous trials are at present underway to evaluate the role of chemotherapy with both single agents and in combination. Also under review is conservative as opposed to more radical surgery, with radiotherapy and hormonal manipulation, both oestrogenic and anti-oestrogenic.

Survival

The overall 5-year survival for breast cancer is 50%. In pregnancy this figure is said to be more than halved, mainly because the instance of positive nodes is greater and metastases have occurred before therapy is commenced. This more advanced stage of presentation is due to various factors: firstly, the enlarged and engorged breast shields the primary mass for a longer period; secondly, the increased vascularity and lymphatic drainage from the gravid or lactating breast aids metastatic spread. An early lesion, present for less than 3 months, and less than 2 cm in diameter with no positive nodes and a moderately well differentiated histopathological picture has a similar prognosis to the non-pregnant state, i.e. 70–80% survival. Involvement of the subareolar region, oedema or ulceration of the skin, medial placed tumours, fixation of the tumour or lymph node involvement worsens the prognosis considerably. Dividing patients into three groups results in the following 5-year survival figures: simultaneous with pregnancy 33%; discovery postpartum 29% and subsequent pregnancy 52%. With positive nodes these figures fall to 21, 15 and 30%, respectively. At the same time the incidence of positive nodes was almost double that in a comparable non-pregnant group (Holleb & Farrow 1962). Clinicians advise that in the first trimester the patient should be treated as if not pregnant.

Whether the pregnancy should be terminated is at present debatable and such a decision is based upon psychological, social and economic reasoning. Operable disease but with positive nodes warrants chemotherapy and this has theoretical teratogenic risks to the fetus, making termination advisable. Later in the pregnancy, there does not appear to be any special risk in treating the patient rather than waiting for the puerperium. A short delay while awaiting fetal viability probably has no significant deleterious effects. Advanced disease may be helped by oophorectomy, but hormonal manipulation by anti-oestrogens is more practical depending on receptor status of the tumour.

Subsequent pregnancy is permissible with a 2-year interval elapsing following treatment. If there is no sign of recurrence then there is no evidence to suggest that pregnancy would alter the prognosis.

Breast feeding is a debatable issue but most emphasize that this should be discouraged. Lactation and subsequent engorgement of the breast would be inadvisable if a second occult primary was present.

'No lady should have a lump in her breast'. This principle must be adhered to at all times if the disease, as with other cancers, is to be stopped at a time when it may be cured in its early stages.

Hodgkin's disease and lymphomas

For the most part, lymphosarcomas, reticulum cell sarcomas, and giant follicular lymphomas affect men in their 40s and 50s. Hodgkin's disease, however, commonly affects young women occurring with a frequency of one in 6000 deliveries. In a series of 364 patients with Hodgkin's disease, 112 were complicated by pregnancy (Barry *et al*. 1962). Of these, many had disease above the diaphragm and could be treated with radiotherapy and suitable shielding of the abdomen. Pregnancy would not appear to adversely affect the disease, although it is advisable to try and delay radiotherapy and chemotherapy until after delivery. This would apply to late second and third trimester pregnancies. Early in the pregnancy this question would have been addressed with careful consideration, however, as encouraging results and better cure rates are being achieved. Therefore continuing the pregnancy may be considered favourably.

Radiation therapy does not appear to affect fertility in Hodgkin's disease patients if the pelvis is spared. When combined with chemotherapy, reproduction may be impaired, however. It should be remembered that oophoropexy performed at the time of staging laparotomy if pelvic irradiation is planned will help to protect the ovaries and developing germinal follicles. Chemotherapy on its own may cause amenorrhoea but this usually spontaneously reverses after therapy. Subsequent fertility and even treatment of infertility is not contraindicated once a cure has been achieved and the patient has been in complete remission for a satisfactory time. Wives of male patients treated with both modalities have a higher incidence of spontaneous abortion (Holmes & Holmes 1978).

Leukaemia

Acute leukaemia is associated with premature labour as well as postpartum haemorrhage. Once the diagnosis is established prompt treatment is advisable to give the best chance of obtaining a remission. Chronic myelocytic leukaemia follows a more insidious course, however. Patients with this variety are less likely to suffer by delaying termination of the pregnancy than those patients with acute types. Patients with this disease may receive both radiotherapy and chemotherapy and still deliver an apparently healthy infant (Lee *et al*. 1965).

Melanoma

Malignant melanomas represent one of the few tumours which are adversely affected by pregnancy. Melanocyte stimulating hormone (MSH) levels increase after the second month of pregnancy and result in increased pigmentation. Metastatic spread would appear to be more rapid in pregnancy but stage for stage there may be no significant difference in the prognosis for the patient (George *et al.* 1960). However, another study (Sutherland *et al.* 1983a) has suggested that melanomas diagnosed initiated or stimulated during pregnancy have a worse prognosis than those presenting in the non-gravid state. Such tumours are clearly hormonally dependent as has been shown by biochemical receptor studies with increasing oestrogen and progesterone levels and the simultaneous stimulation of the melanoma, which subsequently regressed following delivery (Sutherland *et al.* 1983b). Other reports have confirmed this for stage I but have demonstrated a much lower survival for pregnant patients with stage II melanoma (Shiu *et al.* 1976). Although melanomas in pregnancy are rare, almost half of the tumours metastasize to the placenta and 95% of those metastasizing to the fetus are from such a primary.

Management is much the same as in the non-pregnant state, so that wide excision with regional lymph node dissection is the treatment of choice. Adequate excision may necessitate a skin graft to close the defect.

Thyroid cancer

Although rare, this cancer affects young women and is reported after radiation therapy (Asteris & de Groot 1976). When occurring in pregnancy, this is another tumour that may be promoted as thyroid stimulating hormone (TSH) is elevated during pregnancy. As in the non-pregnant state, total thyroidectomy and either unilateral or bilateral block dissection of the lymph nodes of the neck are required. Thyroid extract is given to limit the output of TSH. Radioactive iodine is contra-indicated. Papillary tumours are commoner than follicular tumours and the prognosis is good.

Brain and central nervous system tumours

These may occur between the ages of 10 and 35 but are commoner between 5 and 10 years of age (cerebellar astrocytomas, medulloblastomas and ependymonas) and between 40 and 60 years (gliomas, meningiomas and adenomas). Presenting symptoms are difficult to be differentiated from those of a normal and routine pregnancy. Toxaemia may subsequently produce symptoms of convulsion, coma, proteinuria, oliguria and oedema and these may confuse the issue (Birnard 1898).

A high index of suspicion is required in patients with headaches, visual disturbances or other cerebral symptoms that do not resolve. A neurological examination followed by computerized axial tomography is indicated accompanied by visual field and acuity testing.

Treatment is as in the non-pregnant state: surgical excision with or without radiotherapy. Although a vaginal delivery is aimed for, elevation of the intracerebral pressure should be avoided. The second stage should be shortened with the use of forceps. An epidural anaesthetic should only be used very cautiously; most anaesthetists decline.

In general, most neurologists advise against continuing a pregnancy in the absence of or shortly after the treatment of a central nervous system tumour.

Physiological enlargement of the pituitary gland occurs in pregnancy and if a microadenoma is present, it may enlarge and so precipitate neurological symptoms and signs. It is impossible to predict which microadenomas will enlarge, so it is safer to treat all patients with hyperprolactinaemia and a suspected pituitary microadenoma before pregnancy is commenced. Neither pretreatment serum prolactin nor radiological changes of the sella turcica can predict tumour development during pregnancy. Treatment with bromocriptine for more than 12 months before conception seems to reduce the risk of tumour progress (Holmgren *et al.* 1986). Whether breast feeding should be encouraged is debatable, but with caution this is reasonable. Bromocriptine may be recommenced after weaning if the serum prolactin remains elevated.

Salivary gland, mouth, tongue, pharynx and larynx

Cancers of the tongue, mouth and upper air and food passages do not appear to affect the course of pregnancy or be aggravated by it. These tumours, therefore, must be treated in their own right independent of the pregnancy.

Cancer of the salivary glands, however, may appear to run a short and fatal course when associated with pregnancy. In a small series reported by Sir Stanford Cade (Cade 1964) two of three patients developed metastases unexpectedly that appeared to have been activated by the pregnancy.

Miscellaneous tumours

Although rare, bone tumours are occasionally seen during childbearing years as mainly Ewing's sarcoma, osteogenic sarcoma and osteocytoma. The bones commonly affected are the clavicle, sternum, spine, humerus and femur. Presenting symptoms are usually local pain or a mass that becomes palpable. After an initial biopsy, surgical excision is the usual treatment followed by chemotherapy. The pregnancy does not affect the growth of the tumour but clearly termination may be indicated because of the effects of the drugs on the developing fetus. Recurrences occur usually within 3 years. Further pregnancies should be delayed until after this time.

Sarcomas arising from soft tissues rarely occur. Some, such as angiosarcoma, may be influenced by the hormonal change (Pack & Ariel 1958). Desmoid tumours may arise during pregnancy. Neurofibromata may enlarge and rarely undergo malignant change. Prompt diagnosis and radical ablative surgery is required to obtain survival (Ginsberg *et al.* 1981).

Phaecromocytomas

These are extremely rare but very dangerous during pregnancy with a 50% maternal and fetal mortality. Alpha block control with phenoxybenzamine is required and surgical removal attempted only after localizing the tumour, preferably postpartum (Coombes 1976).

Placental and fetal transmission of cancer

Patients and relatives will always worry and ask about transfer of cancer to the fetus. This is in fact extremely rare with 53 cases documented in the literature from 1866 to the present time (Dildy *et al.* 1989). Cancer may induce abortion and some cases may go unreported. However, in most instances of maternal cancer, there is no metastatic spread to the fetus; it is possible that the types of cancer associated with pregnancy and the types of cancers reported to metastasize to the products of conception differ (Potter & Schoeneman 1970). Breast cancer and cervical cancer each account for 26% of the total number of cancers reported in pregnant women. To date, however, only seven cases of breast cancer and one of cervical cancer have been reported to have spread to placental or fetal tissue. The most common cancer to metastasize is malignant melanoma with 16 cases reported, 12 of which have metastasized to the placenta and seven to the fetus. The next most common malignancies to metastasize are leukaemias and lymphomas. Eight such cases have been reported, five involving the placenta and four the fetus. Seven cases of breast cancer metastasizing have been reported, six of lung cancer, five of various sarcomas and two gastric cancers. All of these involved the placenta and not the fetus. One hepatic carcinoma has been reported (Friedreich 1866) but no further report since this early date. A solitary report of squamous cell carcinoma of the cervix metastasizing to the placenta has been recorded (Cailliez *et al.* 1980). This is surprising as it is one of the most frequent cancers coexisting with pregnancy and in the reported case there was no tumour in the fetus but invasion of the trophoblast occurred with tumour involvement of the intervillous space of the placenta. The mother had a stage IIB poorly differentiated tumour and died 9 months postpartum.

The mode of transmission may be by arterial haematogenous metastases in view of the fact that the uteroplacental blood flow is increased at term up to 500 ml/min, which is 10% of the maternal cardiac output. Haematogenous emboli of cancer cells may therefore become trapped in the placental intervillous space which acts as a filter for the fetus. In the solitary reported case of pulmonary carcinoma transmission to the placenta there was also maternal brain metastases (Dildy *et al*. 1989). It may be that fetal metastases are prevented by the placental barrier (Rothman *et al*. 1973) but animal data does not support this (Pang 1957; Retik *et al*. 1962). A functioning fetal immune system must play a major role dealing with neoplastic cells that do cross the placental barrier.

The advice as to whether the pregnancy should be continued in the presence of coexisting cancer is very controversial. Even with malignant melanoma there is no conclusive evidence regarding the effect of pregnancy on the course of the malignancy (Donegan 1983). Fatal progression of malignant melanoma during pregnancy with dissemination to the products of conception has been reported (Moller *et al*. 1986) and these authors recommended that a woman should not become pregnant within 5 years of treatment of malignant melanoma. Nonetheless, the risk of fetal involvement is minimal and therefore therapeutic abortion is not recommended for fetal indications, although it may be for maternal nonmedical reasons. This concept is supported by the fact that only 53 cases of malignancy have been reported metastasizing to the products of conception with 13 of these to the fetus. Nevertheless, close follow up of the infant is advised, especially for maternal melanoma, leukaemia or lymphoma.

Clearly, it is important to examine the placenta of all cases where maternal cancer is known to have existed and any metastases should be reported in the literature.

Conclusion

Although uncommon, cancer complicating pregnancy does occur and is reported with an accepted frequency on average of one case of cancer in every 1000 births. The effects may be devastating for both the mother and the family. The management requires individualization with careful thought as to whether termination is necessary or whether continuing with the pregnancy is possible prior to definitive treatment. This is one occasion when a joint decision must be reached between the obstetrician, surgeon, medical oncologist and any other specialist involved. The disease must be assessed and treated in the full light of its exact location and stage. An understanding of the natural history within the context of the pregnancy with a potentially viable unborn child is of crucial importance. Nevertheless, the immediate and foremost duty is to treat the cancer of the pregnant patient with the object of controlling the disease (Cade 1964).

References

Asteris G.T. & de Groot L.J. (1976) Thyroid cancer: relationship to radiation exposure and to pregnancy. *J. Repro. Med.*, **17**, 209.

Barber H.R. & Brunschwig A. (1963) Gynaecologic cancer complicating pregnancy. *Am. J. Obstet. Gynecol.*, **85**, 156–64.

Barber H.R. & Brunschwig A. (1968) Carcinoma of the bowel. *Am. J. Obstet. Gynecol.*, **100**, 926–33.

Barclay D.L. (1970) Surgery of the vulva, perineum and vagina in pregnancy. *In*: Barber H.R.K. & Graber E.A. (eds), *Surgical Disease in Pregnancy*. W.B. Saunders Co., Philadelphia. pp. 310–35.

Barry R.M., Diamond H.D. & Craver L.F. (1962) The influence of pregnancy on the course of Hodgkin's disease. *Am. J. Obstet. Gynecol.*, **84**, 445−54.

Beischer N.A., Buttery B.W., Fortune D.W. *et al.* (1971) Growth and malignancy of ovarian tumours in pregnancy. *Aust. NZ J. Obstet. Gynecol.*, **11**, 208−20.

Benedet J.L., Boyes T.A. & Nichols T.M. (1977) Colposcopic evaluation of patients with abnormal cervical smears. *Br. J. Obstet. Gynaecol.*, **84**, 517−21.

Birnard M.H. (1898) Sarcome cerebrale: un evaluation rapide au cours la grossesse et pendant les suites des couches. *Soc. Obstet. Paris*, **1**, 296.

Cade, Sir Stanford (1964) Cancer in pregnancy. *J. Obstet. Gynaecol. Br. Commonwealth*, **71** (3), 341−47.

Cailliez D., Moirot M.H., Fessard C. *et al.* (1980) Localisation placentaire d'un carcinome du coluterin. *J. Gynecol. Obstet. Biol. Reprod. (Paris)*, **9**, 461.

Collins G.G. & Barclay D.L. (1973) Cancer of the vulva and cancer of the vagina in pregnancy. *Clin. Obstet. Gynecol.*, **6**, 927.

Coombes J.B. (1976) Phaeochromocytoma presenting in pregnancy. *Proc. R. Soc. Med.*, **69**, 224−25.

Dildy G.A., Mouse K.J., Carpenter R.J. & Klima J. (1989) Maternal malignancy metastatic to the products of conception: a review. *Obstet. Gynecol. Surv.*, **44**, 535−40.

Donegan W.L. (1983) *Cancer and Pregnancy*. CA 33, 194.

Friedreich N. (1866) Beitrage zür Pathologicdes Krebses. *Virchows Arch. (Pathol. Anat.)*, **36**, 30, 465.

George P.A., Fortner J.G. & Pack G.T. (1960) Melanoma with pregnancy. A report of 115 cases. *Cancer*, **13**, 584−89.

Ginsburg D.S., Hernandez E. & Johnson J.W. (1981) Sarcoma complicating von Recklinghausen's disease in pregnancy. *Obstet. Gynecol.*, **58**, 385−87.

Hacker N.F., Berek J.S. & Legasse L. (1982) Carcinoma of the cervix associated with pregnancy. *Obstet. Gynecol.*, **59**, 735−46.

Hannigan E.V., Whitehouse H.H., Atkinson W.D. & Becker S.N. (1982) Cone biopsy during pregnancy. *Obstet. Gynecol.*, **60**, 450−55.

Herbst A.L., Ulfelder H. & Poskanzer D.C. (1971) Adenocarcinoma of the vagina. *New Engl. J. Med.*, **284**, 878−81.

Holland E. (1949) A case of transplacental metastasis of malignant melanoma from mother to fetus. *J. Obstet. Gynaecol Br. Emp.*, **56**, 529−36.

Holleb A.I. & Farrow J.H. (1962) The relation of carcinoma of the breast and pregnancy in 283 patients. *Surg. Gynecol. Obstet.*, **115**, 65−71.

Holmes G.E. & Holmes F.F. (1978) Pregnancy: outcome of patients treated for Hodgkin's disease: a controlled study. *Cancer*, **41**, 1317−22.

Holmgren U., Bergstrand K., Hagenfeldt K. & Werner S. (1986) Women with prolactinoma — effect of pregnancy and lactation on serum prolactin and on tumour growth. *Acta Endocr.*, **111**, 452−59.

Karlen J.R., Stunburg L.D. & Abbotts J.N. (1972) Carcinoma of the endometrium co-existing with pregnancy. *Obstet. Gynecol.*, **40**, 334−39.

Kempers R.D. & Symonds R.E. (1965) Invasive carcinoma of the vulva in pregnancy. Report of 2 cases. *Obstet. Gynecol.*, **26**, 749−51.

Kistner R.W., Gorbach A.L. & Smith G.V. (1957) Cervical cancer in pregnancy. Review of the literature and presentation of 30 additional cases. *Obstet. Gynecol.*, **9**, 554−60.

Lee R.A., Johnson C.E. & Hanlon G.G. (1965) Leukemia during pregnancy. *Am. J. Obstet. Gynecol.*, **84**, 455−58.

Lee R.A., Neglia W. & Park R.C. (1981) Cervical carcinoma in pregnancy. *Obstet. Gynecol.*, **58**, 584−89.

Lutz M.H., Underwood P.B., Rozier J.C. & Putney J.W. (1977) Genital malignancy in pregnancy. *Am. J. Obstet. Gynecol.*, **129**, 536−42.

McLean D.W., Arminski T.C. & Bradley G.T. (1955) Management of primary carcinoma of the rectum diagnosed during pregnancy. *Am. J. Surg.*, **90**, 816−25.

Moller D., Ipsen L., Asschenfeldt P. (1986) Fatal course of melignantmelanoma during pregnancy with dissemination to the products of conception. *Acta. Obstet. Gynecol. Scand.*, **65**, 501.

Novak E.R. (1975) Ovarian tumours in pregnancy. An ovarian tumour registry review. *Obstet. Gynecol.*, **46**, 401−6.

Pack G.T. & Ariel I.M. (1958) *Tumours of the Somatic Soft Tissue*. Hoeber, New York.

Pang C. (1957) Transplacental metastases of the Brown-Pearce rabbit tumour. *Bull. Tulane Med. Fac.*, **17**, 31.

Plauché W.L., Gruich F.G. & Bourgeois M.O. (1981) Hysterectomy at the time of Caesarian section: analysis of 108 cases. *Obstet. Gynecol.*, **58**, 459−64.

Potter J.F. & Schoeneman M. (1970) Metastasis of maternal cancer to the placenta and fetus. *Cancer*, **25**, 380−88.

Rahman M.S., Rahman J. & Al-Sibaimh (1982) Carcinoma of the vulva in pregnancy. Case Report. *Br. J. Obstet. Gynaecol.*, **89**, 244−46.

Retik A.B., Sabesin S.M., Hume R. *et al.* (1962) The experimental transmission of malignant melanoma cells through the placenta. *Surg. Gynecol. Obstet.*, **114**, 485.

Ribeiro G.G. & Palmer M.K. (1977) Breast carcinoma associated with pregnancy. A clinician's dilemma. *Br. Med. J.*, **2**, 1524−27.

Rothman L.A., Cohen C.J. & Astarlo J. (1973) Placental and fetal involvement by maternal malignancy: a report of rectal carcinoma and review of the literature. *Am. J. Obstet. Gynecol.*, **116**, 1023−34.

Shiu M.H., Schottenfeld D., MacLean B. & Fortner J.G. (1976) Adverse effect of pregnancy on melanoma: a reappraisal. *Cancer*, **37**, 181−87.

Stander R.W. & Lein J.N. (1960) Carcinoma of the cervix and pregnancy. *Am. J. Obstet. Gynecol.*, **79**, 164−67.

Sutherland C.M., Loutfi A., Mather J., Carter R.D. & Krementz M.D. (1983a) Effect of pregnancy upon malignant melanoma. *Surg. Gynecol. Obstet.*, **157**, 443−45.

Sutherland C.M., Wittliff J. & Mabie W.C. (1983b) The effect of pregnancy on hormone levels and receptors in malignant melanoma. *J. Surg. Oncol.*, **22**, 191−92.

17

Radiotherapy of the Cervix, Uterine Corpus and Ovary

CHARLES A.F. JOSLIN

Introduction

The presentation of any woman with a clinically invasive cancer of the cervix is a sad reflection of an opportunity lost to detect and cure at the preinvasive and microinvasive stage of disease.

Approximately 5000 new patients present with invasive cervical cancer in England and Wales each year. The number dying of the disease is showing signs of falling and is currently about 2000 per year. However, the pattern of mortality is changing and fewer women are dying in the 40–55-year age group. Unfortunately, more women are now dying under the age of 35 and this trend is increasing. A similar pattern is also seen in the frequency of the disease and Paterson et al. (1984) have shown, for a given population, how the frequency rates have increased from 1957 to 1982 for patients under 35 years of age.

A further change has also occurred in the number of patients presenting at each clinical stage of disease, with a steady decline in stage III disease and an increase in stage I disease. These changes have resulted in an alteration in workload although the type of treatment used for each stage has not changed.

Preclinical cancer

A diagnosis of preclinical cancer of the uterine cervix is usually made by cervical cytology and colposcopy, followed by some form of biopsy in order to achieve histological classification. Once discovered the treatment for preclinical disease is a dilemma which was highlighted by Younge et al. (1949) when they described eleven ways of treatment ranging from simple cauterization to radium, followed by hysterectomy and external beam irradiation, despite the fact that for the majority of patients treated, the disease process did not extend deeper than 1.0 cm from the surface epithelium.

The major difficulty with this group of patients is in classifying lesions as occult or microinvasive cancer. The depth of penetration from the surface epithelium is the most critical factor. In practice, it is not known at which depth the chance of lymph node involvement begins. The recommendations made for this distance range from 1–7 mm. Averette et al. (1976) reported no involvement of lymph nodes at depths not exceeding 1 mm, but 3.5% were involved between

1 and 5 mm. A review of the literature makes it apparent that neither histology alone nor morphological appearances, as shown by colposcopy, provide adequate assessment of possible spread to pelvic nodes. Unfortunately, the tendency is to take no risks and some will treat on a radical basis with pre- and postoperative radiotherapy. However, Creasman & Weed (1979), after reviewing the literature, advised that vaginal or abdominal hysterectomy with conservation of the ovaries, if indicated, is probably sufficient when stromal invasion is less than 3 mm with limited foci. For invasion to between 3 and 5 mm, particularly if confluent, a radical hysterectomy and pelvic lymphadenopathy is probably indicated and where lymphatic or vascular invasion has occurred, regardless of depth of invasion, radical treatment should be considered. In the latter situation the depth of invasion and/or invasion of vessels may not become apparent until histologically assessed following a radical hysterectomy, such patients not having had a lymphadenectomy. Since the incidence of nodal metastases (Van Nagell *et al.* 1977; Boyce *et al.* 1984) is increased in such cases external beam irradiation should be considered.

Clinically invasive cancer

The primary lesion

The primary lesion invariably originates in the anterior or posterior lip of the cervix below the adenosquamous junction and less frequently from within the endocervical canal. It may spread along the endocervical canal into the uterine cavity and infiltrate the muscular tissues of the cervix or the vaginal epithelium. Provided extension is restricted to within about 2 cm of the endocervical canal, the lesion will be within the range for radical treatment by intracavitary irradiation or, alternatively, radical surgery.

As it continues to grow, the primary lesion may ulcerate or infiltrate the cervical tissues. Some lesions expand into the vagina originating from a well defined base, others infiltrate the cervix itself and expand to produce a barrel shaped tumour. These usually develop from within the endocervix, with a tendency to behave in an aggressive fashion being frequently found in the younger patient. Histologically they are usually adenocarcinomas but in the younger patient squamous celled cancers may also behave in a similar manner (Ashby & Smales 1987).

Involvement of adjacent viscera

Spread from the primary tumour to adjacent tissues is usually determined by vaginal and rectal examination, combined with abdominal palpation. Vaginal examination will reveal the extent of the vaginal spread but rectal examination is vital to establish lateral spread and possible spread into the cardinal or sacral ligaments. Vaginal and rectal examination including cystoscopy and sigmoid-oscopy may be necessary to determine possible rectal or vesical involvement.

Supportive investigations include an intravenous pylogram, lymphan-giography and, more recently, computed tomography and magnetic resonance imaging. An assessment of the value of lymphangiography by Smales *et al.* (1986) advised that lymphography is a reliable method of assessing lymph node status and was preferable to laparotomy for staging.

Clinical classification

In order to allow for a comparison of results between different centres, or to compare the results of one treatment to another, it is necessary to use a standard system of staging. The one used by the author is that of the International Federation of Gynaecology and Obstetrics (FIGO). Assessment is routinely carried out in the clinic and confirmed under anaesthesia for the majority of cases, taking into consideration routine radiological and cystoscopic findings. Once the stage is determined it should stand and not be modified as a result of other investigations such as CT scanning. However, an intravenous pyelogram is part of routine staging. FIGO staging is described in Chapter 4.

Histological classification

Histological classification and grading is important and does have prognostic value. Squamous celled lesions make up 90% of all cancers of the cervix and adenocarcinomas the remainder. About 20% of the squamous celled cancers are well differentiated (large cell keratinizing type) and approximately 60% are moderately differentiated (large cell non-keratinizing). The remainder are poorly differentiated (small cell non-keratinizing).

From a prognostic point of view, opinions differ regarding the effect of grading on prognosis. Joslin (1976) reported a series of 301 patients treated by radical radiotherapy (Table 17.1). The results indicate that histological grade has little bearing on prognosis following radical radiotherapy, although the disease control rates were lower for the anaplastic lesions. Van Nagell *et al.* (1978) found that stage IB small round celled lesions metastasize in about 50% of cases. Radiation therapy was associated with 31% recurrence and surgery with 54%. They suggested radiotherapy was the superior treatment for this group of patients. Swan & Roddick (1972) reported distinct differences in survival for various cell types following radiation therapy. The large cell non-keratinizing tumours had the best prognosis but this difference did not apply when surgery was the sole treatment.

More recently the relationship between the DNA profile of cervical tumours and prognosis has been studied. The results remain equivocal, possibly because survival times are long and cure rates high for early stage disease. Dyson *et al.*

Table 17.1. Disease control rates and histology

5-year state	No	Squamous cancer (differentiated)	Anaplastic cancer	Adenocarcinoma	Other
Alive	209	120	58	13	4
Cancer death	85	22	19	0	3
Intercurrent death	7	3	4	1	0
	301	145	81	14	7

(1987) from this department have suggested that aneuploid tumours metastasize sooner than diploid tumours for early disease and that local recurrence rates are higher for diploid tumours in advanced disease when treated by radiotherapy.

Lymph-vascular involvement

The involvement of lymph-vascular space has been studied by Van Nagell *et al.* (1978) reporting that involvement is associated with a 30% increase in recurrence rate although they did not propose that this made a case for radical radiotherapy.

The whole subject is complex since Pagnini *et al.* (1980) reported that the prognostic factors change, depending upon therapy. For radiotherapy, cell type predominates but for surgery depth of invasion is more important.

Lymph node involvement

Lymphatic spread may take place along the stromal lymphatics, then to the obturator, internal iliac, external iliac and common iliac nodes. These groups, together with the presacral nodes, drain into the lower para-aortic nodes at the bifurcation of the iliac vessels. In general the chance of involvement increases with the size of the primary tumour. One large series of patients carefully assessed for lymph node involvement is that of Plentl & Friedman (1971). Involvement of pelvic lymph nodes ranged from 15% in stage IB to 47% in stage IIB, the most commonly involved group being the external iliac group.

Unfortunately lymphangiography does not provide visualization of lymphatic drainage from the cervix but follows the external iliac chain of nodes. Any filling of the internal lymphatics is by anastomosis. However, Piver *et al.* (1971) report that lymphangiography in carcinoma of the cervix is 87% efficient. Douglas *et al.* (1972) have shown that lymphangiography is particularly valuable in early stages of disease when unsuspected metastases are not infrequent, requiring modification of radiotherapy treatment fields in patients with enlarged nodes.

Kolbenstvedt (1974) reported on 300 patients given preoperative irradiation and, following lymphangiography, a hysterectomy and lymphadenectomy carried out 6 weeks later. A total of 9187 nodes were removed. Ninety-seven contained no contrast media. Postoperative films showed 659 nodes remaining of which 302 were common iliac and 234 internal iliac. Only 87 patients could be said to have had a satisfactory lymphadenectomy. Lymphangiography was considered not sufficiently accurate to be solely relied upon to determine choice of treatment.

On balance, lymphangiography seems justified in identifying patients with involved nodes for stage IB lesions in order that they should be included in a high risk group for whom it is planned to give radical regional radiotherapy. Its routine use by those who carry out a Wertheim hysterectomy does not seem justified.

Tumour size and lymph node status

The size of the primary lesion has been shown to affect survival rates (Corscaden 1962). However, this seems more likely to be related to difficulties in controlling lymph node spread rather than to controlling the primary tumour. This is supported by Piver & Chung (1975) who reported lymph node metastasis in 31% of patients with tumours greater than 3 cm diameter and 21% for smaller lesions. Van Nagell et al. (1977) reported lymph node involvement in 6% of tumours less than 2 cm diameter and 18% in larger lesions. In terms of tumour response to radiotherapy Montana et al. (1983) reported that failure rate was greater in patients who had lesions 4 cm or more in diameter. This is also the experience of the author.

Treatment of early invasive cancer

The curative treatment of stage IB, IIA and early IIB carcinoma of the cervix faces two major problems:
1 The control of the primary tumour.
2 The control of involved pelvic nodes. Where disease has extended to involve the para-aortic nodes the chance of cure is greatly reduced.

The curative treatment of cervical cancer started about 100 years ago with surgical removal of the primary tumour and a block dissection of the pelvic nodes. Since that time extensive efforts have been made to improve the surgical results all of which are based on the Wertheim hysterectomy (Wertheim 1907).

The use of radiotherapy began in 1901 when roentgen rays were directed onto the cervix by an intravaginal cone. In 1903 radium was first used by Cleaves. However, this form of radiotherapy does no more than treat the primary tumour and the chance of total disease control will be limited to those patients without pelvic node involvement. In contrast it has to be proven that either a radical Wertheim hysterectomy or total pelvic irradiation using external beam therapy with or without intracavitary irradiation, is superior to local treatment alone. The different treatment methods used include:

1 Treatment limited to the uterus and vaginal vault tissues using either intra-cavitary irradiation, abdominal hysterectomy or a combination of both.
2 Treatment on a regional basis provided by either Wertheim hysterectomy or combined intracavitary radiation and external beam therapy.
3 A combination of Wertheim hysterectomy with or without preoperative intracavitary irradiation and followed by postoperative external beam irradiation in node positive patients.

As one might expect, such a range of treatments suggests that the cure rates are likely to be similar, although morbidity levels may differ considerably. Radical regional therapy has been defended on the grounds of providing a chance of cure for the 15 to 20% of patients said to have pelvic lymph node involvement.

The 5-year cure rates for stage IB cancers, taken from the 16th Stockholm Report covering 109 institutions in 27 countries ranged from 70–90% whether radiotherapy or surgery predominated (Kottmeier 1976).

The results for institutions performing mainly surgery range from 70–90%. Those performing mainly radiotherapy range from 70–86%. This compares with 79% for the total of 35 480 patients irrespective of treatment method.

These results tend to confirm that there is little difference in disease control rates and in fact one centre, Manchester, exclusively used intracavitary radium. In particular the use of preoperative intracavitary irradiation is a technique which has been used for many years but its value never proven. Pearcey *et al.* (1988) in a comparative review of 224 patients in which 113 had preoperative radiotherapy and 111 did not, reported that preoperative radiotherapy made no difference to survival, the incidence of vaginal vault recurrence, distant metastases or complications.

The control of lymph node disease

When radical surgery is used alone to treat patients reported as lymph node positive, the cure rate is 40–50% for most series whereas it is 80–90% if the nodes are reported as negative; among the best results are those of Morley & Seski (1976) but the difference for the two groups remains similar. Unfortunately there is little evidence to indicate that the prognosis of the surgically proven node positive patients improves with postoperative irradiation (Morrow 1980). Fuller *et al.* (1982) reported no difference in survival for stage IB and IIA node positive patients whether they received postoperative irradiation or not. A recent study by Kinney *et al.* (1989) also reports no significant difference in survival rates where radiotherapy was given to node positive cases when compared to a matched group not receiving radiation. However, the fact that radiotherapy given before surgery can effectively treat pelvic lymph nodes has been shown by Rutledge & Fletcher (1958), Gorton (1964) and Lagasse *et al.* (1974). The latter reported that in a randomized study one group of patients receiving preoperative irradiation were found to have nodal involvement in 12% of cases compared to

22% who received surgery alone. The latter group then had postoperative irradiation, producing a 5-year survival of 74% compared with 88% in the former group. The place for preoperative external beam therapy therefore needs further consideration and evaluation. Despite this and the fact that the number of nodes involved at the time of surgery has been shown to affect survival (Pilleron *et al.* 1974), and until such time as further clinical studies confirm the place for radiotherapy following surgery in node positive patients, many will continue to use it. The author does not subscribe to this approach but does use external beam and intracavitary irradiation to treat the whole pelvis on a composite basis. A prospective comparison of radical hysterectomy and lymphadenectomy against external beam irradiation and intracavitary radium by Newton (1975) showed no significant difference in 5- and 10-year survival.

Also, a study by Papavasiliou *et al.* (1980) which compared total hysterectomy and postoperative external irradiation with the Wertheim—Meigs operation and postoperative external irradiation revealed similar survival rates with a lower morbidity for the former. On balance it seems that the majority of patients with stage IB disease are over treated. Treatment limited to radical surgery for the primary tumour and external beam radiotherapy for the pelvic lymph nodes has much to commend it, even on the grounds of reduced morbidity alone which is a subject demanding attention for all of the above described techniques and which in general is not reported in a consistent fashion.

Treatment of advanced cervical cancer

The commonest cause of death from advanced cancer of the cervix is failure to control disease within the pelvis, with a small number dying from distant metastases.

In general, the following patients are regarded as having advanced disease:

1 All stage IV cases where treatment is normally indicated on a strictly individualized basis, often combined with surgery.

2 All stage IIIA and stage IIIB cases.

3 Stage IIB cases in which the disease has progressed to, at least, half the distance to the pelvic wall on one or both sides.

4 Stage IB cases which present as large barrel-shaped tumours extending at least half the distance to the pelvic wall.

Our classification of advanced disease has been brought about by a common approach to management. In general, this implies treating a large invasive primary cancer with a combination of external and intracavitary irradiation. However, the extent of disease within the pelvis goes beyond the limits of the primary tumour since the chance of lymph node involvement has been reported as high as 50% for bulky ($\geq$6 cm) stage IB tumours (Piver & Chung 1975) to over 60% for stage IIIb tumours (Graham & Graham 1955). Thus, the majority of patients can be considered as having regional disease. The problem is even greater because for stage III cancers the chance of para-aortic nodes being involved has been reported as high as 30% of cases, assessed by surgical laparotomy, although the results by lymphangiographic assessment are lower. With such a depressing picture of extensive disease for the stage IIIB cases, it is surprising that as many as 40% of cases are reported as disease free at 5 years. In fact, the Stockholm Reports indicate an increasing improvement in cure rates following the advent of high energy X-ray irradiation.

Treatment options

Whatever the treatment the problem is one of controlling both local disease and lymph node spread within the pelvis. Where disease has spread to the para-aortic nodes the chance of cure is considerably reduced and this is discussed later. One major radiotherapy difficulty is in achieving an optimal dose distribution throughout the volume of the primary tumour and any extension to pelvic lymph nodes without causing unacceptable morbidity. While intracavitary and external beam irradiation have been used as individual treatments, each has distinct limitations. For intracavitary irradiation alone the fall off in dose within the primary tumour volume may cause the peripheral portion to be undertreated. For external beam irradiation alone treatment is limited by the size of the treatment volume and the damage to normal tissue structures occurring before an adequate cancericidal effect can be achieved. For many years advanced disease was treated in a fashion similar to early disease, using intracavitary treatment alone. It is perhaps hardly surprising that the reported results for stage IIB disease were only 35% and for stage III 20%. This particular treatment is still practised by some, but there is little excuse for such restricted treatment now that high energy teletherapy machines are available.

Combined treatment using intracavitary and external beam irradiation is now normal practice for advanced disease. The exact combination chosen varies for different centres and accounts for the considerable debate about the best method.

Originally our technique used combined treatment for all stages of disease, the predominant component being biased to intracavitary treatment using a high activity after-loaded remote-controlled system. This was supported by external beam irradiation, given by using parallel opposed fields with a central wedge to allow a build up of dose toward the lateral pelvic walls and to protect the central organs as bladder and rectum. The 5-year disease control rates improved from 35 to 57% for stage IIB and from 20 to 42% for stage IIIB (Joslin 1976).

Reasons for failure

Failure to control disease can occur either within the primary site, the regional nodes or because of spread to some distant site.

Table 17.2 shows for the combined radiotherapy regime described above that

Table 17.2. Sites of recurrence for stage IIb and IIIb cancer of the cervix at up to 15 years

Stage	No. treated	Recurrence			Total failing RT	Distant metastases only
		Local	Regional	Distant		
II	170	25	28	36	45	28
III	107	29	34	28	48	16

failure to control disease was of a similar order for local and regional disease. In an attempt to improve our results, the programme was altered so that external beam therapy became the predominant modality and the intracavitary treatment was used to boost treatment centrally depending upon the primary tumour response following external beam irradiation. The external beam irradiation was given over 28 days following which the patient was rested for two weeks to allow tumour shrinkage to take place, following which an assessment of treatment response was made. When the response was poor, additional external beam irradiation was given. When the response was good, intracavitary irradiation was given on two separate occasions spaced one week apart.

The results did not show a significant improvement in 5-year survival. Stage IIB results were 56% and stage IIIB 32% compared with the first regime of 57 and 42%, respectively. Results published by others using various combinations of intracavitary and external beam irradiation are similar. Residual disease is included with recurrent disease supporting the view that, in general, current treatment techniques are not dramatically improving disease control rates and some other means of producing improved results needs to be found.

Metastatic spread

While our previous impression has been that distant metastases have been more commonly associated with local recurrence our most recent assessment, after following patients for 15 years, is that this is not the case and similar metastatic rates occur for patients with or without pelvic recurrence. The metastatic rate for the different stages is also similar in the long term with 21% of stage IIb cases and 26% of stage IIIb cases developing metastases. The subject of para-aortic spread of disease and treatment improving patient survival has been studied by Haie et al. (1988) who reported on a controlled clinical study of prophylactic para-aortic irradiation for advanced cervical cancer carried out by the EORTC group. They found, in a series of 441 patients, that the development of para-aortic disease was three times higher in patients who did not receive para-aortic irradiation but the numbers were not sufficient to show any effect on survival. The question of whether metastatic disease is influenced long term as a result of irradiating para-aortic nodes will remain an open one for the present and more data are necessary.

Other factors affecting radiotherapy results

Age of patient

Advanced disease occurs more often in women over 50 years of age. However, within each stage, the author's experience is that the prognosis is worse for the younger woman, particularly for the stage IIIb cases. This is supported by the published data of Benstead *et al.* (1986). Lybeert *et al.* (1987) found the effect of age to be highly significant in women under 28 years compared with women aged 28 to 45 years.

Hyperbaric oxygen (HBO) therapy

Watson *et al.* (1978) reported results for the Medical Research Council (MRC) Trial of radiotherapy in hyperbaric oxygen for carcinoma of the cervix and reported a significant improvement in disease control for stage IIIb patients treated in HBO, compared with treatment in air. However, when compared with the best published treatment results for conventional treatment in air, there was no significant difference between the two methods.

Radiosensitizers

The failure of treatment in hyperbaric oxygen led to the development of radio-sensitizers (electron affinic agents). The results for misonidazole were reported by Dische (MRC Working Party Report 1984) and do not reveal any worthwhile improvement over conventional therapy. In fact, misonidazole can increase patients' problems by causing neurotoxicity. Unless the problems of neurotoxicity are resolved by using less toxic agents, further progress is unlikely. For further information the reader is referred to Dische (1985).

Combining chemotherapy with radiotherapy

The reported results for combined chemotherapy with radiotherapy for cancer of the uterine cervix have been generally disappointing. However, these combined treatments have in general involved giving the chemotherapy before radiotherapy is started, or following completion of radiotherapy. More recently interest has centred on concomitant chemotherapy with radiotherapy. In a phase II study Khoury *et al.* (1989) have reported that when 5-fluorouracil and mitomycin C are given during irradiation for advanced cervical cancer the pelvic disease control rates are 85% at a median follow up of 11 months and we suggest that this warrants a prospective randomized study. Other groups are also engaged with similar assessments of concomitant therapy and a final decision of the value of this form of treatment is awaited.

Morbidity due to radiotherapy

The reported morbidity resulting from radiotherapy to the pelvis is generally underestimated and often overlooked. This is due, in part, to the major emphasis being placed on curing the patient. However, if the results of cure are the same for two different regimes, it does become important to give serious consideration as to which regime provides the least morbidity. Also for a particular technique, the type of morbidity which occurs will depend upon the extent of dose distribution, the quantity of irradiation to the various structures and the volume of tissue irradiated.

Morbidity in radiotherapy

Attempts have been made to standardize a method of reporting morbidity (Sismondi *et al.* 1989) and to provide definitions and a classification. When radiotherapy is being considered it is important to relate morbidity to the treatment method used. To provide some guidance on this the ICRU Report 38 (1985) provides a method of reporting dose specification for intracavitary therapy and Report 29 (1978) for reporting external beam therapy with photons and electrons.

In general, morbidity can be described as acute when it occurs during or shortly following irradiation, with recovery occurring during the next two to three weeks.

An acute reaction which fails to heal may lead to a chronic condition and functional impairment which can seriously affect the quality of life. This situation is brought about where the ability of a tissue to repair itself is exhausted. Late tissue damage may develop months or even years following irradiation and is usually the result of devitalized tissues suffering secondary damage such as minor trauma, which fails to heal and produces a necrotic ulcer or haemorrhage. It has been shown by Turesson (1989) that the rate of progression of late radiation damage is dose dependent and time dependent; consequently late complication rates should be specified at a fixed time of follow-up.

Bladder morbidity

This may take one of several forms ranging from recurrent nonspecific cystitis to a contracted bladder. The latter is now rarely seen and principally the result of a high dose of irradiation to the whole bladder. When it occurs treatment invariably entails urinary diversion which to most patients is acceptable as opposed to suffering severe frequency of micturition. One problem which may cause serious concern and is frightening to the patient is haematuria. This is usually due to telangiectasia of the capillary vessels within the bladder base. It is often associated with some degree of atrophy of the bladder wall which unfortunately tends to be biopsied as part of the routine investigation. This may lead to a necrotic ulcer which can take a long time to heal and, rarely, may progress to produce a vesico–vaginal fistula. However, the commonest cause of a radio necrotic ulcer is where a small part of the bladder base has become avascular due to a high dose of irradiation. If the tissues become hypoxic, necrosis may follow to produce a vesico–vaginal fistula. If the fistula is small and surrounded by tissues with a good blood supply they can occasionally be closed, but often progress and require urinary diversion.

Large bowel injury

The commonest long term injury is to the rectum. This may take the form of chronic proctitis or ulceration, with bleeding. With modern techniques it only occurs in a small percentage of cases, but unfortunately, when it does occur, can lead to a recto–vaginal fistula. The basic cause of the fistula is an endarteritis obliterans of the intrinsic blood vessels supplying the anterior rectal wall. This causes ischaemic changes in the recto–vaginal septum and in turn may lead to a fistula. With the modern techniques for delivering intracavitary irradiation, recto–vaginal fistulae are infrequent. However, they do more commonly occur either as a result of recurrent tumour or following irradiation of tumour which is invading the rectal wall at presentation. A defunctioning colostomy is the usual method of treatment and should always be done preparatory to irradiating stage IV disease in which the rectum is involved.

The sigmoid colon can suffer late morbidity which is usually due to a narrowing of a short length of bowel or to ulceration, although the latter is not often seen. When it is present the patient may lose considerable quantities of blood and not only require repeated blood transfusions but also a defunctioning colostomy.

Small bowel injury

Small bowel epithelium is extremely sensitive to the effect of irradiation and quite low doses can produce permanent flattening of the villi. This form of injury has become more common since external beam irradiation has been more frequently used for treating pelvic disease. The commonest symptomatic problem is the onset of infrequent bouts of abdominal colic due to narrowing of the gut lumen. The narrowing usually affects only a short length of gut and appears as a stricture on X-ray barium studies. The lesion usually affects the terminal ilium close to the iliocaecal junction. A classical picture of subacute obstruction may occur with the patient being admitted for acute surgical attention. They often settle down with conservative measures but invariably recur and a bypass operation or resection becomes necessary (Russell & Welch 1979). Once surgically treated it is unusual for a patient to have further problems. However, one other effect of irradiation on the terminal ilium is to reduce vit. B12 and fat absorption (Tankel *et al*. 1965). Fortunately, malabsorption syndromes are extremely rare.

Radiotherapy techniques

Intracavitary irradiation

The various systems available have been exhaustively described in the literature and each is claimed to have some specific advantage over the others. Joslin & Peel (1982) and Kjellgren (1981) are but two publications which deal with the classical methods of Stockholm and Paris on which all other techniques are based. The major concept relating to these systems is that they were originally designed in order that a quantity of milligrams of radium, loaded into a particular source configuration, was used for a specified time in hours. This milligram hours dose concept was crude but under the conditions used, whereby only small changes in either parameter were permitted, the clinical effects could be reproduced from one case to another despite the rapid change of dose rate which occur with distance from the source of irradiation within the treated volume.

Compared with external beam irradiation where a treatment volume is planned to include a defined target volume (consisting of the tumour volume and an allowance for possible spread), the intracavitary therapy treatment volume is largely determined by the configuration of the sources. In turn it is hoped this will result in a cancericidal dose within the target volume. Some target volumes are too large to be satisfactorily treated by intracavitary irradiation alone and require combined intracavitary and external beam irradiation.

Source configurations

Essentially all systems which have been developed to provide a radical treatment to the primary tumour can be separated into two components: the intrauterine source and the intravaginal source(s). The design of these systems has to take into account the tolerance of the vaginal vault tissues to irradiation, which is fortunately higher than the cancericidal dose by a factor of about 3 to 1. However, despite this it is still necessary to take some precautions by enclosing the vaginal sources in a suitable carrier to provide a distancing effect between the source and the vaginal vault tissues (e.g. a Manchester Ovoid). The same situation exists in relation to providing protection to the anterior rectal wall and to the base of the bladder. Other limiting tissues include the vasculature of the rectum which will usually only tolerate doses of less than 60% of the standard cancericidal dose before morbidity starts to become a problem.

Dose specification and prescription

In the early systems the intrauterine and vaginal sources were separated and the positions of the two sets of sources varied according to the anatomy and the size of tumour being treated. The strength of sources available provided for treatment times ranging from 20–190 hours. Treatment was prescribed in milligram hours, and varied somewhat depending upon the rate at which the dose was delivered. The Stockholm method (Forsell 1917) provided for treatment in two parts each of 20–24 hours with a 3-week gap in between. This delivered a treatment of 7000–8000 milligram hours. Likewise, the Paris method (Regaud 1926) delivered in a single treatment 7000–8000 milligram hours in 5 days. These methods of prescribing radiotherapy were effective since they provided a means of producing a dose response relationship for the different tissues included in the treatment.

An alternative technique, developed from the Paris system, was the Manchester technique (Tod & Meredith 1938). This essentially provided a means of using a number of predetermined source sizes and radioactive loadings such that a constant dose rate would be delivered to the Manchester point A within about 10%, provided certain criteria were followed. Point A was defined as a point 2 cm lateral to the central axis of the uterus and 2 cm up from the mucous membrane of the lateral fornix now normally measured from the intrauterine flange. A second point (B) lying in the same plane 3 cm lateral to point A, later changed to 5 cm from the patient's midline, was used to determine the dose to the parametrial tissues (Fig. 17.1).

There have been further changes in dose specification and many now calculate the dose at other fixed points in the pelvis (Chassagne & Horiot 1977; Fletcher 1980) and more recently the concept of an isodose volume has been proposed (ICRU 38) which is that volume of tissue included within a 60 Gy isodose envelope and expressed in terms of its length in the plane of the intrauterine canal, its maximal width and maximal thickness.

In general, the current systems available are described by the source activities used, the geometrical position of the sources for a typical insertion and the time required to deliver an expected dose to a fixed point. There are two alternative methods of treatment:

1 Following insertion of the sources for each patient a dose distribution is calculated for their particular treatment following check radiographs (Fig. 17.2). The dose to a particular point can then be calculated as a product of dose rate and treatment time. When a dose is prescribed to this point the treatment time can be adjusted to deliver the prescribed dose. Since treatment may be from 15–70 hours there is time to carry out these calculations.

2 The initial physical dosimetry is carried out in a physics department using a system where the source applicators are placed in a standard position so that dose rates at set points are predictable. For any prescribed dose, therefore, the treatment time can be calculated from the standard measurements. No individual calculations are made and the method is essentially similar to the concept of milligram hours. This system applies particularly to high dose rate afterloading systems because of the short treatment times.

In general, current practice is to specify a prescribed dose of radiation at a specific point, usually the Manchester point A. Also, the absorbed dose at other points related to organs at risk and bony structures is used. The latter will

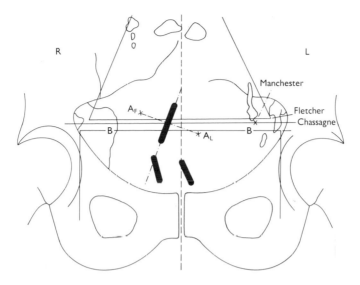

Fig. 17.1. Three alternative systems available for determining the dose received to the pelvic nodes; namely, the Manchester, Fletcher and Chassagne systems. In addition the Manchester system provides for a prescribed dose at point A.

provide an indication of the dose to the various lymph node groups. The two principle methods are:

1 The lymphatic trapezoid (Fletcher 1980) The upper points provide an estimation of the dose to the lower para-aortic nodes, the mid and lower points to the common iliac and mid external iliac nodes, respectively (Fig. 17.1).

2 The pelvic wall reference point (Chassagne *et al.* 1977). This provides an indication of the dose to the distal parametrium and obturator nodes (Fig. 17.1).

These systems provide a means whereby the intracavitary treatment can be combined with external beam therapy. When external beam irradiation is combined with intracavitary therapy the intracavitary treatment times will need to be reduced to compensate for the external beam treatment otherwise severe overdosing may occur. Unfortunately, the problem can be complicated due to the different radiobiological efficiency factors which apply and are dependent on dose rate, dose per treatment fraction and overall treatment time (Orton 1985, 1986).

Afterloading systems

The methods discussed so far were originated during the era of radium which for gynaecological application could only be safely and satisfactorily handled by using small quantities. With the availability of man-made radioactive nuclides of high specific activity it became possible to produce small source capsules. A further advance has been the technical development of 'afterloading' devices to automatically move the radioactive sources from a storage safe to the patient.

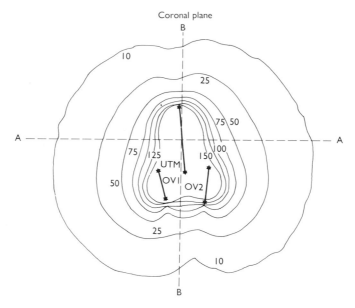

Fig. 17.2. This illustrates the dose distribution around an intrauterine and two vaginal sources. The isodoses can be constructed in terms of dose rate per minute or hour. The time to achieve a given dose at any defined point or isocurve can thus be calculated.

Thus, empty source carriers are inserted into the treatment position within the patient. These are, in turn, connected to hollow tubes — usually rigid — which project down the vagina and can be held in the treatment position by a suitable clamping system, external harness or vaginal packing. The vaginal tubes are then connected to a protected storage safe which contains the active sources used. Overall control is automated from a central control panel to provide a fully radiation protected system. However, the early systems, many of which are still in use, were manually afterloaded. The simplest and best known of these was described by Henschke (1960) and Suit (1963). A number of remote loaded machines have been developed since Walstam (1965) described a system for automated afterloading for low activity sources and O'Connell *et al.* (1967) described a system for high activity sources. For most systems using low activity sources ^{137}Cs has replaced radium and for high activity sources ^{60}Co or ^{192}Ir are used. The use of these latter sources has allowed a reduction in treatment times to only a few minutes. However, to maintain an adequate therapeutic advantage of tumour damage against normal tissue damage, an increased number of treatment fractions are necessary. For further information the reader is referred to Mould (1988).

Combined intracavitary and external beam therapy

As already discussed a problem with intracavitary therapy alone is that it can only provide a cancericidal effect to a small volume of tissue centred on the uterine cervix. When bulky tumours and lymph node disease are to be treated solely by radiotherapy it is necessary to add external beam irradiation to the treatment schedule. Unfortunately it is difficult to achieve a cancericidal effect on large bulky tumours with external therapy alone and doses of 60 Gy and more are necessary. This would entail giving the same dose to vital structures such as small gut, bladder and rectum with ensuing morbidity. It is usual, therefore, to follow a course of external beam therapy of 45–50 Gy with a reduced dose of intracavitary therapy to treat the residual central tumour. The intracavitary ir-radiation will deliver a high dose to any residual tumour with a rapid fall off in dose outside the tumour volume. Because of the slow rate of shrinkage of most tumours it is usual to wait for 1–2 weeks between giving external and intracavitary irradiation.

For early cancers the management differs because intracavitary therapy alone is capable of controlling and curing the primary tumour. However, where nodes are involved they can be effectively treated by external irradiation. The two treatments can be combined but it is necessary to shield the midline structures from the effects of external irradiation with a suitable combination of treatments. This will permit a high dose of irradiation to be delivered to the pelvic lymph nodes (45–50 Gy) and by increasing the amount of intracavitary irradiation

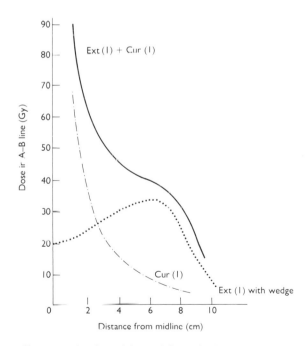

Fig. 17.3. This figure illustrates the dose delivered from the intracavitary source(s) — Cur (1); the external beam irradiation — Ext (1), and the combined treatment, with distance from the mid-line of the pelvis. It can be seen that the technique provides a very high localized dose of irradiation to tissues within 2.0 cm of the mid-line.

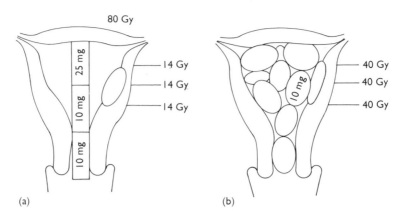

Fig. 17.4. The figure above illustrates the dose delivered from the intracavitary source(s) (Cur [1]), the external beam irradiation (Ext [1]) and the combined treatment, with distance from the midline of the pelvis. It can be seen that the technique provides a very high localized dose of irradiation to tissues within 2.0 cm of the midline.

a very high dose (60−65 Gy) can be delivered to the cervix. Figure 17.3 is an illustration of one such method.

When the overall results for these new radiotherapy techniques are assessed, the cure rates for each individual stage of disease have shown a steady progressive improvement over the past 20 years of some 10−15% which is most probably due to the introduction of machines which deliver high energy photons rather than any other single cause.

Endometrial cancer

Adenocarcinoma of the endometrium represents about 45% of all uterine cancer. Approximately 4000 new cases present in England and Wales each year and the incidence rates are slowly increasing. This is possibly due to the loss of endocrine protection brought about by a reduction in the number of pregnancies, or due to an irregularity of endocrine function (Chamlian & Taylor 1970; Maas 1987).

The age-specific rates indicate that the disease occurs in an older age group than cervical cancer.

The primary lesion

The classical presentation of postmenopausal bleeding occurs early enough in the natural history of the disease for approximately 80% of patients to present with stage I carcinoma.

In a series treated by the author (1974−83), of 197 patients, 160 presented with stage I carcinoma, 18 with stage II, 10 with stage III and nine with stage IV.

The primary tumour may originate at any part of the uterine cavity which with time it proceeds to fill. It originates either from a discrete focus growing as a polypoidal mass or has a multifocal origin, initially spreading to cover the endometrium.

The primary lesion usually enlarges slowly and may invade the lower uterine segment as far as the cervix and the vagina. Myometrial invasion may extend as far as the serosa but does not usually penetrate it. As with carcinoma of the cervix spread may involve adjacent viscera when the prognosis becomes extremely poor. Fortunately, most cases present with disease limited to the uterus and the majority of these are curable.

Preclinical cancer

The chance of diagnosing microinvasive carcinoma of the endometrium is extremely low. It is usually diagnosed as the result of careful pathological assessment following a routine hysterectomy in the older woman. It may also be occasionally detected as a result of an endometrial curettage.

Clinical classification

The International Federation of Gynaecology and Obstetrics system of classification of corpus cancer is the one in most general use (see Chapter 6, p. 124).

Stage 0   Preinvasive cancer
Stage I   Carcinoma confined to the corpus
     IA   Uterine cavity measures 8 cm or less
     IB   Uterine cavity measures more than 8 cm
Stage II   The carcinoma also involves the cervix
Stage III   The carcinoma has extended outside the uterus but not outside the pelvis. This may include spread into the vagina
Stage IV   The carcinoma has extended outside the true pelvis and has involved the mucosa of the bladder or rectum (bullous oedema of the bladder base is not sufficient evidence)

Clinical staging involves an examination under anaesthesia, careful fractional curettage and measurement of length of the uterine cavity. An IVP and chest X-ray should also be done as part of a routine work-up. The case for surgical staging is still controversial but its place and value are becoming established (Gastaldi et al. 1985).

Lymph node involvement

The lymphatic drainage of the body of the uterus follows the same route as for the cervix with the exception of the fundal part which drains to the inguinal nodes via the inguinal canal and along the ovarian vessels to the para-aortic nodes. The value of lymphangiography has been studied as an aid to preoperative assessment by many being reported as unreliable by Jackson (1976) but being defended by others (Douglas et al. 1972). Also as an aid to surgical lymphadenectomy it has been reported as having limitations (Kolbenstvedt & Kolstad 1973) and in general is not done.

Lymph node spread has a considerable effect on prognosis. A particularly important relationship to lymphatic involvement is histological grading and depth of myometrial invasion. The author has found that myometrial invasion by tumour can be related to pelvic recurrence rate and metastases (Table 17.3). Others, such as Creasman *et al.* (1976), have shown a relationship between depth of myometrial invasion and metastases. In a recent series the author has found that only 12.5% of cases have disease limited to the endometrial tissue without myometrial invasion. Thus, the majority of stage I cases have some degree of myometrial involvement. These high risk patients should be separated from the

Table 17.3. Incidence of pelvic node involvement in stage I corpus cancer in relation to myometrial invasion

	Myometrial invasion	
Reference	Superficial (%)	Deep (%)
Javert (1952)	6.2	50
Liu & Meigs (1955)	4.0	45
Delclos & Fletcher (1969)	7.0	18
Lewis (1971)	—	36
Creasman *et al.* (1976)	11.5	43

	Tumour grade		
	GI	GII	GIII
Lewis *et al.* (1970)	5.5	10.0	26.0
Creasman *et al.* (1976)	3.0	10.0	36.0
Boronow *et al.* (1984)	2.2	11.4	26.8

Table 17.4. Endometrial carcinoma — stage I depth of myometrial invasion vs. disease failures. Patients were treated by surgery followed by intravaginal irradiation in 28 cases and with the addition of external beam therapy in 132 cases

Depth of myometrial invasion	Total cases	Disease failures					
		Vag. rec.	Pel. rec.	Vag. + pel. rec.	Met. only	Met. + pel. rec.	Total failures
No invasion	20	0	0	0	0	0	0
Less than one-third	45	0	0	0	0	0	0
One-third to two-thirds	33	2	0	0	3	0	5
More than two-thirds	51	2	3	1	7	0	13
Not known	11	0	0	0	0	1	1
Total	160	4	3	1	10	1	19

group as a whole as radical regional therapy is needed. This is supported by our results in Table 17.4.

Tumour size

The size of the primary tumour related to prognosis has been studied by Trotnow *et al.* (1978). They showed, in a series of 441 evaluated patients, that the size of the primary lesion in the surgically removed uterus was prognostically important. They separated patients into three groups; lesions $\leqslant 1$ cm in any greatest dimension, lesions $\leqslant 1.5$ cm and lesions > 1.5 cm. The 5-year survival rates were 91.9, 78.5 and 20.6%, respectively.

This seems a better system than measuring the size of the uterus using the length of the cavity, which forms part of the FIGO staging system first introduced by Healy & Brown (1939), which is now being reviewed (see Chapter 6).

Treatment of early endometrial cancer (stage IA and IB)

Treatment policies

Intrauterine irradiation alone with or without external beam therapy has not been greatly used because the results are generally inferior to those for surgery. A survey by Jones (1975) showed that the result for surgery alone was 75% irrespective of whether Wertheim hysterectomy or an abdominal hysterectomy and bilateral salpingo-oophorectomy were carried out. These results are better than those reported by Kottmeier (1959) in which a corrected radium cure rate of 63% was obtained. Most reports for radium alone irrespective of technique used produce results which are around 60%. A further alternative is to use a combination of preoperative intrauterine therapy or postoperative intravaginal therapy. Whichever method is used the results are around 75%. However, when external beam therapy is added either pre- or postoperatively a further improvement has been reported (Joslin *et al.* 1977; Salazar *et al.* 1978).

Some patients who present with early disease are technically operable but unfortunately are not fit enough to withstand the procedure. For such patients some form of radiotherapy is preferable, and intracavitary treatment with or without external beam therapy can be used. In general the results are not as good as those for surgery with or without irradiation.

Radiotherapy alone

A number of intrauterine treatment methods exist, most of which were fully developed between 1930 and 1950. These developments were concerned with two aspects:

1 An evenly distributed dose of radiation throughout the uterine volume.
2 An adequate dose of radiation to the periphery of a deeply invasive tumour.

SOURCE DISTRIBUTION

The positioning of the sources is extremely important in order to provide an adequate distribution of radiation to what is often an irregularly shaped intra-uterine carcinoma. There are three basic types of intrauterine insertion.

1 *The tandem.* This takes the form of a single line of sources contained within a semi-flexible carrier. This forms the basis of the Manchester system and consists of a differentially loaded system (Fig. 17.4). A 25 mg radium source or 75 mCi of ^{137}Cs are placed at the fundal end and two or more 10 mg radium sources or 30 mCi ^{137}Cs in tandem below it. Vaginal ovoids loaded with 10 mg of radium or 30 mCi ^{137}Cs are used during one of two insertions lasting 72 hours spaced 7 days apart. This delivers a dose of 80 Gy 2 cm from the central tube.

2 *Hysterostats.* These are designed to position the radioactive sources into a preconceived triangular shape in order to fit the uterine cavity. A modern counterpart of this technique has been described by Strickland (1965). This uses a helical spring of flexible steel to form a loop to fit the uterine cavity.

3 *A system of uterine packing.* This method was greatly advocated and developed by Heyman (1947). The technique depends upon tightly packing the uterine cavity with radium or ^{137}Cs capsules (Heyman capsules). The source carriers are attached to steel threads which are used to retrieve the sources. The number of sources which can be introduced on the first occasion varies from about 5 up to 12. A second insertion 2–3 weeks later will usually result in a lower number of capsules being inserted due to shrinkage of the uterus. A total dose of 30 Gy at 1.5 cm deep to the endometrial surface is given on each occasion. It is also worthwhile using two vaginal ovoids on the first occasion. The 5-year cure rates are around 60%.

For poorly differentiated tumours and particularly for stage II cases external beam therapy can be used initially to deliver 40 Gy in 20 fractions over 28 days followed by one application of Heyman's capsules 2 weeks later to deliver 20–26 Gy at 1.5 cm deep to the endometrial surface.

DEPTH DOSE CONSIDERATION

A major advantage of the Heyman technique is that the introduction of the capsules can, with care, bring about a stretching of the walls of the uterus and provide for a greater depth dose within the myometrium. An illustration of the dose at different points for a single line source and Heyman system is shown in Fig. 17.3. This is reflected in the increase in 5-year cure rates, reported by Kottmeier (1953), of 45 to 61% when changing from a tandem system to a packing technique. In 1971 Simon *et al.* reported an afterloading method for Heyman's applicators in an attempt to reduce the amount of exposure to staff. More recently this technique has been developed for high activity sources but remains unpublished.

COMBINED EXTERNAL BEAM AND INTRAUTERINE IRRADIATION

This form of therapy is not routinely used for stage IA or IB patients. However, in patients medically unfit for surgery who have a large uterus and a poorly differentiated cancer, the chance of lymph node involvement will be high and a case for external beam therapy combined with intracavitary treatment can be made. While the results do not match those for surgery with external beam therapy a 50% 5-year cure rate can be achieved. The dose required is 40−50 Gy by external irradiation in 4−5 weeks followed by intrauterine therapy 2 weeks later to deliver a dose of 20 Gy 1.5 cm deep to the endometrium.

PREOPERATIVE INTRAUTERINE OR POSTOPERATIVE INTRAVAGINAL IRRADIATION COMBINED WITH SURGERY

While many who have experience of this form of management consider one or other of these approaches as the best treatment, there is no proven case that either is the better. Indeed there is no continuing evidence that combined radiotherapy and surgery is superior to surgery alone in terms of survival as shown in a review by Jones (1975).

Graham (1971) carried out a randomized clinical trial comparing hysterectomy versus preoperative intracavitary radium versus postoperative intravaginal radium. The results are not significantly different for a P value of 0.05. A study by Piver (1980) compared surgery alone against preoperative intrauterine radium and postoperative vaginal radium. The overall 10-year survival rate was 93%, the individual rates being 90% for surgery alone, 93% for preoperative radium and 96% for postoperative radium. However, the vaginal vault recurrence rates were 7.5% for cases having surgery alone as against 4.5% in those having preoperative radium and none in the postoperative radium group. The other important finding was that grade III lesions had a survival rate of only 70% against 94% for grades I and II.

The major fact resulting from these studies is that vaginal recurrence rates are reduced when surgery is supported by radiotherapy. On these grounds alone the additional therapy is worthwhile when one considers the misery that this sort of recurrence produces.

The advantages and disadvantages claimed for each of the supporting radiotherapy procedures have little substantiation apart from vaginal recurrence rates. However, for the sake of completeness they are listed below:

Preoperative intrauterine radiation:

Advantages	Disadvantages
Reduced vaginal recurrence rate	Delays definitive treatment
Shrinks the primary tumour making	Makes assessment of myometrial

it more operable
Reduces vascular dissemination at
surgery

invasion difficult
Depending upon technique
complication rates can be high
(Boronow 1969)

Postoperative vaginal irradiation:

Advantages

Disadvantages

Reduced vaginal recurrence rate
Does not delay definitive primary
management
Reduces sub-urethral recurrence

Morbidity can be high producing
vaginal stenosis, recurrent proctitis
and recurrent cystitis

The case for preoperative intrauterine irradiation or postoperative intravaginal irradiation is a reduction in vaginal recurrences (Table 17.5). There is no evidence which shows that the overall survival is improved although the quality of life may be enhanced. Whilst there are some who disagree (Price *et al.* 1973), there are those who would argue that an extended vaginal cuff at the time of surgery would produce similar results, despite it not protecting the suburethral region.

The place for pre- or postoperative external beam therapy

The case for external beam therapy can be made on the high incidence of lymph node involvement in those cases which are either stage IB, poorly differentiated cancers or particularly those in which the myometrium is invaded to a depth greater than one-half of the overall thickness.

PREOPERATIVE EXTERNAL BEAM THERAPY

Little attention has been given to the value of external beam therapy on a

Table 17.5. Vaginal vault recurrence rates in relation to treatment

Reference	Surgery alone (%)	Preop intrauterine (%)	Postop intravaginal (%)	Postop ext. irrad. ±intravaginal (%)
Rutledge *et al.* (1958)	20.0	1.5	—	—
Dobbie (1953)	5.5	0	1.8	—
Onsrud *et al.* (1976)	—	—	4.6	2.1
Graham (1971)	12.0	3.0	—	—
Beiler *et al.* (1972)	12.0	1.6	—	—
Joslin *et al.* (1977) Series (1)	—	—	3.6	3.3
Joslin (1985) Series (2)	—	—	< 1.5	—

preoperative basis and yet the results that have been published show considerable promise. Wintz (1941) was among the first to report a cure rate of 69% in operable cases, but as discussed by Corscaden (1962) no one else had such success although it was suggested that external radiation could have a definite role based on indirect evidence. Lampe (1963) reported giving 40 Gy deep X-ray therapy 4 weeks before surgery in stage IB cases and getting a 90% 5-year survival as opposed to a group having postoperative intravaginal therapy which gave a 69% survival. Ritcher et al. (1981) also reported good results when surgery followed a range of doses of irradiation averaging 35 Gy. Salazar et al. (1978) used a combination of intrauterine and external therapy depending upon the size of the uterus with 5-year results of 82% but with surgical complications in 10% and chronic radiation problems in 5%.

Salazar et al. (1978) also reported on a literature review of some 362 cases with a survival of 87% compared with 80% for pre- or postoperative intrauterine or intravaginal therapy. These results were significant ($P > 0.05$) with the pelvic recurrence rates in particular being low. More recently Vaeth et al. (1988) reported on the use of preoperative irradiation for stage I disease and recommended its use for all stage I cancers based on treating 185 patients. As was said of the experience of Wintz by Corscaden, 'we must review this experience critically before tossing it out'.

POSTOPERATIVE EXTERNAL BEAM THERAPY

The use of external beam therapy following surgical removal of the uterus is based on the experience of radiotherapy curing involved lymph nodes within the pelvis. Delclos & Fletcher (1969) reported on disease control of 77% in unresectable cases receiving more than 30 Gy in 3 weeks. Previously, Masson & Gregg (1940) and Corscaden (1962) found that the addition of X-ray therapy to postoperative cases improved survival for unfavourable cases. Joslin et al. (1977) reported using postoperative intravaginal irradiation combined with external beam irradiation. Treatment was given by either telecobalt or 6 MeV X-rays to a dose of 35 Gy in 15 fractions followed by intravaginal high dose rate therapy to a dose of 20 Gy in four fractions over 3 days at a depth of 0.5 cm from the applicator surface. This was later reduced to 16 Gy in four fractions for a 3 cm diameter obturator and 12 Gy in four fractions for a 2.5 cm obturator. The results showed a significant improvement in pelvic recurrence rates and in survival (91%) when compared to surgery alone.

An important trial carried out by Onsrud et al. (1976) compared postoperative intravaginal radiotherapy with and without external beam therapy in 386 patients. A vaginal vault dose of 60 Gy was given by intravaginal therapy and 40 Gy by external beam therapy. The vaginal recurrence rates were less in the patients having external beam therapy (Table 17.5) but the 5-year survival rates were the same for both groups.

Stage II disease

This occurs much less frequently than stage I disease. From 1974–83, the author treated only 18 cases of stage II disease. Most cases were suitable for surgery and where possible this should be carried out. Postoperative external beam therapy to 45 Gy in 20 fractions over 4 weeks, with additional intravaginal treatment, was given to 15 patients. Of these 18, one developed pelvic recurrence although four developed distant metastases. These five patients died within 18 months and two others died of intercurrent disease. The remaining 11 were disease free at periods ranging from 12–98 months. Gagnon *et al.* (1979) reported on 24 stage II cases receiving 45–50 Gy radiation followed by surgery after about 5 weeks. Surgery in 23 of these cases revealed local disease in 14. The adjusted survival rate at 5 years was 81%. Of the four recurrences one was vaginal and three had distant metastases.

Aalders (1982) reported on a clinical trial carried out on 174 patients. All but 39 patients had preoperative intrauterine Heyman's capsules with an abdominal hysterectomy and bilateral salpingo-oophorectomy (BSO) 6 weeks later. Following surgery all patients had intravaginal therapy to 60 Gy and were then randomized to either no further treatment or 40 Gy external beam therapy. The 5-year survival rates were similar for each group at just over 80%. There were more local recurrences in the irradiated group but the cancer free interval to first recurrence was longer at 39 months in the irradiated as opposed to 21 months in the non-irradiated group. More recently Larson *et al.* (1987) reported on the results of giving preoperative external beam irradiation followed by an extrafascial hysterectomy in 69 patients. They reported a 5-year actuarial survival rate of 67% together with a lower incidence of pelvic lymph node metastases for this group of patients.

These results, of a combined approach using surgery and radiotherapy, appear to be similar to those having preoperative intrauterine irradiation but for most other published series the results reported for surgery alone, with or without preoperative intrauterine therapy, are around 40–60%.

Advanced disease

From 1974–83, 10 cases of stage III disease and nine cases of stage IV were seen by the author. Of the 10 stage III cases six were treated by external therapy alone to a minimum dose of 45 Gy in 4 weeks, one had external beam and two intrauterine insertions. Four cases died within 9 months with pelvic disease and one lived for 54 months dying of metastatic disease. Three cases had a total hysterectomy, two had postoperative external beam radiotherapy and one had intravaginal therapy only. Only the latter case survived more than 9 months but had a pelvic recurrence 16 months later. More promising results have been published by Mackillop & Pringle (1985) who concluded from a series of 90 patients that surgery was the treatment of choice for operable cases. However, 13 of 36 cases with inoperable disease who completed radiotherapy were alive and free of disease at 5 years.

Stage IV disease is treated on an individual basis and includes surgery, radiotherapy and hormones. Of the nine cases treated, four had surgery to remove the uterus and bulk tumour followed by radiotherapy and progestogens. One died at 4 months from lung metastases and one at 36 months with pelvic recurrence. The remaining two cases remain alive with a clear pelvis at 4 and 8 months. The remaining five cases could only be palliated and all died within 1 year.

It is clear that once endometrial cancer has reached stage III or IV the prognosis is very poor with 5-year reported results for stage III disease of around 30% and for stage IV disease 10%. Also, as discussed by Aalders (1982) a radical surgical approach to these patients is important. When successful and followed by radiotherapy, a 5-year actuarial survival rate of 41% can be achieved. However, without complete surgical clearance of disease the results are only 11%.

Recurrent disease

Radiotherapy has little to offer for local recurrence in a patient previously treated by radical external beam radiotherapy. For those who have had preoperative intrauterine or postoperative intravaginal therapy, external beam irradiation can be considered.

Suburethral deposits in particular may be suitable for an interstitial implant using radium, ^{137}Cs or ^{192}Ir. Radiotherapy may also be of benefit in bringing about pain relief from bone metastases or to restrict the growth of soft tissue lesions particularly in situations such as the left supraclavicular fossa and, although rare, for brain metastases.

Ovarian cancer

Introduction

Cancer of the ovary is a sinister cancer, remaining silent until well advanced in many cases, at which stage it is difficult to control. However, despite this some patients do extremely well with minimal treatment. The incidence of the disease is slowly increasing and the overall cure rates are much the same now as they were 20 or more years ago.

Ovarian cancer is one of the most difficult cancers for the oncologist to manage and often produces a frustrated doctor and a disillusioned, distressed patient. Barber (1982) summed up the situation by stating, 'Those therapeutic nihilists who plead that the patient should be left to die with dignity, must face a dilemma when forced to apply their philosophy to a woman dying with advanced ovarian cancer'.

The primary lesion

Tumours of the ovary are either benign or malignant. They usually start in one ovary but they may be bilateral. They tend to remain localized for a time and can grow to an enormous size. The malignant variety may, as they enlarge, spread by direct infiltration along peritoneal surfaces. This can cause pain, but very often the only symptoms are vague abdominal discomfort and a feeling of lassitude and intestinal upset.

A specific diagnosis and estimate of spread can only be accurately carried out at laparotomy and it is on the basis of these findings, coupled with the histological grading, that management is determined.

Prognostic indicators

The subject of prognosis and prognostic indices is covered elsewhere in this book. However, a major problem with prognostic factors in ovarian cancer is that they may change depending on the situation, e.g. in the case of epithelial tumours a careful assessment by Sigurdsson (1982) found that the histologic type only affected prognosis in stage III patients who had large residual disease when mucinous tumours had the best prognosis. The tumour grade has significance only in patients with no or small residual tumours ($\leq$2 cm) postoperatively. Residual tumour postoperatively has a marked effect on prognosis when >2 cm in diameter. More recently Rodenberg *et al.* (1987) have reported on the tumour ploidy being a major prognostic factor in advanced ovarian cancer.

The value of steroid receptors as a prognostic indicator has not produced the same promising results (Quinn *et al.* 1982) as the ploidy studies have shown, but this work is continuing (Leake *et al.* 1987).

Involvement of other tissues

Malignant ovarian tumours commonly spread to other intra-abdominal structures. Peritoneal deposits may occur at any site and in particular may involve the greater omentum. Pelvic masses, discrete from the primary lesion, may occur and this can involve viscera. Other intra-abdominal sites of spread include the sub-diaphragmatic areas and around the ascending and descending colon. Spread to the fallopian tubes, uterus, pelvic regional nodes and extension to the periaortic nodes may also occur. The assessment of possible spread within the abdomen is a vital step in furthering more information about the behaviour of the disease and developing the best form of management. The methods used are discussed further in Chapter 10.

Clinical classification

A number of staging systems have been described and are particularly important when discussing treatment, although it is often what is left following surgery which is more important than the original stage.

The FIGO system (1971) is the one most commonly used, and is shown in Chapter 10.

Histological types

This chapter is concerned with the place for radiotherapy and will only concern itself with those ovarian tumours where radiotherapy is normally considered.

1 Epithelial tumours:
   serous cystadenocarcinomas
   pseudomucinous cystadenocarcinomas
   unclassified adenocarcinomas
   undifferentiated carcinomas
   clear celled carcinomas
   endometrial carcinomas
2 Gonadal stromal tumours:
   granulosa cell tumours
3 Germ cell tumours:
   dysgerminomas
   malignant teratomas
4 Others such as:
   lymphoreticular tumours
   secondary carcinomas

Treatment

The first essential requisite is surgical diagnosis and staging followed by surgical excision of all operable disease. The staging procedures are dealt with elsewhere but from the radiotherapy point of view the less disease left within the patient the greater the chance of radiotherapy bringing the disease under control with the chance of cure being greatest for occult metastases. The evidence available to support this view includes the reports of Delclos & Quinlan (1969) who found that when the abdomen was irradiated following surgery, the tumour recurrence rates increased with the amount of disease left within the abdomen. This was further substantiated by Dembo *et al.* (1979) who reported that radiotherapy only benefited those patients who had small or no macroscopic residual disease. It is advocated, therefore, that a bilateral salpingo-oophorectomy, total hysterectomy and omentectomy should be carried out in all cases including appropriate resection and removal of all other bulk disease if radiotherapy is to be considered. The one exception would be a young woman with a stage IA(I) tumour who does not wish to become sterile (Disaia & Creasman 1981). It is also questionable whether omentectomy is necessary in these cases. With modern high energy photon machines there is no case for retaining the uterus to act as a carrier for an intrauterine irradiation.

Current practice is to use one of two techniques when either irradiation is given to the whole abdomen with additional pelvic irradiation or irradiation is restricted to the pelvis alone.

Pelvic irradiation

When disease is localized to the pelvis some still consider that radiotherapy has a part to play in treatment. However, others would disagree and the results of two randomized controlled studies reported by Dembo *et al.* (1983) and Hreshchyshyn *et al.* (1980) showed no improvement in intra-abdominal recurrence rates whether patients were watched, received postsurgical pelvic irradiation or, in the case of Hreshchyshyn, alternatively received melphalan. In a further trial Dembo (1984) reported for stages I, II and III significantly better results for abdomino—pelvic irradiation compared with pelvic irradiation plus chlorambucil.

The case for pelvic irradiation alone now seems difficult to make except in selected cases on a palliative basis with concomitant chemotherapy.

Whether given as a special situation or as part of abdomino—pelvic irradiation, with the availability of high energy photon therapy machines patients can be treated by parallel opposed fields. Adequate coverage can be achieved by fields measuring 15 × 15 cm although the author tends to use fields 16—17 cm wide and 14 cm high. The field should extend up from the lower level of the obturator foramen and the lower corners can usually be leaded off. The upper border should reach the lower border of L5 and laterally should extend to between 1.0 and 2.0 cm external to the bony pelvic brim. To achieve a radical effect a dose of 40—50 Gy, given at a rate of 1.8 to 2 Gy each day, is standard practice. In some patients, depending on whether they are receiving or have recently received chemotherapy, the daily dose may require reducing to 1.7 or 1.8 Gy per fraction.

When the pelvis is being irradiated in conjunction with abdominal irradiation, the pelvic treatment has to be reduced to stay within the 5% morbidity tolerance for small gut. Depending upon the technique used, the additional pelvic treatment should be reduced to about 20 Gy in 10 fractions over 2 weeks. Readers requiring further information are referred to Dembo (1984).

Abdomino—pelvic irradiation

There are two basic techniques in current use:

1 *Large parallel opposed fields.* These fields are set up to cover the abdomen from above the dome of the diaphragm on each side to the pelvic floor and extend laterally to outside the peritoneal reflection. The kidneys are carefully located by means of a planning pyelogram and protected from irradiation so that a maximum dose of 20 Gy is received by each kidney. Many also protect the liver after 20 Gy. A total abdominal dose of 30 Gy in 25—30 fractions over 5—6 weeks is normally given but it may be difficult to maintain daily treatments during the last 2 weeks due to a low blood count and systemic upset. Largely to overcome these problems many switched to using a moving strip technique only to find, as has the author, that bowel morbidity is high and have therefore returned to wide field irradiation. Also it is important to reduce the dose used if patients have received chemotherapy, the effect of which can last for several months.

2 *Moving strip technique.* This was first developed by Paterson (1948); later, using telecobalt therapy, by Delclos *et al.* (1963) and more recently by Dembo *et al.* (1979). This technique delivers a high radiobiologically effective dose to the abdomen by arranging treatment in a series of strips, each of 2.5 cm width. Parallel opposed strips are treated daily and the number of strips treated increased by one width every 2 days. Once a total width of 10 cm is reached the process is moved down 2.5 cm and the first strip is left off. Treatment starts from the diaphragmatic level following initial treatment to the pelvis. The pelvic irradiation is usually given in 10 fractions to a total dose of 22 Gy. For the abdominal field each strip receives 12 treatments and a total dose of 22 Gy although some give doses as high as 26 Gy.

The aim of the strip field is to provide a better therapeutic ratio, but the author's experience is that it produces an unacceptably high small gut morbidity as reported by Perez *et al.* (1978). Dembo *et al.* (1983) reported a significantly ($P < 0.05$) greater morbidity for the moving strip technique compared with open fields, which applied to basal pneumonitis, hepatitis (biochemical) and enteritis. Also, the reported results of disease control vary; Perez found that this treatment did not improve results as was also reported by Fazekas & Maier (1974).

Treatment

Stage 1 disease

IA(I) AND IB(I)

These tumours are invariably cured by surgery alone and it is difficult to argue a case for adjuvant therapy. Certainly the well differentiated primary tumours do well following conservative surgery without supportive chemotherapy or radiotherapy and cure rates of 95% and more have been reported (Munnell 1969; Webb et al. 1973; Hreshchyshyn et al. 1980; Sigurdsson 1982).

Sigurdsson also showed in a prospective randomized study that the non-mucinous tumours did as well whether they received postoperative melphalan or radiotherapy. Unfortunately, there was no control group of surgery only.

STAGE IC

This group of patients carry a high risk of recurrent disease particularly for grade III lesions. Recurrence can occur anywhere in the abdomen and the place for adjuvant radiotherapy needs considering. Delclos & Smith (1975) reported that for stage I disease postoperative radiotherapy to the whole abdomen, with additional treatment to the pelvis, gave a 5-year disease free rate of 76%. Dembo (1985) in a stratified randomized trial reported a survival gain of 25% at 10 years for stages IB, II and III, in patients with no or minimal residual disease following surgery. The group which did best received pelvic–abdominal irradiation compared with a second group receiving pelvic irradiation and chlorambucil. They suggested, from this study, that provided special care is taken with abdomino–pelvic irradiation, results are superior to pelvic irradiation alone or combined with chlorambucil. Sigurdsson (1982) also reported that for advanced stages I and II the results for postoperative radiotherapy were not improved when melphalan was added, which makes for a strong case in favour of irradiation alone. However, Barber (1978) sees no place for radiotherapy when used routinely in stages I, II or III, but does support the use of colloidal ^{32}P. Morrow (1981) in an excellent review of the published results from different centres draws attention to the fact that postoperative radiotherapy appears to make no difference to 5-year survival rates for stages I, II or III. However, for many of the series quoted, irradiation was limited to the pelvis. More recently Macbeth et al. (1988), in a prospective study of 57 women with early stage disease (49% were stage I), were not convinced of the efficacy of total abdomino–pelvic irradiation using a similar treatment regime to Dembo. However, they suggested that a higher dose of irradiation would probably achieve better results as found by Fuller et al. (1987) and Martinez et al. (1985).

The value of pelvic–abdominal irradiation must still remain an open question but since tumour control is much more probable when the volume of tumour is minimal, it seems reasonable to expect the results to be particularly beneficial for stage IC cancers.

An alternative to chemotherapy and external beam radiotherapy is the use of colloidal ^{32}P as described by Clarke et al. (1976) which improved survival rates from 65% to 90%. These results are impressive and cannot easily be ignored especially as the morbidity from ^{32}P is reported as low (Alderman 1977). Kolstad

(1981) reported that the 5-year survival results using colloidal ^{198}Au with 30 Gy pelvic irradiation in treating stage I cases was 84% compared to 63% for 50 Gy or high energy external irradiation to the pelvis alone. However, he reported a high morbidity for the ^{198}Au because of its gamma component and also advised changing to ^{32}P. This particular study did not give external beam irradiation to the whole abdomen and a controlled clinical trial would be well worthwhile.

While the management for stage I disease might be considered controversial it is chiefly because of the difficulty in evaluating the effects of different forms of therapy on the different subgroups of patients. In particular for grade III lesions irrespective of substaging an aggressive approach seems advisable.

STAGES IIA, IIB AND IIC

While many would include stage IIC with stage III for management purposes, it is still a situation where extrapelvic disease is occult rather than overt with a better prognosis. Prognosis will be particularly dependent upon whether any overt residual disease remains within the pelvis following surgery, with a prognosis similar to that for stage I disease when no or small residual lesions remain, particularly for the well differentiated cancers (Dembo et al. 1982). There really can be no case for pelvic irradiation alone in these patients, although there are some who treat with systemic cytotoxic agents, in combination with pelvic irradiation, the case for pelvic irradiation being that this is the region at greatest risk of recurrence. Certainly for patients with a poor prognosis either by grade of tumour or because of residual disease there may be some value in adopting this procedure.

An alternative method of treatment is to instil colloidal ^{32}P into the abdominal cavity.

However, Barber (1978) advises it is for the stage I cases that the results of ^{32}P are most successful and that its application in stage II cases is less dramatic. It is also suggested that omentectomy should be carried out before instilling ^{32}P as this reduces the amount of omental tissues present to which the ^{32}P fixes and also improves the distribution of ^{32}P. A major problem is in the attention required to ensure an adequate spread of the isotope, since any localization may cause radionecrosis with disastrous results. Also, current regulations for handling and using unshielded radionuclides make them difficult to use. However, it is a much neglected technique and has never been fully evaluated.

Morrow (1981) advised from his review of seven published series that the addition of radiotherapy following surgery improved the 5-year survival from 23.5 to 37.0%. However, there are no controlled clinical trials to evaluate postoperative radiotherapy for these patients. Sjovall & Einhorn (1985) report on the use of preoperative irradiation in carefully selected patients with fixed bulky tumours, stages II–IV. When the tumour mass remaining after radiotherapy was less than 2.0 cm and followed by surgery, the 5-year survival was 52% compared with 44% in patients receiving primary surgery whose residual disease was also less than 2.0 cm and then followed by radiotherapy.

A technique used by the author is to give chemotherapy following surgery. Before commencing treatment a CT scan of the whole abdomen is done, following which chemotherapy is given (usually a cisplatin regime) for about 4 months. Following this a second CT scan is done and in selected patients, showing evidence of localized recurrent disease, a second look operation is carried out with the aim of achieving further cytoreduction. If no evidence of residual disease is found then full abdominal irradiation is given as for stage I disease although some reduction in dose may be necessary. The reason for this approach is that chemotherapy alone rarely cures and radiotherapy only seems to cure the occult.

The evidence for using postoperative abdominal irradiation as compared to systemic chemotherapy using cisplatin based schedules remains to be proven. One difficulty is the small number of patients in any one institution available for assessment. However, the morbidity following full abdominal irradiation is such that many have given it up in favour of chemotherapy alone. Alternatively, there may well be a case following bulk reduction by surgery to follow with chemotherapy and if clear 6 months later to give radiotherapy. The major problem with this latter situation is the increased morbidity and it is this which limits treatment. Finally, the place for preoperative irradiation with or without chemotherapy for fixed tumours requires further study.

STAGES III AND IV

The current philosophy of management points towards getting the maximal amount of tumour bulk reduction as possible by surgery. This is followed by some form of chemotherapy which may extend for 6 months. In the group of patients found to have minimal or no residual disease, the case for postoperative irradiation is one which has its supporters (Delclos & Quinlan 1969; Dembo 1985). In particular Dembo reports on a lower relapse rate in grade I serous and clear celled tumours with stage III disease and this also applied to mucinous and endometrioid types provided there was no evidence of residual disease. These findings are supported by Goldberg & Peschel (1988) who also refer to the poor prognosis for the undifferentiated lesions. An assessment of postoperative chemotherapy, radiotherapy and repeat laparotomy has been carried out by Sigurdsson (1982). The clear message seems to be that tumour bulk reduction provides the best prognosis whichever method is used and no clear superiority of radiotherapy over chemotherapy alone or chemotherapy plus radiotherapy can be made. In recent years, however, the trend has been towards chemotherapy and a number of randomized trials have now been completed. Also, it is important that maximal tumour bulk reduction is achieved at the initial laparotomy.

Vogl *et al.* (1984) reported that after chemotherapy further partial resection was followed by prompt relapse despite further chemotherapy and abdominal irradiation.

In inoperable patients radiotherapy has been shown to bring about operability (Frick *et al.* 1978; Sigurdsson *et al.* 1982). Sigurdsson reported that re-laparotomy could be performed in 41% of patients resulting in the same operative radicality and survival as those patients primarily submitted to extensive surgery.

Granulosa cell tumours

While these tumours can occur at any age they tend to have a long natural history and are sometimes hormone producing. They are sometimes associated with theca celled tumours. One of the better reviews of these tumours is by Stenwig *et al.* (1979) who reported that 78% of patients present as stage I lesions. However, there is a tendency for local recurrence even after 10 or 20 years. Stenwig *et al.* report a 5-year survival rate of 80.5% and at 15 years 56.8%.

Treatment is essentially surgical with removal of the encapsulated tumour and the ovary. A wedge biopsy of the other ovary is performed by some. The malignancy rate is low but if proven to be malignant or spread has occurred, an abdominal hysterectomy and BSO are advisable.

Radiotherapy in these patients is indicated when spread has occurred but particularly where residual or recurrent tumour is present. For these patients abdominal irradiation with protection of the kidneys and liver and a boost to the pelvis is recommended. The dose regime is the same as that for the epithelial tumours, but they are generally more radiosensitive although not as sensitive as dysgerminomas.

For stage I patients who are beyond childbearing age bilateral oophorectomy is desirable followed by pelvic irradiation.

Dysgerminoma

These tumours tend to affect women before the age of 30 years. Despite the fact that the primary lesion can be large, they usually present as stage IA cases. They can, however, be IB which may require histological evidence from the contra-lateral ovary since 10% of them are bilateral. Stage IA cases are probably satis-factorily treated by conservative surgery but there is a tendency for these tumours to spread to the omentum and para-aortic nodes. In view of this all cases should have routine node biopsy and lymphography carried out.

Where disease has extended to stage IB and beyond, a radical hysterectomy and BSO should be performed, perhaps with an omentectomy.

In a review of 33 cases over a 34-year period, Lucraft (1979) reported an 85% 5-year survival. She advised that young patients with stage IA disease should have total resection and no supplementary treatment. All other cases should have radical surgery and complete abdominal irradiation. It was also recommended that bulk reduction in stage III was important and that radiotherapy should not be less than 30 Gy in 20 fractions over 28 days. The kidneys and liver should be protected and a boost dose to the pelvis should be considered where residual tumour is known to be present.

When para-aortic nodes are positive or lymphography suggests mediastinal nodes are involved irradiation should be extended to the mediastinum and left supraclavicular fossa starting 1 month after completing abdominal irradiation. A dose of 30 Gy in 20 fractions in 28 days is recommended although lower doses are used by many because of the high radiosensitivity of these tumours.

Other ovarian cancers

The lymphoreticular tumours are usually radiosensitive and treatment is planned as for lymphoreticular tumours of other sites.

The teratomas are usually radioresistant and treatment is with surgery and cytotoxic therapy.

Endodermal sinus tumours are treatable by radiotherapy but its role is essentially palliative or supportive to chemotherapy (Ungerleider *et al*. 1978). Krukenberg tumours are radioresistant and not suitable for radiotherapy.

References

Cancer of the cervix

Ashby M.A. & Smales E. (1987) Invasive carcinoma of the cervix in young women: clinical data and prognostic features. *Radiother. Oncol.*, **10**, 167–74.

Averette H.F., Nelson J.H., Ng A.B.P., Hogkins W.J., Boyce J.G. & Ford J.H. (1976) Diagnosis and management of microinvasive (stage IA) carcinoma of the uterine cervix. *Cancer* (Suppl.1), **38**, 414.

Benstead K., Cowie V.J., Blair V. & Hunter R.D. (1986) Stage III carcinoma of the cervix. The importance of increasing age and extent of parametrial infiltration. *Radiother. Oncol.*, **5**, 271–76.

Boyce J.G., Fruchter R.G., Nicastri A.D. *et al*. (1984) Vascular invasion in Stage I carcinoma of the cervix. *Cancer*, **53**, 1175–80.

Chassagne D., Gerbaulet A., Dutreux, A. *et al*. (1977) Utilisation pratique de la dosimetrie par ordinateur en curietherapie gynaecologique. *J. Radiol. Electrol.*, **58**, 387.

Chassagne D. & Horiot J.C. (1977) Propositions pour une definition commune de points de reference en curietherapie gynaecologique. *J. Radiol. Electrol.*, **57**, 371.

Cleaves M.A. (1903) Radium: With a preliminary note on radium rays in the treatment of cancer. *Med. Rec.*, **64**, 601.

Corscaden J.A. (1962) *Gynecological Cancer*. Williams & Wilkins, Baltimore.

Creasman W.T. & Weed J.C. (1979) Micro invasive cancer vs. occult cancer. *Int. J. Rad. Oncol. Biol. Phys.*, **5**, 1871–72.

Dische S. (1984) The MRC trial of Misonidazole in carcinoma of the uterine cervix. A report from the MRC Working Party on Misonidazole for cancer of the cervix. *Br. J. Radiol.*, **57**, 491–99.

Dische S. (1985) Chemical sensitizers for hypoxic cells: a decade of experience in clinical radiotherapy. *Radiother. Oncol.*, **3**, 97–115.

Douglas B., MacDonald J.A. & Baker J.W. (1972) Lymphography in carcinoma of the uterus. *Clin. Radiol.*, **23**, 286.

Dyson J.E.D., Joslin C.A.F., Rothwell R.I., Quirke P., Khoury G.G. & Bird C.C. (1987). Flow cytofluorometric evidence for the differential radioresponsiveness of aneuploid and diploid cervix tumours. *Radiother. Oncol.*, **8**, 262–72.

Fletcher G.H. (1980) Squamous cell carcinoma of the uterine cervix. *In*: Fletcher G.H. (ed.) *Textbook of Radiotherapy*. Lea & Febiger, Philadelphia.

Forsell G. (1917) Uebersicht uber due resultate die Kreksbehandling am Radiumhemmet. Stockholm, 1910–15. *Fostschr. a.d. Geb. D. Rontgenstrohlen*, **25**, 142–49.

Fuller A.F., Elliott N., Kosloff C. & Lewis J.L. (1982) Lymph node metastases from carcinoma of the cervix, stages IB and IIA; Implications for prognosis and treatment. *Gynecol. Oncol.*, **13**, 165–77.

Gorton G. (1964) Radiation therapy and excision of the lymph nodes in cervical cancer. *Acta Obstet. Gynaecol. Scan.* (Suppl. 2), **43**, 49.

Graham J.B. & Graham E.R. (1955) Curability of regional lymph node metastasis in cancer of the uterine cervix. *Surg. Gynaecol. Obstet.*, **100**, 149–55.

Haie C., Pejovic M.H., Gerbaulet A., Horiot J.C. *et al.* (1988) Is prophylactic para-aortic irradiation worth while in the treatment of advanced cervical carcinoma? Results of a controlled clinical trial of the EORTC Radiotherapy Group. *Radiother. Oncol.*, **11**, 101–11.

Henschke U.K. (1960) Afterloading application for radiation therapy of carcinoma of the uterus. *Radiology*, **74**, 834.

ICRU (1978) Dose specification for reporting external beam therapy with photons and electrons. *ICRU Report No. 29*, ICRU. Bethesda, USA.

ICRU (1985) Dose specification for reporting intracavitary therapy in gynaecology. *ICRU Report No. 38*, ICRU. Bethesda, USA.

Joslin C.A.F. (1976) Management of cervical malignant disease—radiotherapy. *In*: Jordan J.A. & Singer A. (eds), *The Cervix*. W.B. Saunders, London.

Joslin C.A.F. & Peel K.R. (1982) Clinical practice—uterus. *In*: Halman K. (ed.), *Treatment of Cancer*. Chapman & Hall, London.

Khoury G.G., Joslin C.A.F. & Rothwell R.I. (1989) Concomitant pelvic irradiation, 5 fluorouracil and mitomycin in the treatment of advanced cervical cancer *(accepted for publication)*.

Kinney W.K., Alvarez R.D., Reid G.C., Schray M.F., Soong S.J., Marley G.W., Podratz K.C. & Shingleton H.M. (1989) Value of adjuvant whole pelvis irradiation after Wertheim hysterectomy for early stage squamous carcinoma of the cervix with pelvic nodal metastasis: a matched—control study. *Gynaecol. Oncol.*, **34**, 258–62.

Kjellgren O. (1981) Clinical invasive carcinoma of cervix: place of radiotherapy as primary treatment. *In*: Coppleson M. (ed.), *Gynecologic Oncology*. Churchill Livingstone, Edinburgh.

Kolbenstvedt A. (1974) Lymphography in the diagnosis of metastases from carcinoma of the uterine cervix stages I and II. *Acta Radiol. Diagn.*, **16**, 81–97.

Kottmeier H.L. (1976) *Annual Report of the Results of Treatment for Carcinoma of the Uterus, Vagina and Onary 16.* Cancer Committee of the International Federation of Gynaecology and Obstetrics, Stockholm.

Lagasse L.D., Smith M.L., Moore J.C., Morton D.G., Jacobs M., Johnson G.H. & Watring W.G. (1974) The effect of radiation therapy on pelvic lymph node involvement in stage I carcinoma of the cervix. *Am. J. Obstet. Gynecol.*, **119**, 328–34.

Lybeert M.L.M., Meerwaldt J.H. & van Putten W.L.J. (1987) Age as a prognostic factor in carcinoma of the cervix. *Radiother. Oncol.*, **9**, 147–51.

Montana G.S., Fowler W.C., Varia M.A., Walton L.A., Kirsch M., Halle J.S. & McCafferty B.B. (1983) Carcinoma of the cervix stage IB; results of treatment with radiation therapy. *Int. J. Radiat. Oncol. Biol.Phys.*, **9**, 45–49.

Morley G.W. & Seski J.C. (1976) Radical pelvic surgery versus radiation therapy for stage I carcinoma of the cervix. *Am. J. Obstet.*, **126**, 785–98.

Morrow P.C. (1980) Moderator of panel report. Is pelvic radiation beneficial in the post-operative management of stage IB squamous cell carcinoma of the cervix with pelvic node metastasis treated by radical hysterectomy and pelvic lymphadenectomy. *Gynecol. Oncol.*, **10**, 105–10.

MRC Working Party Report (1984) The Medical Research Council trial on misonidazole in carcinoma of the uterine cervix. *Br. J. Radiol.*, **57**, 491–9.

Newton M. (1975) Radical hysterectomy or radiotherapy for stage I cervical cancer. *Am. J. Obstet. Gynecol.*, **123**, 535.

O'Connell D., Joslin C.A., Howard N. *et al.* (1967) The treatment of uterine carcinoma using the Cathetron. *Br. J. Radiol.*, **40**, 882–87.

Orton C.G. (1985) Bio-effect dosimetry in radiation therapy. *In*: Orton C. (ed.), *Radiation Dosimetry: Physical and Biological Aspects*. Plenum Press, New York. pp. 1–71.

Orton C.G. & Wolf-Rosenblum S. (1986) Dose dependence of complication rates in cervix cancer radiotherapy. *Int. J. Rad. Oncol., Biol. Phys.*, **12**, 37–44.

Pagnini C.A., Palma P.D. & De Laurentiis G. (1980) Malignancy grading in squamous carcinoma of uterine cervix treated by surgery. *Br. J. Cancer*, **41**, 415–21.

Papavasiliou C., Yiogarakis D., Pappas J. & Keramopoulos A. (1980) Treatment of cervical carcinoma by total hysterectomy and post-operative external irradiation. *Int. J. Radiat. Oncol. Biol. Phys.*, **6**, 871–74.

Paterson M.E.L., Peel K.R. & Joslin C.A.F. (1984) Cervical smear histories of 500 women with invasive cervical cancer in Yorkshire. *Br. Med. J.*, **289**, 896–98.

Pearcey R.G., Peel K.R., Thorogood J. & Walker K. (1988) The value of pre-operative intracavitary radiotherapy in patients treated by radical hysterectomy and pelvic lymphadenectomy for invasive carcinoma of the cervix. *Clin. Radiol.*, **39**, 95–98.

Pilleron J.P., Durrand J.C. & Hamelin J.P. (1974) Prognostic value of node metastasis in cancer of the uterine cervix. *Am. J. Obstet. Gynecol.*, **119**, 458–62.

Piver M.S. & Chung W.C. (1975) Prognostic significance of cervical lesion size and pelvic node metastases in cervical carcinoma. *Obstet. Gynecol.*, **46**, 507–12.

Piver M.S., Wallace S. & Castro J.R. (1971) The accuracy of lymphangiography in carcinoma of the uterine cervix. *Am. J. Roentgenol. Radium Ther. Nucl. Med.*, **111**, 278–83.

Plentl A.E. & Friedman E.A. (1971) *Lymphatic System of the Female Genitalia*. Saunders, Philadelphia.

Regaud C. (1926) Traitment des cancer du col et l'uterous par les radiations: idee sommaire des methodes et des resultats; indications therapeutique. *Rapp VIIc. Cong. Soc. Int. Chirurg.*, **35**.

Russel J.C. & Welch J.P. (1979) Operative management of radiation injuries of the intestinal tract. *Am. J. Surg.*, **137**, 433–42.

Rutledge F.N. & Fletcher G.H. (1958) Trans peritoneal pelvic lymphadenectomy following super-voltage irradiation for squamous cell carcinoma of the cervix. *Am. J. Obstet. Gynecol.*, **76**, 321.

Sismondi P., Siniestrero G. & Zola P. (1989) Complications of uterine cervix carcinoma treatments: the problem of a uniform classification. *In*: Mould R.F. (ed.), *Proceedings of the 5th International Selectron Users' Meeting 1988*. Nucletron International B.V.

Smales E., Perry C.M., Macdonald J.S. & Baker J.W. (1986) The value of lymphography in the management of carcinoma of the cervix. *Clin. Radiol.*, **37**, 19–22.

Suit H.D. (1963) Modifications of the Fletcher system for afterloading using standard size radium tubes. *Radiology*, **81**, 126–31.

Swan D.S. & Roddick J.W. (1972) A clinico-pathological correlation of cell type classification for cervical cancer. *Am. J. Obstet. Gynecol.*, **116** (5), 666–70.

Tankel M.I., Clark D.H. & Lee F.D. (1965) Radiation enteritis with malabsorption. *Gut*, **6**, 560–69.

Tod M.C. & Meredith W.J. (1938) A dosage system for use in the treatment of cancer of the uterine cervix. *Br. J. Radiol.*, **11**, 809–24.

Turesson I. (1989) The progression rate of late radiation effects in normal tissue and its impact on dose–response relationships. *Radiother. Oncol.*, **15**, 217–26.

Van Nagell J.R., Donaldson E.S. & Gay E.C. (1978) Evaluation and treatment of patients with invasive cervical cancer. *Surg. Clin. North Am.*, **58**, 67–85.

Van Nagell J.R., Donaldson E.S., Parker J.C., Van Dyke A.H. & Wood E.G. (1977) The prognostic significance of cell type and lesion size in patients with cervical cancer treated by radical surgery. *Gynecol. Oncol.*, **5**, 142–51.

Van Nagell J.R., Donaldson E.S., Wood E.G. & Parker J.C. (1978) The significance of vascular invasion and lymphocytic infiltration in invasive cervical cancer. *Cancer*, **41**, 228–34.

Walstam R. (1965) Remotely-controlled afterloading radiotherapy apparatus. *Phys. Med. Biol.*, **7**, 225–28.

Watson E.R., Halnan K.E., Dische S., Cade I.S., Wiernick G. & Sutherland I. (1978) Hyperbaric oxygen and radiotherapy: a Medical Research Council Trial in Carcinoma of the Cervix. *Br. J. Radiol.*, **51**, 879−87.

Wertheim E. (1907) The radical abdominal operation in carcinoma of the cervix uteri. *Surg. Gynaecol. Obstet.*, **4**, 1.

Younge P.A., Hertig A.T. & Armstrong D. (1949) A study of 135 cases of carcinoma *in situ* of the cervix at the Free Hospital for Women. *Am J. Obstet. Gynecol.*, **58**, 867.

Endometrial cancer

Aalders J.G. (1982) *Prognostic Factors and Treatment of Endometrial Cancer. A Clinical and Histological Study.* Rijksuniversiteit Te Groningen, Drukkerij Dijkstra Niemeyer Bv, Groningen.

Beiler D.D., Schmutz D.A. & O'Rourke T.L. (1972) Carcinoma of the endometrium: radiation and surgery versus surgery alone. *Radiology*, **102**, 159−64.

Boronow R.C. (1969) Carcinoma of the corpus: Treatment at M.D. Anderson Hospital. *Cancer of the Uterus and Ovary, Year Book*, Chicago. pp. 35−61.

Boronow R.C., Morrow C.P., Creasman W.T., Disaia P.J., Silverburg S.G., Miller A. & Blessing J.A. (1984) Surgical staging of endometrial cancer: 1. Clinico-pathological findings of a prospective study. *Obstet. Gynecol.*, **63**, 825−38.

Chamlian D.L. & Taylor H.B. (1970) Endometrial hyperplasia in young women. *Obstet. Gynecol.*, **36**, 659.

Corscaden J.A. (1962) *Gynecologic Cancer*. Williams & Wilkins, Baltimore.

Creasman W.T., Boronow R.C., Morrow C.P., Disaia P.J. & Blessing J. (1976) Adenocarcinoma of the endometrium: its metastatic lymph node potential. *Gynecol Oncol.*, **4**, 239−43.

Delclos L. & Fletcher G.H. (1969) Malignant tumours of the endometrium: evaluation of some aspects of radiotherapy. M.D. Anderson Hospital. *Cancer of the Uterus and Ovary, Year Book*, Chicago. pp. 62−72.

Dobbie B.M.W. (1953) Vaginal recurrences in carcinoma of the body of the uterus and their prevention by radium therapy *J. Obstet. Gynaecol. Br. Commonwealth*, **60**, 702−5.

Douglas B., MacDonald J.S. & Baker J.W. (1972) Lymphography in carcinoma of the uterus. *Clin. Radiol.*, **23**, 286−94.

Gagnon J.D., Moss W.T., Gabourel L.S. & Stevens K.R. (1979) External irradiation in the management of stage II endometrial carcinoma. *Cancer*, **44**, 1247−51.

Gastaldi A., Zotti L., Cavagnini A., Brighenti R. & Bianchi U.A. (1985) Surgical staging in endometrial cancer. New surgical trends in integrated therapies in endometrial, vulva, trophoblastic neoplasias. *Eur J Gynaecol. Oncol. Ser.*, **59** 66.

Graham J. (1971) The value of pre-operative or post-operative treatment by radium for carcinoma of the uterine body. *Surg. Gynecol. Obstet.*, **132**, 855−60.

Healy W.R. & Brown R.L. (1939) Experience with surgical and radiation therapy in carcinoma of the corpus uteri. *Am. J. Obstet. Gynecol.*, **38**, 1.

Heyman J. (1947) Improvement of results in the treatment of uterine cancer. *J. Am. Hosp. Ass.*, **135**, 412−16.

Jackson R.J.A. (1967) Lymphographic studies related to the problem of metastatic spread from carcinoma of the female genital tract. *J. Obst. Gynaecol Br. Commonwealth*, **74**, 339−52.

Javert C.T. (1952) The spread of benign and malignant endometrium in the lymphatic system with a note on co-existing vascular involvement. *Am. J. Obstet. Gynecol.*, **64**, 780−806.

Jones H.W. (1975) Treatment of adenocarcinoma of the endometrium. *Obstet. Gynecol. Surv.*, **30**, 147.

Joslin C.A.F. (1985) The place for radiotherapy in endometrial cancer. *Proceedings of International Meeting of Gynaecological Oncology, Venice-Lido (Italy), 21−24 April 1985.* pp. 53−5.

Joslin C.A.F., Vaishampayan G.V. & Mallik T. (1977) The treatment of early cancer of the corpus uteri. *Radiology*, **50**, 38−45.

Kolbenstvedt A. & Kolstad P. (1973) Pelvic lymph node dissection under pre-operative lymphographic control. *Gynecol. Oncol.*, **2**, 39−59.

Kottmeier H.L. (1953) *Carcinoma of the Female Genitalia.* Williams & Wilkins, Baltimore.

Kottmeier H.L. (1959) Carcinoma of the corpus uteri: diagnosis and therapy. *Am. J. Obstet. Gynecol.*, **87**, 1127.

Lampe I. (1963) Endometrial carcinoma. *Am. J. Roentgenol.*, **90**, 1011−15.

Larson D.M., Copeland L.J., Gallagher S.H., Kong J.P., Wharton T.J. & Stringer C.A. (1987) Stage II endometrial carcinoma. *Cancer*, **61**, 1528−34.

Lewis B.V. (1971) Nodal spread in relation to penetration and differentiation. *Proc. R. Soc. Med.*, **64**, 406−7.

Lewis B.V., Stallworthy J.A. & Cowdell (1970) Adenocarcinoma of the body of the uterus. *J. Obstet. Gynaecol. Br. Commonwealth*, **77**, 343−84.

Liu W. & Meigs J.V. (1955) Radical hysterectomy and pelvic lymphadenectomy: a review of 473 cases including 244 for primary invasive carcinoma of the cervix. *Am. J. Obstet. Gynecol.*, **69**, 1−32.

Maas H. (1987) Epidemiology and Etiology. *In*: Schulz K.D. *et al.* (eds), *Endometrial Cancer*. (Intl. Symposium Marburg 1986). Zuckschwedt Verlag, San Francisco.

Mackillop W.J. & Pringle J.F. (1985) Stage III endometrial cancer. *Cancer*, **56**, 2519−23.

Masson J.C. & Gregg R.O. (1940) Carcinoma of the body of the uterus: experience of the Mayo Clinic for 24 years. *Surg. Gynecol. Obstet.*, **70**, 1083.

Onsrud M., Kolstad P. & Normann T. (1976) Post operative external pelvic irradiation in carcinoma of the corpus stage I: a controlled clinical trial. *Gynecol. Oncol.*, **4**, 222−31.

Piver M.S. (1980) Stage I endometrial carcinoma: the role of adjunctive radiation therapy. *Int. J. Radiat. Oncol. Biol. Phys.*, **6**, 367−68.

Price J.J., Hahn G.A. & Rominger C.J. (1973) Vaginal involvement in endometrial cancer. *Am. J. Obstet. Gynecol.*, **88**, 1063−68.

Ritcher N., Lucas W.E., Yon Jr J.L. & Sanford F.G. (1981) Preoperative whole pelvic external irradiation in stage I endometrial cancer. *Cancer*, **48**, 58−62.

Rutledge F.N., Tan S.K. & Fletcher G.M. (1958) Vaginal metastasis from adenocarcinoma of the corpus uteri. *Am. J. Obstet. Gynecol.*, **75**, 167−74.

Salazar O.M., Feldstein M.L., De Papp E.W., Bonfiglio T.A., Keller B.E., Rubin P. & Rudolph J.H. (1978) The management of clinical stage I endometrial carcinoma. *Cancer*, **41**, 1016−26.

Simon N., Silverstone S.M. & Roach C.C. (1971) Afterloading Heyman Applicators. *Acta Radiol.*, **10** (2), 231.

Strickland P. (1965) Carcinoma corpus uteri: a radical intracavitary treatment. *Clin. Radiol.*, **16**, 112−18.

Trotnow S., Becker H. & Paterok E.M. (1978) Tumour volume of endometrial cancer. *In*: Brush M. & Taylor R.W. (eds), *Endometrial Cancer*. Bailliere Tindall, Eastbourne.

Vaeth J.M., Fontanesi J., Tralius A.H. & Chauser B. (1988) External radiation therapy of stage I cancer of the endometrium: a need for reappraisal of this adjunctive modality. *J. Rad. Oncol., Biol. Phys.*, **15**, 1291−97.

Wintz H. (1941) Ergebrisse der Behandling von unterleibkrebsen mit Röntgenstrahlen. *Strahlentherapie*, **69**, 3.

Ovarian cancer

Alderman S.J. (1977) Post-operative use of radioactive phosphorus in stage I ovarian carcinoma. *Obstet. Gynecol.*, **49** (6), 659−62.

Barber H.R.K. (ed.) (1978) *Ovarian Cancer, Etiology, Diagnosis and Treatment*. Masson, USA.

Barber H.R.K. (1982) Cancer of the ovary: *In*: Van Nagell J.R. & Barber H.R.K. (eds), *Modern Concepts of Gynecologic Oncology*. John Wright PSG Inc, USA.

Clarke D.G.C., Hilaris B.S. & Ochoa M. (1976) Treatment of cancer of the ovary. *Clin. Obstet. Gynaecol.*, **3**, 159−79.

Delclos L., Braun E.J., Herrera J.R., Sampiere V.A. & Van Roosenbeck E. (1963) Whole abdominal irradiation by Cobalt−60 moving-strip technique. *Radiology*, **81**, 632−41.

Delclos L. & Quinlan E.J. (1969) Malignant tumours of the ovary managed with post operative megavoltage irradiation. *Radiology*, **93**, 659−63.

Delclos L. & Smith J.P. (1973) Tumors of the ovary. In: Fletcher G.H. (ed.), *Textbook of Radiotherapy.* 2nd Edn. Lea & Febiger, Philadelphia. pp. 690–702.

Delclos L. & Smith J.P. (1975) Ovarian cancer, with special regard to types of radiotherapy. *Natl. Cancer Inst. Monogr.* **42**, 129–35.

Dembo A.J. (1985) Abdominopelvic radiotherapy in ovarian cancer: A 10-year experience. *Cancer,* **55**, 2285–90.

Dembo A.J. (1984) Radiotherapeutic management of ovarian cancer. *Semin. Oncol.,* **11**, 238–50.

Dembo A.J., Bush R.S., Beale F.A., Bean H.A., Brown T.C. et al. (1983) A randomized trial of moving-strip versus open field whole abdominal irradiation in patients with invasive epithelial cancer of the ovary. *Int. J. Rad. Oncol. Biol. Phys.,* (Suppl.), **9**, 97.

Dembo A.J., Bush R.S. & Brown T.C. (1982) Clinico-pathological correlates in ovarian cancer. *Bull. Cancer. (Paris),* **69**, 292–98.

Dembo A.J., Van Dyk J., Japp B., Bean H.A., Beale F.A., Pringle J.F. & Bush R.S. (1979) Whole abdominal irradiation by a moving-strip technique for patients with ovarian cancer. *Int. J. Rad. Oncol. Biol. Phys.,* **5**, 1933–42.

Disaia P.J. & Creasman W.T. (1981) *Clinical Gynecologic Oncology.* C.V. Mosby, St Louis.

Fazekas J.T. & Maier J.G. (1974) Irradiation of ovarian carcinomas. A prospective comparison of the open-field and moving-strip techniques. *Am. J. Roentgenol. Radium. Ther. Nucl. Med.,* **120**, 118–23.

Frick G., Johnsson J.E., Landberg T. & Snorradottir M. (1978) Relaparotomy in advanced ovarian carcinoma. *Acta Obstet. Gynecol. Scand.,* **57**, 165.

Fuller D.B., Sause W.T., Plenk H.P. & Menlowe R.L. (1987) Analysis of post operative radiation therapy in stage I through stage III epithelial ovarian cancer. *J. Clin. Oncol.,* **5**, 897–905.

Goldberg N. & Peschel R.E. (1988) Postoperative abdomino pelvic radiation therapy for ovarian cancer. *Int. J. Oncol. Biol. Phys.,* **4**, 441–43.

Hreshchyshyn M.M., Park R.C., Blessing J.A., Norris H.J., Ley D., Lagosse L.D. & Creasman W. (1980) The role of adjuvant therapy in stage I ovarian cancer. *Am. J. Obstet. Gynecol.,* **138**, 139.

Kolstad P. (1981) Malignant tumours of the ovary: Norwegian experience and management protocols. In: Coppleson M. (ed.), *Gynecologic Oncology.* Churchill Livingstone, Edinburgh.

Leake R.E., Cowan S.V., Kaye S.B. & Kennedy J.H. (1987) Steroid receptors and prognosis. In: Sharp F. & Soutter W.P. (eds), *Ovarian Cancer — The Way Ahead.* Royal College of Obstetricians and Gynaecologists, London.

Lucraft H.H. (1979) A review of thirty-three cases of ovarian dysgerminoma emphasising the role of radiotherapy. *Clin. Radiol.,* **30**, 585–89.

Macbeth F.R., McDonald H. & Williams C.J. (1988) Total abdominal and pelvic radiotherapy in the management of early stage ovarian carcinoma. *Int. J. Rad. Oncol. Biol. Phys.,* **15**, 353–58.

Martinez A., Schray M.F., Howes A.E. & Bagshaw M.A. (1985) Postoperative radiation therapy for epithelial ovarian cancer: the curative role based on 24 years experience. *J. Clin. Oncol.,* **3**, 901–11.

Morrow C.P. (1981) Malignant and borderline epithelial tumours of ovary: clinical features, staging, diagnosis, intra-operative assessment and review of management. In: Coppleson M. (ed.) *Gynecologic Oncology.* Churchill Livingstone, Edinburgh.

Mould (1988) *Brachytherapy 2.* Proceedings Brachytherapy Working Conference 5th International Selection Users' Meeting. The Hague, The Netherlands. Nucletron International B.V., Leersum, The Netherlands.

Munnell E.W. (1969) Is conservative therapy ever justified in stage Ia cancer of the ovary. *Am. J. Obstet. Gynecol.,* **103**, 641.

Paterson R. (1948) *The Treatment of Malignant Disease by Radium and X-rays: Being a Practice of Radiotherapy.* Edward Arnold, London.

Perez C.A., Korba A., Zivnuska F., Prasad S. & Katzenstein A. (1978) ^{60}Co moving-strip technique in the management of carcinoma of the ovary: analysis of tumour control and morbidity. *Int. J. Rad. Oncol. Biol. Phys.,* **4**, 379–88.

Quinn M.A., Pearce P., Rome R., Finder J.W., Fortune D. & Pepperell R.J. (1982) Cytoplasmic steroid receptors in ovarian tumours. *Br. J. Obstet. Gynaecol.,* **89**, 754–59.

Rodenburg C.T., Cornelisse C.J., Heintz P.A.M., Hermans J. & Fleuren G.J. (1987) Tumour ploidy as a major prognostic factor in advanced ovarian cancer. *Cancer,* **59**, 317–23.

Sigurdsson K. (1982) Malignant epithelial tumours. A study of prognostic factors and the effects of combined treatments from the Gynecologic Section, Dept of Oncology, University Hosp, Lund, Sweden.

Sigurdsson K., Johnsson J.E. & Tropé C. (1982) Carcinoma of the ovary, stages I and II. A prospective randomised study of the effects of post-operative chemotherapy and radiotherapy. *Ann. Chir. Gynaecol.*, **71**, 321−29.

Sjövall K. & Einhorn N. (1985) Preoperative radiation therapy in advanced carcinoma of the ovary. *Radiother. Oncol.*, **4**, 329−33.

Smith J.P., Rutledge F. & Delclos L. (1975) Postoperative treatment of early cancer of the ovary: a random trial between postoperative irradiation and chemotherapy. *Natl. Cancer Inst. Monogr.*, **42**, 149−53.

Stenwig J.T., Hazekamp J.T. & Beecham J.B. (1979) Granulosa cell tumours of the ovary. A clinico-pathological study of 118 cases with long-term follow-up. *Gynecol. Oncol.*, **7**, 136−52.

Ungerleider R.S., Donaldson S.S., Warnke R.A. & Wilburn J.R. (1978) Endometrial sinus tumour. *Cancer*, **41**, 1627−34.

Vogl S.E., Seltzer V., Calanog A., Moukhtar M., Camacho F., Kaplan B.H. & Greenwald E. (1984) 'Second effort' surgical resection for bulky ovarian cancer. *Cancer*, **54**, 2220−25.

Webb M.J., Decker D.G., Mussey E. & Williams T.J. (1973) Factors influencing survival in stage I ovarian cancer. *Am. J. Obstet. Gynecol.*, **116**, 222.

18

Nutrition and Nutritional Support in Gynaecological Cancer

MICHAEL J.G. FARTHING & BRYAN J. FEHILLY

During the last decade there has been increasing interest in diet and nutritional status of patients with gynaecological cancer. There is now persuasive epidemiological evidence that environmental factors, particularly dietary factors, play a major role in the aetiopathogenesis of many tumours, including those of the female genital tract. In addition, women with certain types of gynaecologic tumours often present at an advanced stage when the patient's nutritional resources may be seriously depleted by a combination of factors including reduced oral intake, direct tumour competition for nutrients, secondary effects on intestinal function and the production of protein-rich serous effusions.

Radical surgery followed by radiotherapy and/or chemotherapy has made long term survival a reality in some gynaecologic tumours. However, each of these treatment modalities can themselves produce deleterious effects on nutritional status which may increase operative morbidity and mortality and reduce tolerance to adjunctive chemo- or radiotherapy.

Diet as an aetiological factor

The importance of diet in the aetiopathogenesis of cancer is now widely recognized. Major public interest was generated in the USA by the publication in 1982 of an extensive review of the role of diet in the aetiology and prevention of cancer (National Academy of Sciences 1982). The recommendations of this committee included a reduction in total dietary fats and further supplementation of the diet with fruit, vegetables and grain.

Environmental factors in the causation of cancer have been variously estimated at 50–90% (Wynder 1976; Willet & MacMahon 1984). Diet has been incriminated in 50% of all female cancers in the Western world and in up to 70% of all cancers (Willet & MacMahon 1984) making diet second only to smoking as a single aetiological determinant of cancer.

Although there are geographical differences in the incidence of gynaecological cancer, immigrants generally acquire the incidence rates of their country of domicile rather than their country of origin. Chinese or Japanese women living in Hawaii for instance have approximately half the incidence of cancer of the ovary when compared to the white women living in North America but on migration they develop similar incidence rates to their American counterparts (Blayney & Longo 1983).

Estimates of dietary habits have revealed interesting differences between countries with high and low incidence of cancer of the ovary. In Sweden, American and western European countries there is a high intake of red meat, dairy products and coffee which at least superficially correlates with the high incidence of ovarian cancer. In Japan and China where the incidence of this disease is low the intake of these foods is also significantly lower.

Despite geographic correlations between coffee consumption and certain cancers, notably ovary, pancreas and urinary bladder, the link remains uncertain although Sweden, which has the highest incidence of carcinoma of the ovary also consumes the world's largest amount of coffee per capita (Lingman 1983).

Carcinoma of the body of the uterus is also a disease of Western civilizations and in some studies has been related to obesity rather than any specific nutritional factors (Lew & Garfinkel 1979). In other studies it has been associated with fat or meat intake (Armstrong & Doll 1975). Many factors have been studied to try to elucidate important environmental factors with carcinoma of the cervix, which remains the second most common cancer in women (Nelson 1982). From a nutritional viewpoint cervical carcinoma has been related in some studies to low intake of vitamin A and vitamin C (Wynder 1969).

There is also convincing laboratory evidence that the contents of our diet may be involved in the initiation of neoplastic change in some tissues. Laboratory analysis of foodstuffs has revealed a huge array of naturally occurring carcinogens (Ames 1983). These substances may occur in a variety of foods such as potatoes, coffee, black pepper, celery and many others. These toxic substances are thought to act as cellular oxidants through the generation of superoxide dismutase and oxygen free radicals and thence cause DNA damage. Rancid fat, for instance, may produce a whole variety of damaging oxidants (Cutler & Schneider 1974). Some of these substances have been shown to be carcinogenic in animals (Toth 1979). The story is fortunately not all gloom, for many naturally occurring foodstuffs appear to oppose these actions and have been termed anticarcinogens. The evidence to support this is often variable but includes such substances as vitamin E (Lew & Garfinkel 1979), beta carotene (Matthews-Roth 1982), selenium (Jacobs 1983) and vitamin C (Magee 1982).

Undernutrition in gynaecological malignancy

There are many reasons why patients with gynaecological malignancy become undernourished and cachectic. These factors may be part of cancer induced debility or the result of intensive treatment by surgery, chemotherapy or radiotherapy. Cachexia is commonly present in patients with advanced cancer, and although particularly prevalent in patients with gastrointestinal tumours (Brown 1954) it also occurs in association with some gynaecological neoplasms. Ovarian cancer often progresses without causing symptoms such that 60—75% of patients have stage III or IV disease at presentation (Blayney & Longo 1983). A review of patients with gynaecological cancers showed that patients with stage III and IV disease had a high prevalence of undernutrition (Tunca 1983) which was not necessarily related to gastrointestinal disturbance following surgery. Table 18.1 summarizes the major causes of malnutrition in gynaecologic malignancy.

Anorexia with diminished intake of food is a major contributing factor. Cachexia results from depletion of protein and fat stores in an attempt to make good a negative nutrient balance which may include protein and non-protein calories and in some cases multiple vitamin deficiencies. Weight loss may be a striking feature and overall the picture bears a close superficial resemblance to simple starvation. Anorexia, nausea and vomiting are common features of malignant disease and may compromise the patient's nutritional intake at an early stage. Hypercalcaemia, for example, is the most commonly reported paraendocrine abnormality associated with carcinoma of the ovary (Hreshchyshyn 1982). Depression and other affective disorders and abnormalities of taste may worsen anorexia (Dickenson 1984). This latter observation concerning taste appears to increase in severity with increase in tumour bulk (De Wys 1978) and has important implications for planning dietary support regimens. Learned food aversions have been described in animals (Berstein & Sigmundi 1980) and in children receiving chemotherapy (Bernstein et al. 1982). Malabsorption, diarrhoea and intestinal obstructive symptoms may occur either from direct spread of pelvic neoplasms or from peritoneal seeding. Interruption of normal nervous control of bowel function by damage to myenteric nerves may result in a form of intestinal pseudo-obstruction.

The above-mentioned causes of nutritional impairment remain the more obvious and understandable causes of cancer and cachexia. If these alone were the cause of wasting then the nutritional and metabolic consequences of malignancy could be reversed by appropriate enteral or parenteral nutritional supplementation. This, however, is not the case for there is evidence that patients with malignancy show an increased basal metabolic rate and an inability to conserve body tissue as would be the usual response to simple starvation. Thus the patient with cancer may show a rapid dissolution of body mass, indeed a negative nitrogen balance has been found in a high proportion of patients with advanced cancer (Watkin 1961). Some of this increased energy expenditure may be the result of metabolic activity of the tumour itself. Tumour substrate consumption has been studied in animals and man. The consumption of glucose by a rat tumour may be as high as 40 mmol min^{-1} per 100 g tumour and studies of tumours sited on limbs in man have shown the tumours to consume as much as 500 g of glucose per 24 h (Brennan 1982).

Apart from direct competition with the host for nutrients, tumours also affect

Table 18.1. Causes of malnutrition in gynaecologic malignancy

Diminished intake	Effects of tumour on metabolism	Inherent tumour metabolism	Treatment
Anorexia, taste abnormalities	Endocrine factors 'Toxohormones'	Anaerobic metabolism, liberating lactic acid, nitrogen trap and reduces available nitrogen for host	Anorexia
Nausea	↑ Energy metabolism		Nausea
Vomiting	↓ Glucose tolerance		Vomiting
Recurrent intestinal obstruction	↑ Lactic acid production		Post-op debility
			↓ intake, ileus, etc.
Pseudo-obstruction from myenteric plexus damage	↑ Gluconeogenesis		Fistula formation
Malabsorption	↑ FFA metabolism		Mucositis ⎫
	↓ Protein synthesis in muscle		Dysphagia ⎬ Radiotherapy
			Diarrhoea ⎭
Depression, pessimism, suicidal ideas	Altered adaptive response to starvation		Mouth ulceration ⎫
	↑ BMR		Taste abnormalities ⎬ Chemotherapy
	↓ Insulin sensitivity		Nausea
	Production of protein-rich effusions		Vomiting
			Diarrhoea ⎭

the metabolism of the host in a variety of ways. These include an increase in basal metabolic expenditure (Bozzetti *et al*. 1980) and changes in glucose metabolism with decreased glucose tolerance and increased whole body glucose turnover rate (Brennan 1981). Increased lactic acid production is also described with increased glucogenesis and diminished insulin sensitivity. Whole body protein turnover appears to be increased in the tumour bearing individual (Scherstein *et al*. 1982) with net loss of skeletal muscle. Fat metabolism is also altered in cancer states with a rise in plasma free fatty acids and increased free fatty acid oxidation which is not readily reduced by glucose administration.

Definition and recognition of malnutrition

The exact definition of malnutrition is difficult and in many ways less important than its recognition and the realization that malnourished patients are prone to many complications such as poor wound healing and increased susceptibility to infection. The rate of weight loss is an important factor and a well recognized prognostic index of disease outcome (Studley 1936); certainly loss of 15% or more of premorbid weight is likely to result in a severely malnourished state. Surveys of hospital patients have shown evidence of malnutrition in a high percentage, up to 48% in some cases and among these the highest incidence was in patients with neoplastic disease (Butterworth & Blackburn 1975).

In practice, a fair estimation of nutritional status can be obtained by clinical observation of the percent body weight loss and low serum albumin (less than 35 g/l). A recent study showed that clinical assessment alone can provide a good estimation of nutrition status (Baker *et al*. 1982). Abnormalities in these simple parameters should certainly arouse suspicion of malnutrition. A whole range of clinical, immunological, biochemical and haematological tests have been devised to aid accuracy of assessment, many of which are also valuable in monitoring the effects of treatment. Some of these measurements can be compared with tables of normal values and expressed as a percentage of normal for individual patients. In some cases a nutritional scoring system has been formulated in an effort to grade overall nutritional status (Klidjan *et al*. 1981). These more sophisticated tests should not, however, replace a good clinical and dietary history. This is an area which is often neglected and can very quickly and simply give an indication of how severely a patient's nutrition has been affected.

Clinical examination may be misleading as even obese patients can be malnourished and many specific nutritional and vitamin deficiency states may not be clinically obvious until a severe deficiency exists. Apart from the parameters shown in Table 18.2, other indices of protein status have been developed including the measurement of 3-methylhistidine excretion in the urine, total body nitrogen and total body potassium estimations, but these are rarely used in clinical practice. Many of the measurements described above reflect body state at only one particular instant and do not reflect functional deficits. Advances such as the

Table 18.2. A range of tests devised to aid accuracy of assessment of nutritional status

Parameter	Body compartment	Level of values suggesting malnutrition
Important anthropometric measurements		
Height in cm		Many parameters vary not only with height but also with age and sex
Weight in kg		Weight *loss* of $\geq$10% of normal weight or $\geq$5 kg in 3/12
Actual weight as % of ideal body weight for height		<80%
Triceps skinfold thickness	Fat stores	♂ <12.5 mm ♀ <16.5 mm (these standards may vary with different communities)
Mid-upper arm circumference (MAC)	Fat and protein stores	[♂ <23 cm, ♀ <22 cm]
Mid-arm muscle circumference (MMC) = MAC − (π × triceps skinfold thickness)		[♂ <19 cm, ♀ <17 cm]
MMC as % standard	Protein stores	
Hand grip dynamometry	Protein mass	<85% of control values for age and sex
Biochemical		
24-h urinary creatinine		Varies with sex and height
Creatinine/height index (CHI)		
$\text{CHI} = \dfrac{\text{Actual urinary creatinine}}{\text{Ideal urinary creatinine}} \times 100$	Lean body mass	<80%
	Protein stores	
Serum albumin		<35 g/l
Serum transferrin		<2 g/l
Serum prealbumin		<200 mg/l
Serum retinol-binding protein		<100 mg/l
Serum vit B$_{12}$ folic acid and red cell folate etc.	Micronutrient pool	Low normal or abnormally low levels
Immunological		
Total peripheral lymphocyte count	Protein–calorie malnutrition	<1200/cm^2
Delayed hypersensitivity skin testing, e.g. *Candida*, tuberculin, mumps		Allergy is induration reaction <5 mm within 48–72 h
Haematological		
Hb, blood film		
Prothrombin time		>17 s

handgrip dynamometer represent an attempt to use function as a parameter and have been shown to be a sensitive and accurate predictor of complications related to nutritional status. A value of less than 85% of normal in one study accurately predicted 87% of serious complications (Karran 1982). The value of anthropometric data has often been questioned (Forse & Shizgal 1980). There is substantial interobserver variation and these indices have been shown to be relatively insensitive during trials of refeeding. There is a wide range of apparently normal values and few data are available on the effects of ageing (Neale 1984).

Attempts to assess the dietary intake of an individual using retrospective dietary analysis is prone to subjectivity and is therefore inaccurate. For monitoring patients prospectively it may be more relevant to study the dynamics of nitrogen balance rather than secondary effects on plasma proteins and body mass. This is carried out mainly by the analysis of 24 h urinary samples for urea and then adding an arbitrary figure for non-urinary nitrogen losses. This of course relies on accurate intake charting and output collecting and from a practical point of view often puts excessive demands on medical and nursing resources.

Rationale and results of nutritional support

Despite the obvious link between cancer and nutrition there are few studies which have attempted to assess nutritional status in women with gynaecological malignancy. Information on the impact of nutritional support in these conditions is also scarce, both with respect to reversal of the metabolic complications of undernutrition and long term survival.

Nutritional status in gynaecologic cancer

It is now clear that 50% of hospitalized medical and surgical patients have some degree of undernutrition (Hill et al. 1975; Bistrian et al. 1976), a large proportion of whom are patients with cancer. A recent study examined the nutritional status of 97 patients with gynaecological cancer, 10% of whom had carcinoma of the vulva, the remaining patients being distributed fairly equally between cervix, endometrium and ovary (Tunca 1983). Nutritional status was assessed by standard techniques (Blackburn et al. 1977), which included loss in body weight, serum albumin and transferrin, total lymphocyte count and delayed hypersensitivity skin testing to recall antigens. The results suggested that patients with all stages of cervical, endometrial and vulval cancer, and patients with stage I and II ovarian cancer had normal or almost normal nutritional status. Patients with stage III and IV ovarian cancer, however, had impaired nutritional status with marked reduction in serum proteins and total lymphocyte count and an almost universal failure to respond to recall antigens. Weight loss was only modest, supporting the view that change in body weight alone may be a poor indicator of overall nutritional status in the cancer patient (Smale et al. 1981). It has been suggested that the reason why advanced ovarian carcinoma has profound effects on nutritional status relates to the clinically silent accumulation of a large tumour burden and its propensity to cause intestinal obstruction and segmental paralytic ileus (pseudo-obstruction).

Possible goals of nutritional support

The aims of nutritional support in any clinical setting are either to (1) restore the anthropometric and/or metabolic disturbances of undernutrition, or (2) maintain adequate nutritional state during an illness or its treatment. Thus in patients with gynaecologic malignancy one might ask whether nutritional support can (1) reverse or ameliorate the metabolic and anthropometric disturbances of cancer, (2) improve patient tolerance of surgery, chemotherapy and radiotherapy, (3) improve quality of life, and (4) enhance survival.

Reversal of metabolic and anthropometric deficits

It is now generally agreed that weight loss in excess of 10% of initial or ideal body weight of surgical patients has a negative effect on operative morbidity and mortality (Müller *et al.* 1982). Preoperative nutritional support can improve biochemical deficits in the short term (10−14 days) and will reduce the prevalence of postoperative complications (particularly major sepsis) and improve survival. Although there are no controlled studies of preoperative nutritional support in patients with gynaecologic malignancy, uncontrolled studies of postoperative support with total parenteral nutrition (TPN) have demonstrated reduction or avoidance of postoperative weight loss (Solassol & Joyeuz 1979; Solassol *et al.* 1979). Whether this was due to increase in lean body mass or merely to fluid retention is not clear, although the latter would seem more likely. A study of TPN as adjunctive therapy in bronchogenic carcinoma has shown quite clearly that, despite provision of adequate nutrition, lean body mass did not increase and the increase in body weight could be attributed solely to increase in body fat (Shike *et al.* 1984).

Nutrition support as adjunctive therapy

Surgery

Nutritional support, particularly TPN, has an important part to play in preparing patients for surgery and in supporting patients through a difficult postoperative period. Although there are no controlled prospective data to support this view, patients undergoing massive resection for advanced ovarian cancer, particularly with bowel resection in whom there is prolonged ileus, can almost certainly be maintained in a better nutritional state by intensive support during the post-operative period (Berman *et al*. 1979; Fuller & Griffiths 1979). Similarly, patients who develop proximal, high output small bowel fistulae or intestinal obstruction often require nutritional support either to maintain good nutritional status or to improve nutritional deficits prior to surgical and/or chemotherapeutic intervention.

Chemotherapy

The role of adjunctive nutritional therapy with chemotherapy is more contentious. There is evidence to suggest that intensive intravenous nutritional support has a protective effect during chemotherapy by reducing the white cell nadir (Issell *et al*. 1978). This effect appears to be most marked when nutritional support is continued for periods of 14–28 days. It is also suggested that intravenous nutritional support can reduce the nausea and vomiting associated with chemotherapy (Issell *et al*. 1978).

The provision of intensive nutritional support during chemotherapy has been put forward as a possible way by which the patient might be able to withstand more intensive or more prolonged drug treatment. Reported experience is largely anecdotal and remains to be confirmed by controlled prospective analysis. Chemotherapy and parenteral nutritional support have been used successfully in the treatment of intestinal obstruction due to ovarian cancer (Tunca 1981). Patients were supported with TPN for an average of 6 weeks during which time they received cisplatinum, doxorubicin and cyclophosphamide. Six of the seven patients responded with complete resolution of bowel obstruction. Clearly this approach may have an important part to play in rendering previously inoperable tumours suitable for surgery and may provide useful palliation in some situations.

Radiotherapy

The nutritional effects of radiotherapy are well described (Donaldson 1977), but possible protective effects of nutritional support during treatment have not been adequately examined. However, one study did suggest that the long term benefit of TPN given before and during the radiotherapy depended largely on the response of the tumour to radiation (Valerio *et al*. 1978). Weight gain was significantly higher in those patients whose tumour responded to radiotherapy than in those who failed to respond. Finally, there has been interest in the value of pulsed nutritional support given alongside each cycle of chemotherapy and continued until the nausea and vomiting has ceased and a normal diet resumed. The value of such an approach with respect to patient tolerance of chemotherapy and nutritional status requires further evaluation.

Improvement in quality of life

TPN pundits have for many years held the opinion that TPN can improve mood and give sense of well being in an otherwise ill and debilitated patient (Rickard *et al*. 1979). Cancer and cancer therapy can have profound effects on mood, emotional drives and 'energy levels' such that day to day living is no longer a pleasure. In addition, the dramatic loss of muscle bulk that occurs as a result of reduced dietary intake, surgery and bed rest probably contributes substantially to the feelings of fatigue that many patients with cancer experience. Whether intensive nutritional support can alter this situation still remains to be evaluated, but it is clearly becoming an important issue as the efficacy of cancer therapy increases and medium and long term survival becomes a reality for more patients. The pressures on women for an early resumption of normal activity both at work and in the home are probably increasing.

Effect on survival

Brennan (1981) reviewed the results of 23 prospective randomized studies which examined the impact of TPN as an adjunctive therapy during chemotherapy, surgery or radiotherapy, particularly with respect to long term survival. Although a number of these studies showed improvement in body weight and biochemical parameters, in none was there clear evidence of improved survival in patients treated with TPN. A preliminary report on patients with ovarian cancer treated by surgery and intensive chemotherapy indicated that survival was improved in patients who received adjunctive TPN. Although statistically significant the patient numbers were small and confidence limits low.

There has been considerable concern in recent years that intensive nutritional support would stimulate tumour growth and reduce host survival. Animal studies certainly support the view that TPN can disproportionately enhance tumour growth although no such observations have been reported in humans (Brennan 1981). Paradoxically, however, one might anticipate that the increase in tumour growth rate might improve its susceptibility to chemotherapy and radiotherapy, thus cancelling out any obvious negative effects of nutritional support.

Indications for TPN in gynaecologic cancer

From the foregoing discussion we must conclude, in the words of Murray Brennan (1981), that 'TPN is a major tool in the management of cancer, not a weapon for anti-cancer warfare'. TPN can also make major contributions to restoration of nutritional status prior to surgery, particularly in those patients who have lost 10% or more of their actual or ideal body weight and may be invaluable in supporting patients in the postoperative period. When tumour resection has been extensive and when bowel or urinary tract anastomoses have been constructed one might argue that TPN is advisable merely to reduce the likelihood of post-operative complications. Similarly TPN may be invaluable in the short term management of intestinal obstruction, pseudo-obstruction or intestinal fistulae, largely to support the patient whilst exposed to other therapeutic modalities. The role of nutritional support during radiotherapy or chemotherapy is unclear although future studies may highlight specific situations where its impact may be important.

Methods of nutritional support

Once the clinical decision has been made that a patient with gynaecological malignancy is malnourished or likely to become so during treatment the most appropriate route for the provision of nutrients must be determined. In most respects these women are no different from patients with non-gynaecological malignancies. Some, however, present with their disease at a relatively young age and many face major surgery. Major elective surgery can increase the basal energy expenditure by 15–20% and energy expenditure may increase further by 20–50% in patients with septicaemia or peritonitis (Silk 1982). Prevention, of course, is always better than cure and it may be that clinicians should offer nutritional support at an early stage to patients likely to be exposed to these forms of stress. In some centres any patient likely to be in hospital for more than 15 days and who is likely to ingest less than 1000 kcal per day is considered appropriate for some form of nutritional support (Brennan 1982). To regain a kilogram of body tissue may require up to 8000 kcal and 50 g of nitrogen (Allison 1984), but problems of supplying this amount to sick patients can be enormous.

Enteral nutrition

Whenever possible the enteral route should be used for nutritional support. The success of this approach is dependent on both the accessibility of the intestinal tract and on its ability to absorb the nutrients presented. Enteral feeding is simpler, safer and cheaper than parenteral feeding and has the major advantage that it is more physiological. There is evidence to suggest that nutrients administered by this route are better assimilated. In addition the continued presence of dietary substrates in the intestine is vital for the maintenance of intestinal mucosal integrity, which tends to diminish in patients supported parenterally. Enteral nutritional support may be provided by (1) oral supplements (oroenteral nutrition), (2) nasoenteral feeding by nasogastric or nasoenteral tube, and (3) jejunostomy feeding.

Simple dietary oral supplementation is often still recommended as an initial step by many clinicians, but more often than not this fails to provide sufficient nutrients, particularly in patients with advanced malignancy, those recovering from major surgery or undergoing intensive anti-cancer chemotherapy. These individuals simply lack the drive to eat for many reasons including profound anorexia, taste disturbance, lassitude and abdominal discomfort. They therefore fail to take adequate quantities of liquid oral supplements which in general are less appetizing than normal food. Many patients dislike the idea of nasogastric feeding and it is often reasonable therefore to allow a 24–48-h trial of oral supplementation if only to demonstrate that this approach to nutritional support is inadequate. Accurate quantification of the volume of feed consumed during this period is essential. Some of the available supplementary feeds and their composition are shown in Table 18.3.

Nasogastric and nasoenteral feeding

The standard Ryles nasogastric tube used for gastric suction and in the past for bolus feeding is now quite unacceptable for providing enteral nutritional support. Use for more than a few days may cause inflammation and ulceration in the oesophagus and is uncomfortable for the patient. The new generation of soft, fine bore nasogastric tubes with internal diameters of 1 mm or slightly more should now be used routinely. A variety of tubes are available made from different materials including polyvinyl chloride (Clinifeed), polyurethane (Dobhoff, Corpak–Silk) and silicone. Some tubes have a flexible guide wire to stiffen the tube during placement while others have mercury weighted tips (Meguid *et al*. 1985). In an alert co-operative patient the tubes can be passed by the conventional technique but in others an endoscopic approach may be necessary (Keohane *et al*. 1983a). There is evidence that gastric atony is significantly more prolonged than ileus of the small intestine and thus a slightly longer weighted duodenal tube can be used early in the postoperative period.

Nasogastric tubes for enteral feeding often become displaced or inadvertently pulled out but this should not be seen as a sign of failure. The tube simply needs to be replaced and feeding recommenced. One study showed that the average time that a tube remained in position was only 3 days.

Jejunostomy feeding has been used for many years traditionally by a large bore tube placed at laparotomy. For patients who are likely to require prolonged postoperative feeding, placement of a fine bore jejunostomy tube should always

Table 18.3. Preparations for oral supplementary feeding*

Feed	Protein (g)	Fat (g)	Carbohydrate (g)	Osmolality (mOsm/kg)
Build Up	114	70	244	675
Complan	80	64	220	420

* Nutrient values for 2 l. Total energy content for 2 l of Build Up is 2000 kcal and for Complan 1800 kcal. Feeds listed in Table 18.4 may also be used as supplementary sip feeds.

be considered at the time of laparotomy (Dunn *et al.* 1980). They produce little if any discomfort to the patient, can be used early in the postoperative period and when no longer required can easily be 'pulled' without significant leakage. These tubes can also be placed at a mini-laparotomy using either local or regional anaesthesia (Fig. 18.1).

Enteral feed should no longer be administered by the bolus technique. Continuous feeding from a large reservoir either by gravity drip or a constant infusion pump has minimized the common side effects of nausea, diarrhoea and vomiting. It is now considered unnecessary to gradually increase the strength of the feed at the beginning of enteral feeding but concomitant antibiotic therapy (oral or parenteral) is commonly associated with diarrhoea in enterally fed patients (Keohane *et al.* 1983b).

Complete enteral feeds

The supplemental feeds shown in Table 18.3 are not suitable for long term enteral nutrition as they do not necessarily contain sufficient nutrients, notably vitamins and trace elements. Complete feeds may be considered according to their composition namely (1) whole protein feeds; (2) partial protein hydrolysates and (3) amino acid based feeds containing either glucose polymer or a combination of polymer and free glucose. Examples of some of these feeds and their composition are shown in Table 18.4. In most situations a whole protein, complex carbohydrate preparation is the feed of choice. These have two major advantages in that they are relatively inexpensive and tend to have lower osmolalities than the hydrolysate or elemental feeds. Ideally an enteral feed should have an osmolality as close as possible to that of human plasma (285 mOsm/kg) as introduction of a hypertonic solution into the intestinal lumen initiates water secretion such that the luminal

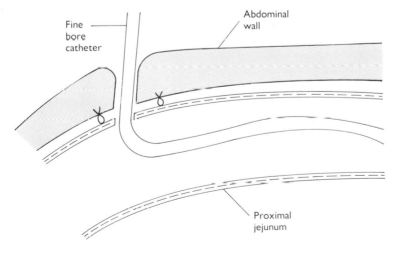

Fig. 18.1. Fine bore jejunostomy tube placed at mini-laparotomy.

Table 18.4a.   Some complete enteral feeds: whole protein*

Feed	Protein (g)	Fat (g)	Carbohydrate (g)	Osmolality (mOsm/kg)
Clinifeed Iso (Roussell)	56	82	261	270
Ensure (Abbott)	70	70	275	380
Osmolite (Abbott)	70	73	274	263
Fortison Std (Cow & Gate)	80	80	240	260
Enteral 400 (SHS)	58	78	288	330
Fresubin (Fresenius)	76	68	276	300–340
Isocal (Mead Johnston)	64	84	252	300
Triosorbon (Merck)	81	81	238	238
Nutrauxil (KabiVitrium)	76	68	276	350

* Nutrient values for 2 l. Total energy content for 2 l of each feed is 2000 kcal.
SHS: Scientific Hospital Supplies.

Table 18.4b.   Some complete enteral feeds: peptide based*

Feed	Protein (g)	Fat (g)	Carbohydrate (g)	Osmolality (mOsm/kg)
Peptisorbon (Merck)	81	26	350	400
Nutranel (Roussell)	80	20	372	410
Reabilan (Roussell)	63	78	263	300
Peptide 2+ (SHS)	56	72	252	288
Salvipeptid (MCP Pharmaceuticals)	67	24	380	450

* Nutrient values for 2 l. Total energy content for 2 l of each feed is 2000 kcal with the exception of Peptide 2+, 1800 kcal.
SHS: Scientific Hospital Supplies.

contents are rendered isotonic. Thus, the hypertonicity of elemental feeds is thought to be an important factor when diarrhoea is a complication. Partial hydrolysate or elemental feeds are really only indicated when hydrolysis of dietary substrates is likely to be impaired. This may occur in severe pancreatic exocrine insufficiency although it might be argued that this could equally well be dealt with by providing pancreatic enzyme supplements. Hydrolysis may be rate

Table 18.4c. Some complete enteral feeds: amino acid based (elemental)*

Feed	Protein (g)	Fat (g)	Carbohydrate (g)	Osmolality (mOsm/kg)
Vivonex Std. (Eaton Lab)	41	3	460	610
Flexical (Mead Johnston)	45	68	304	550
Elemental 028 (SHS)	40	27	312	450

* Nutrient values for 2 l. Total energy content for 2 l of each feed is 2000 kcal.
SHS: Scientific Hospital Supplies.

limiting in some patients with the short bowel syndrome. This can occur in patients with gynaecological malignancy after extensive resection for radiation enteritis or possibly when a substantial proportion of the small intestine has either been resected or bypassed in advanced ovarian cancer.

Complications of enteral feeding

Incorrect tube placement and inappropriate delivery of enteral feed must be avoided at all cost. The position of the tube should always be checked radiologically before enteral feeding is begun. The majority of modern fine bore tubes are radio-opaque and can be localized either by fluoroscopy or plain X-ray. Enteral feeds have inadvertently been administered intravenously but this is now totally avoidable if enteral administration sets with reversed luer-locks are used, thus ensuring that enteral and parenteral systems are totally incompatible. Oesophageal damage has been dramatically reduced by the use of fine bore tubes made of softer materials. However, after extended periods of feeding oesophagitis, gastro-oesophageal reflux and peptic stricture can occur. Aspiration of feed is a potential danger, particularly in debilitated patients. Fine bore tubes may become blocked but this is now uncommon, with commercially available liquid feeds administered at an appropriate rate.

The most frequent clinical side effects of enteral feeding are nausea, abdominal distension and diarrhoea. These symptoms are generally attributed to the rapid delivery of hypertonic solutions into the intestine and may occur in up to 25% of patients. Concurrent antibiotic therapy has also been implicated and *Clostridium difficile* enterocolitis should always be considered as a possible cause. Bacterial contamination of feeds is no longer a significant problem when commercially available sterile liquid preparations are used. Many patients gain weight during the initial phase of enteral feeding and this is almost invariably due to fluid retention. Metabolic complications include hyperglycaemia, hypokalaemia and hypophosphataemia all of which are avoidable by regular monitoring. A third or more of patients may develop abnormalities of liver biochemistry, usually minor elevations of alkaline phosphatase and the transaminases. This is usually due to fatty infiltration of the liver which rapidly reverts to normal when feeding is stopped.

Parenteral nutrition

Since the observation that normal growth of dogs could be sustained with total parenteral nutrition (TPN) (Dudrick *et al.* 1968), this technique has been widely accepted for the management of intestinal failure and for pre- and postoperative support of patients with a variety of other disorders. It is expensive and potentially hazardous and is demanding with respect to nursing and hospital pharmacy resources. It is thus essential that the indication for TPN in an individual patient is clearly established before treatment is begun. It must be agreed by all involved in the patient's care that nutritional support cannot be achieved by the enteral route, having given full consideration to endoscopic placement of tubes, gastrostomy and jejunostomy. Brief periods of TPN of less than one week duration should be avoided as it exposes the patient to many of the risks with little, if any, measurable benefits. When providing nutritional support for patients with malignant disease the use of TPN must be considered as part of the overall management strategy of the patient. This is particularly important in patients with advanced disease in whom cure is unlikely.

Indications for TPN

Intestinal failure due to the short bowel syndrome (usually massive intestinal resection for mesenteric infarction, Crohn's disease or radiation enteritis), extensive destructive intestinal disease (Crohn's disease, radiation enteritis), high output enterocutaneous fistulae and advanced motility disorders (idiopathic intestinal pseudo-obstruction) are all well established indications for TPN some of which may ultimately require long term TPN at home. Radiation enteritis and intestinal pseudo-obstruction occur in patients with gynaecologic malignancy as does true mechanical intestinal obstruction.

Probably the most important and most frequently used indication for TPN in gynaecologic malignancy is before and after major surgery. Following surgery, continued parenteral support may be required for patients undergoing intensive anti-cancer chemotherapy particularly if there has been preoperative intestinal obstruction or bowel-associated metastases.

Administration of TPN

The success of TPN depends heavily on (1) central venous catheter placement and management, (2) delivery of appropriate nutrients, and (3) monitoring to avoid metabolic complications.

Central venous catheter placement and management

The majority of modern central venous catheters are now made of silicone elastomer which is softer and less thrombogenic than polyvinyl chloride. The most commonly used catheters for TPN are those with detachable hubs (such as the Vygon Neutricath S) which makes insertion and tunnelling considerably easier. These catheters can be placed under local anaesthesia using a percutaneous Seldinger technique and the infraclavicular approach into the subclavian vein. There are larger catheters (Broviac & Hickman catheters) with a Teflon cuff which serves to fix the catheter in its subcutaneous tunnel and may limit retrograde spread of microorganisms. These large catheters are generally inserted by a surgical cut-down technique rather than blind puncture, often under general anaesthesia. More recently totally implanted catheters have been developed which incorporate a stainless steel chamber with latex injection port, all of which is located subcutaneously. This development should reduce the incidence of catheter sepsis and gives patients more freedom. Some individuals dislike percutaneous needle insertion which is necessary for administration of parenteral fluids.

Catheter insertion should always be carried out under full aseptic conditions either in an operating theatre or another designated room with an image intensification radiographic facility. It is common practice to tunnel the catheter 7–10 cm away from the site of vein entry. This was initially developed to reduce catheter sepsis although recent studies have shown that with appropriate nursing care there is no difference in the incidence of sepsis between tunnelled and non-tunnelled catheters (Keohane et al. 1983). Nevertheless, the practice has continued because the tunnel provides better anchorage for the catheter and at the same time makes catheter management easier. The technique of catheter insertion has been extensively described (Peters et al. 1984) and is relatively straightforward in expert hands. Complications of insertion include arterial puncture and dissection (subclavian and carotid arteries), pleural and mediastinal injuries (pneumothorax, haemomediastinum), embolism (air or catheter), lymphatic damage and neurological problems such as brachial plexus damage and rarely, fatal cerebro-vascular accidents. Care should be taken to ensure that the catheter tip is in the superior vena cava as right atrial or ventricular placement can cause cardiac dysrhythmias or rarely pericardial tamponade following catheter perforation of the right ventricle.

Once placed the most important catheter related complication is that of infection (Cooper & Hopkins 1985; Pettigrew et al. 1985). Infection may be localized, usually beginning at the catheter exit site in the skin with retrograde extension along the skin tunnel. This produces reddening and skin tenderness sometimes associated with discharge from the exit site. Infection may become disseminated to produce bacteraemia or even septicaemia. Traditionally it has been thought that catheter colonization by bacteria occurred by retrograde spread from the skin exit sites. However, recent work suggests that colonization of the catheter hub most commonly accounts for catheter related sepsis (Linares et al. 1985). The most common infecting organisms are *Staphylococcus aureus, Staphylococcus epidermis, Escherichia coli* and *Candida* sp. Diagnosis of catheter related sepsis requires the taking of several peripheral and central (blood is drawn back through the catheter) blood cultures and if it is decided to remove the catheter, the tip of the catheter should be sent for culture (Bozetti *et al.* 1984; Cooper & Hopkins 1985).

Faced with catheter related sepsis, the main decision centres around whether to remove the catheter or to leave it in place and treat with appropriate antibiotics. This decision will depend on the availability of other venous access sites, the patient's immune status and the immediate requirements for parenteral therapy. A balance has to be obtained between the risk of catheter infection and the loss of venous access in these often difficult patients. Many units have developed a modified Seldinger technique where a catheter can be removed and replaced with a new one over a guide wire, thus preserving the access site (Brennan 1981). However, fever and infection are very common in patients who are debilitated particularly those receiving cytotoxic chemotherapy. Many studies have failed to significantly incriminate venous catheters in the aetiology of infections and fever, unless there is obvious involvement of the site of catheter entry. A large study showed that 97 of 335 (27%) catheters were removed for suspicion of catheter sepsis; of these only 20 (5%) showed clear bacteriological and clinical agreement of infection (Ryan *et al.* 1974).

Superior vena caval thrombosis is a potential complication and has been reported in up to 25% of autopsy studies (Ryan *et al.* 1974). Fibrin sleeve formation around the catheter appears to be a common finding and in one study was reported in 37 of 38 silicone rubber catheters after a mean catheter life of 55 days. There was however, no evidence in this study of venous thrombosis (Laidlaw *et al.* 1983). Management involves either catheter removal or temporary withdrawal of TPN followed by treatment with heparin alone or after initial treatment with streptokinase. Other important catheter complications include occlusion and both air and catheter embolism.

Parenteral solutions and their administration

Since the need for TPN virtually excludes nutrient intake by any other route, all nutrient requirements must be supplied by this route including amino acids, electrolytes, vitamins, trace elements, water and an energy source (glucose, lipid). Current practice is to administer approximately 50% of the energy source as dextrose and the remainder as lipid. The latter has the advantage of increased calorie density compared to carbohydrate and avoids the excessive hyperosmolality associated with glucose infusions. Some of the available amino acid solutions are shown in Table 18.5. Nitrogen requirement is best calculated from analysis of body secretions in the form of urine, faeces, fistula losses, etc. In practice this can often be difficult but the nitrogen output can be derived from the 24 h urine urea (mmol/24 h) multiplied by 0.028 which converts millimoles of urea to grams of

Table 18.5. Some amino acid preparations for TPN

Preparation		Nitrogen content (g/l)	Na (mmol/l)	K (mmol/l)
Synthamin	9	9.1	73	60
(Travenol)	14	14.0	73	60
	17	16.5	73	60
Vamin	9	9.4	50	20
(KabiVitrium)	14	13.5	100	50
Aminoplex	12	12.4	35	30
(Gelstlich)	14	13.4	35	30
	25	24.9	35	30

nitrogen. To this figure is added an arbitrary amount, usually 2–4 g to allow for non-urinary nitrogen losses. Nitrogen requirements will usually be satisfactory if given as 0.2 g/kg (14 g nitrogen for 70 kg person) although this may need to be increased to 0.3 kg/g nitrogen in hypercatabolic patients. Energy requirements are often calculated on the basis of 40 kcal/kg/24 h which would provide 2800 kcal/24 h for a 70 kg person. Energy and nitrogen sources can be combined together with appropriate electrolytes, trace elements and vitamins in a collapsible 3-l bag prepared under sterile conditions in the hospital pharmacy or through a commercial compounding service. These bags must be prepared under strict aseptic conditions and no additions should be made to the bag once it leaves the pharmacy.

In recent years it has become clear that TPN prescriptions should be simplified and many hospitals now prepare two or three standard TPN formulations with respect to energy and nitrogen contents. Typically these might contain 14 g nitrogen and 1200 kcal as glucose to which a further 500 or 1000 kcal can be added as intralipid. A second regimen might consist of 9 g nitrogen and 800 kcal as glucose to which 500 or 1000 kcal intralipid could be added. Electrolyte requirements need close attention particularly when there are increased losses. If losses are extremely high additional water and electrolytes can be given as a separate infusion following the administration of the 24 h requirements of TPN.

At the start of TPN, nutrients are generally infused continuously using a volumetric pump over 18–24 h. Once patients are stabilized the infusion time can be reduced such that the majority of the TPN is given at night allowing the patient to have several hours free during the day. Catheter patency can be preserved by filling the catheter in the interim period with heparinized saline.

Complications

Early complications of TPN include hyperglycaemia and dehydration, hypoglycaemia usually if the infusion is stopped abruptly, abnormalities of water and

electrolyte balance particularly salt and water retention and hyper- or hypocal-
caemia, hypomagnesaemia and hypophosphataemia. Metabolic acidosis is now
relatively uncommon since the introduction of buffered amino acid solutions and
the virtual disappearance of fructose and ethanol as energy substrates. After
prolonged TPN there are often abnormalities of liver biochemistry, particularly
elevations of alkaline phosphatase and the transaminases. Care must be taken to
avoid micronutrient deficiency, notably vitamins D and K.

Monitoring of patients on TPN is essential and a simplified approach is
outlined in Table 18.6.

Nutritional support at home

With the increasing pressure on hospital beds and the economic strictures in the
health service there are incentives for patients to receive as much of their
treatment as is possible at home. In reasonably fit and well motivated patients
who have supportive friends and relatives, enteral nutrition via nasogastric tube
can be performed safely and effectively at home. Patients can be taught to pass
their own nasogastric tube on a daily basis if they do not wish to maintain the
tube *in situ* throughout the day. This approach has been used to give nocturnal
nutritional supplements and could also be used for improving nutritional status
before surgery.

There is likely to be an increasing demand for home TPN in women with
intestinal obstruction due to advanced and incurable gynaecological malignancy.
Other than the intestinal obstruction, the woman can be otherwise well. This is a
substantial undertaking requiring not only the financial approval of the patient's

Table 18.6. A patient monitoring schedule for TPN

	Parameter	Frequency*
Clinical	Temp, pulse, blood pressure	4-hourly
	Body weight Fluid balance Catheter inspection	Daily
Blood tests	Urea, electrolytes glucose, blood count	Daily
	Biochemistry, including Mg^{++} and Zn^{++}	Twice weekly
	Prothrombin time	Twice monthly
Urine	Glucose, urea	Daily

* In patients receiving long term TPN either in hospital or at
home, the frequency of testing would be reduced significantly
once stabilized on a particular feeding regimen.

District General Manager (yearly cost approximately £30 000) but a considerable input from the patient and relatives, since it is they who will carry out the day to day running of TPN. Nevertheless in selected patients who have been adequately trained, home TPN can increase both the survival time and quality of life. However, before entering into such a situation all the implications of such a venture need to be clearly discussed, not only with the hospital team but with the general practitioner and other health workers in the community.

References

Allison S.P. (1984) Univers. Hosp. Nottingham. Ent. Parent. Feed. *Prescriber's Journal*, **24** (1), 2−11.

Ames B.N. (1983) Dietary carcinogens and anti-carcinogens. *Science*, **221**, 1256−64.

Armstrong B. & Doll R. (1975) Environmental factors and cancer incidence and mortality in different countries with special reference to dietary practises. *Int. J. Cancer*, **15**, 617.

Baker J.P., Detsky A.S., Wesson D.E., Walman S.L., Stewart S., Whitewell, J., Langer B. & Jejeebhoy K.N. (1982) Nutritional assessment − a comparison of clinical judgement and objective measurement. *N. Engl. J. Med.*, **306**, 969−72.

Berman M.L., Hamrell C.E., Lagasse L.D., Ballon S.C., Watring W.G., Schlesinger R.E. & Donaldson R.C. (1979) Parenteral nutrition by peripheral vein in the management of gynecologic oncology patients. *Gynecol. Oncol.*, **7**, 318−24.

Bernstein I.L. & Sigmundi R.A. (1980) Tumour anorexia: a learned food aversion? *Science*, **209**, 416−18.

Bernstein I.L., Webster M.M. & Bernstein I.D. (1982) Food aversions in children receiving chemotherapy for cancer. *Cancer*, **50** (12), 2961−63.

Bistrian B.R., Blackburn G.L., Vitale J., Cochran D. & Naylor J. (1976) Prevalence of malnutrition in general medical patients. *JAMA*, **235**, 1567 70.

Blackburn G.L., Bistrian B.R., Maini B.S., Schlamm H.T. & Smith M.F. (1977) Nutritional and metabolic assessment of the hospitalized patient *JPEN*, **1** (1), 11−22.

Blayney D.W. & Longo D.L. (1983) Ovarian cancer: epidemiology, diagnosis and management. *Comprehensive Therapy*, **9**, 50−58.

Bozzetti F., Pognoni A.M. & Del Veichio M. (1980) Excessive calorie expenditure as a cause of malnutrition in patients with cancer. *Surg. Gynecol. Obstet.*, **150** (2), 229−34.

Bozzetti F., Terno G. & Bonfanti G. (1984) Blood culture as a guide for the diagnosis of central venous catheter sepsis. *J. Parent. Ent. Nutr.*, **8**, 396−98.

Brown M.J. (1954) Symposium on total care of surgical patients; nutritional problems in surgery. *S. Clin. North America*, **34**, 1239−48.

Brennan M.F. (1981) Total parenteral nutrition in the cancer patient. *N. Engl. J. Med.*, **305**, 375−82.

Brennan M.F. (1982) Supportive care of the cancer patient. *In*: De Vita *et al. Principles and Practice of Oncology*. Plymouth: Lippincott. pp. 1628−40.

Butterworth C.E. & Blackburn G.L. (1975) Hospital malnutrition and how to assess the nutritional status of patients. *Nutr. Today.*, **10**, 818.

Cooper G.L. & Hopkins C.C. (1985) Rapid diagnosis of intravascular catheter associated infection by direct gram staining of catheter segments. *N. Engl. J. Med.*, **312**, 1142−47.

Copeland E.M., MacFadyen B.V., Lanzotti V.J. & Dudrick S.J. (1975) Intravenous hyperalimentation as an adjunct to cancer chemotherapy. *Am. J. Surg.*, **129** (2), 167−73.

Cutler M.G. & Schneider R. (1974) Tumours and hormonal changes produced in rats by subcutaneous injections of linoleic acid hydroperoxide. *Food Cosmet. Toxicol.*, **12**, 451−97.

De Wys W.D. (1978) Changes in taste sensation and feeding behaviour in cancer patients: a review. *J. Hum. Nutr.*, **32**, 447−53.

Dickerson J.W.T. (1984) Nutrition in the cancer patient: a review. *J. Roy. Soc. Med.*, **77**, 309−15.

Donaldson S.S. (1977) Nutritional consequences of radiotherapy. *Cancer Res.*, **37**, 2407−13.

Dudrick S.J., Wilmore D.W., Vars H.M. & Rhoads J.E. (1968) Long term total parenteral nutrition with growth, development and positive nitrogen balance. *Surgery*, **64**, 134 42.

Dunn E.L., Moore E.E. & Bohus R.W. (1980) Immediate post-operative feeding following massive abdominal trauma: the catheter jejunostomy. *J. P. E. N.*, **4**, 393—95.

Forse R.A. & Shizgal H.M. (1980) The assessment of malnutrition. *Surgery*, **80**, 17—24.

Fuller A.F. & Griffiths C.T. (1979) Ovarian cancer cachexia—surgical interactions. *Gynecol. Oncol.*, **8**, 301—10.

Hatfield A.R.W. (1982) Hyperalimentation. *Br. J. Hosp. Med.*, **28**, 220—33.

Hill G.L., Blackett R.L., Burkinshal L. *et al.* (1975) Proceedings: high incidence of malnutrition in hospitalised surgical patients. *Br. J. Surg.*, **63** (8), 663—64.

Hreshchyshyn M.M. (1982) Gynaecologic cancer. *In*: Holland J.F. & Frei III E. (eds), *Cancer Medicine*. 2nd Edn. Lea & Febiger. pp. 1957—2056.

Issell B.F., Valdivieso M., Zaren H.A., Dudrick S.J., Freireich E.J., Copeland E.W. & Bodey G.P. (1978) Protection against chemotherapy toxicity by intravenous hyperalimentation. *Cancer Treat. Rep.*, **62**, 1139—43.

Jacobs M.M. (1983) Selenium inhibition of 1,2-dimethylhydrazine-induced colon carcinogenesis. *Cancer Res.*, **43**, 1646—49.

Karran S. (1982) Who needs nutritional support? *In*: Lumley J.S.P. & Craven J.L. (eds), *Surgical Review 3*. Pitman, London. pp. 25—61.

Keohane P.P., Attrill H. & Silk D.B.A. (1983a) Endoscopic placement of fine bore naso-gastric and naso-enteral feeding tubes. *Clin. Nutr.*, **1**, 245—47.

Keohane P.P., Atterill H., Jones B.J.M., Brown I., Frost T. & Silk D.B.A. (1983b) The role of lactose intolerance and Clostridium difficile infection in the pathogenesis of enteral feeding-associated diarrhoea. *Clin. Nutr.*, **1**, 259—64.

Klidjan A.M., Russell L. & Karran S.J. (1981) A malnutrition score for rapid nutritional assessment. *In*: *Proceedings Surgical Research Society*.

Laidlaw J.M., McIntyre P.B., Wood S.R., Bartram C.I. & Lennard-Jones J.F. (1983) A radiological study after parenteral nutrition through silicone rubber catheters: fibrin sleeves without thrombosis. *Clin. Nutr.*, **1**, 305—11.

Lew E.A. & Garfinkel L. (1979) Variations in mortality by weight in 750 000 men and women. *J. Chronic Dis.*, **32**, 563—76.

Linares J., Sitges-Serra A., Garass J., Percz J.L. & Martin R. (1985) Pathogenesis of catheter sepsis: a prospective study with quantitative and semi-quantitative culture of hub and segments. *J. Clin. Microbiol.*, **21**, 357—60.

Lingman C.H. (1983) Environmental factors in the etiology of carcinoma of the human ovary: a review. *Am. J. Indust. Med.*, **4**, 365—79.

Magee P.N. (ed.) (1982) *Banbury Report 12. Nitrosamines and Human Cancer: Cold Spring Harbor Laboratory. Cold Spring Harbor*, NY.

Matthews-Roth M.M. (1982) Anti-tumour activity of beta-carotene, Canthoxanthin and phytoene. *Oncology*, **39**, 33—37.

Meguid M.M., Eldar S. & Wahba A. (1985) The delivery of nutritional support. A pot-pourri of new devices and methods. *Cancer*, **55**, 278—89.

Müller J.M., Dienst C., Brenner U. & Pichlmaier H. (1982) Preoperative parenteral feeding in patients with gastrointestinal carcinoma. *Lancet*, **i**, 68—71.

National Academy of Sciences (1982) *Diet, Nutrition & Cancer. Assembly of Life Sciences*. National Research Council, Washington DC. National Academy Press.

Neale G. (1984) Clinical assessment of nutritional status. *Hospital Update*, **10** (10), 825—33.

Nelson J.R. (1982) Gynaecologic cancer. *In*: Holland J.F. & Frei III E. (eds), *Cancer Medicine*, 2nd Ed. Lea & Febiger. pp. 1957—2056.

Peters J.L., Belsham P.A., Taylor B.A. & Watt-Smith J.A. (1984) Vascular access—long term venous access. *Br. J. Hosp. Med.*, **32** (5), 230—42.

Pettigrew R.A., Lang S.D.R., Haydock B.A., Parry B.R., Bremner D.A. & Hill G.L. (1985) Catheter related sepsis in patients on intravenous nutrition: a prospective study of quantitative catheter cultures and guidewire changes for suspected sepsis. *Br. J. Surg.*, **72**, 52—55.

Rickard K.A., Grosfeld J.L., Kirksey A., Ballantine T.V.N. & Baehner R.L. (1979) Reversal of protein—energy malnutrition in children during treatment of advanced neoplastic disease. *Ann. Surg.*, **190**, 771—81.

Ryan J.A., Abel R.M., Abbott W.M., Hopkins C.L., Clesney T., McColley R., Phillips K. & Fishcer J.E. (1974) Catheter complications in total parenteral nutrition. *N Engl. J. Med.*, **290** (14), 757−61.

Scherstein T., Bennegard K., Ekman I., Karlberg I., Svaninger G., Teinell M. & Lundholm K. (1982) *In*: Wesdap R.I.C. & Soeters P.B. (eds), *Clinical Nutrition.* pp. 143−52.

Shike M., Russell D.McR., Detsky A.S., Harrison J.E., McNeill K.G., Shepherd F.A., Feld R., Evans W.K., Khursheed N. & Jeejeebhoy K.N. (1984) Changes in body composition in patients with small-cell lung cancer. The effect of total parenteral nutrition as an adjunct to chemotherapy. *Ann. Int. Med.*, **101**, 303−9.

Silk D.B. (1982) Enteral nutrition. *Med. Int.*, **1** (15), 668−73.

Silk D.B. (1983) *Nutritional Support in Hospital Practice.* Blackwell Scientific Publications, Oxford. p. 12.

Smale F.B., Mullen L.J., Buzby P.G. & Rosato F.E. (1981) The efficacy of nutritional assessment and support in cancer surgery. *Cancer*, **47**, 2375−81.

Solassol C. & Joyeuz H. (1979) Artificial gut with complete nutritive mixtures as a major adjuvant therapy in cancer patients. *Acta. Chir. Scand.* (Suppl.), **494**, 186−87.

Solassol C., Joyeuz H. & Dubois J.B (1979) Total parenteral nutrition (TPN) with complete nutritive mixtures: an artificial gut in cancer patients. *Nutr. Cancer*, **I**, 13−18.

Studley H.O. (1936) Percentage of weight loss, a basic indicator of surgical risk. *JAMA*, **106**, 458−60.

Toth B. (1979) *In*: Miller E.C., Miller J.A., Hirono I., Sugimura T. & Tokayam S. (eds), *Naturally Occurring Carcinogens-Mutagens and Modulators of Carcinogens* (Japan Scientific 1979). Societies Press & University Park Press, Tokyo & Baltimore. pp. 57−65.

Tunca J.C. (1981) Impact of Cisplatin multiagent chemotherapy and total parenteral alimentation on bowel obstruction caused by ovarian cancer. *Gynecol. Oncol.*, **12**, 219−21.

Tunca J.C. (1983) Nutritional evaluation of gynecologic cancer patients during initial diagnosis of their disease. *Am. J. Obstet. Gynecol.*, **147** (8), 893−96.

Valerio D., Malcolm A. & Blackburn G.L. (1978) Nutritional support for cancer patients receiving abdominal and pelvic radiotherapy: a randomized prospective clinical experiment of intravenous versus oral feeding. *Surgical Forum*, **29**, 145−48.

Wassertheil-Smaller S., Romney S.L., Wylie-Rosset J. *et al.* (1981) Dietary Vit C and uterine cervical dysplasia. *Am. J. Epidemiol.*, **114**, 714−24.

Watkin D.M. (1961) Nitrogen balance as affected by neoplastic disease and its therapy. *Am. J. Clin. Nutr.*, **9**, 446−60.

Willet W.C. & MacMahon B. (1984) Diet & cancer−an overview−first of two parts. *N Engl. J. Med.*, **310**, 633−38.

Wynder E.L. (1969) Epidemiology of cancer *in situ* of the cervix. *Surg. Obstet. Gynaecol.*, **24**, 697−711.

Wynder E.L. (1976) Nutrition & cancer. *In*: W.H. Griffith Memorial Symposium, presented by American Institute of Nutrition at the 59th Annual Meeting of the Federation of American Societies for Experimental Biology. Atlantic City, New Jersey. April 15 1975. *Fedn. Proc.*, **35**.

19

Gynaecological Malignancy: Care of the Terminally Ill

MICHAEL KEARNEY

Terminal care must not be seen as some 'soft option' heralded by the phrase 'there is nothing more we can do', but as a positive form of treatment which can be both demanding and rewarding to those practising it. Terminal care implies a continuation of treatment but with a different emphasis from treatment of the earlier stages of malignant disease. Saunders (1984) has described it as a 'facet of oncology concerned with the control of symptoms instead of with the control of the tumour' but stresses that the aim of terminal care is 'not merely the absence of symptoms but that the patient and family might live to the limits of their potential' (Saunders & Baines 1983).

Bates (1985) has pointed out that the overall 'cure rate' of cancer is no more than 20–30% and that 55% of all cancer patients are incurable from time of diagnosis. These patients obviously require treatment with palliative rather than curative intent and terminal care is the final phase and logical continuation of this palliative care. In comparison to these figures there are, as outlined in previous chapters, grounds for optimism in the treatment of gynaecological malignancy. Carcinoma of the cervix and body of the uterus are often diagnosed early and with stage I disease of both tumours, 5-year survival rates of 75–90% can be expected following radical treatment (Souhami & Tobias 1986). However, carcinoma of the ovary is often diagnosed late when stage III–IV disease has (even with radical treatment) a 5-year survival rate of only 3–5% (Tobias & Griffiths 1976). It causes approximately 4000 deaths annually in the UK, making it the commonest fatal gynaecological malignancy (Baker & Diggory 1982). These patients, together with the approximately 4000 patients who die with various other forms of gynaecological malignancy in the UK each year, can present the clinician and the rest of the caring team with many challenging and often intractable problems which are examined in this chapter.

Appropriate treatment

The concept of appropriate treatment is crucial in a discussion of terminal care (Saunders 1984). It refers to a treatment regime that is tailored to each individual patient and is referenced by a number of factors including the aim of treatment (cure or palliation), the physical and emotional state of the patient and the wishes of both patient and family. While radical treatment with major side effects is appropriate for the patient with potentially curable malignancy, a similar regime will be inappropriate and unjustified in the patient whose cancer is incurable. The concept of appropriate treatment underlines the value in pausing before embarking on a new line of treatment to carefully consider the full implications of· such a treatment decision, including patient and family in such discussion.

Symptom control

The control of symptoms associated with gynaecological malignancy is obviously important from the time of diagnosis. However, when the cancer is no longer curable and the main aim is to improve the quality of the patient's remaining life, symptom control takes priority (Baines 1987a). Whatever the symptom the approach should be along the following lines.

ASSESSMENT

In essence this means diagnosis of the specific pathology underlying the symptom. A carefully taken history and detailed clinical examination will often provide this information. This clinical assessment is more important than time consuming and often distressing investigations although occasionally simple investigations are needed.

TREATMENT

Choice of the most appropriate treatment requires an understanding of the precise aetiology of the symptom (Baines 1981). Where possible one should make a single therapeutic move at a time so that it is clear whether this move has been effective or not. As part of the treatment plan it may be useful to incorporate a simple goal setting approach where the patient can be included in the planning of objectives (Lunt & Jenkins 1983).

REVIEW

Treatment must be closely monitored which means frequent reassessments so that the symptoms are controlled quickly with minimal side effects.

Pain

The incidence of pain in patients with advanced gynaecological malignancy is high — e.g. cervix 85% (Foley 1979). Severe chronic pain occurs in approximately

60% of patients with advanced terminal cancer of all sites (Twycross & Lack 1983) and although there is encouraging evidence that this pain is now being better controlled than previously (Parkes & Parkes 1984), many patients still die with uncontrolled pain (Wilkes 1984). This perpetuates the myth among remaining family and involved medical and nursing personnel that terminal cancer and pain are inseparable. Saunders (1984) has underlined the need to distinguish acute pain — 'the postoperative or post-trauma event with its built in meaning' from chronic terminal pain — 'the situation which holds the patient prisoner with no meaning other than an unnamed threat'. She has also usefully emphasized the concept of 'total pain' (Saunders & Baines 1983) which reminds us that we are not just dealing with an unpleasant sensation but a complex and dynamic situation involving not only the patient but those around her (Table 19.1). Successful pain control can only be achieved by appreciating the different components of the 'total pain' and treating each in an appropriate manner while never losing sight of the whole person.

Control of physical pain

Patients with gynaecological malignancy can have pain of many different aetiologies. The therapeutic approach will vary depending on the underlying pain mechanism (Table 19.2). Pelvic pain is common and often intractable in these patients (Baines & Kirkham 1984). The mechanism is involvement of pelvic nerves and soft tissues by tumour. Although pain of this origin is usually experienced in the pelvis itself, it may be referred elsewhere in the abdomen, in the back or legs. Patients may describe pelvic pain as 'a bearing down pain' or 'a sickening, dragging ache'. When there is invasion of or pressure on the rectum by tumour the patient may describe tenesmus, or liken the discomfort to 'sitting on a tennis ball'.

Diagnose the cause of pain

As part of the initial assessment it is helpful to use a body chart (Twycross & Lack 1983). This records the site(s) of pain, its severity as well as duration, aggravating and relieving factors and the patient's own verbatim description (Fig. 19.1). The chart, possibly used in conjunction with a simple 10 cm visual analogue scale, can be used subsequently as a baseline against which to monitor therapy.

Table 19.1. Components of total pain

Physical		
Mental		
Social	}	Total pain
Staff		
Spiritual		

Table 19.2. Treatment of pain depending on cause

Cause of pain	Primary treatment	Secondary treatment	To consider
Visceral (from involvement of pelvic or abdominal organs)	Analgesics	Steroids may help	Epidural opioids Nerve block (e.g. intrathecal for pelvic pain, coeliac plexus for abdominal pain)
Bone pain (direct spread or distant metastases)	1 Palliative radiotherapy 2 Non-steroidal anti-inflammatory drugs 3 Immobilization (e.g. pinning)	Analgesics	Nerve block Steroids may help
Soft tissue infiltration	Analgesics	NSAID or steroids may help	Nerve block
Nerve compression	Analgesics	High dose steroids	Nerve block
Deafferentation pain	Anticonvulsants (e.g. carbamazepine) Centrally active drugs (e.g. tricyclics and phenothiazines)	Steroids	Epidural steroids or local anaesthetic
Secondary infection Deep	Systemic antibiotics Local surgery	Analgesics	Nerve block
Superficial	Systemic antibiotics Local applications (e.g. povidone, iodine)	Analgesics	Nerve block
Colic in bowel obstruction	Stop peristaltic drugs Faecal softeners Antispasmodics	Analgesics	Nerve block (coeliac plexus)
Chronic oedema	Intermittent positive pressure machine Pressure bandage, sleeve or stocking	Diuretics Analgesics	Palliative radiotherapy High dose steroids may help
Ascites	1 Oral diuretics 2 Paracentesis	Analgesics	Cytoxic chemo-therapy Slow intravenous infusion of diuretic
Pain in para-lysed limb(s)	Physiotherapy and frequent passive movement	NSAID	Muscle relaxants

Adapted from Saunders C.M. & Baines M. (1983) *Living with Dying* (published by Oxford University Press, Oxford, with permission).

Simple procedures

Simple pain relieving procedures must be thought of at an early stage. Faecal disimpaction is the appropriate treatment for rectal discomfort, spasms of rectal pain or abdominal colic caused by constipation. Barrier creams or catheterization may ease the pain from excoriated skin in a patient with urinary incontinence. Steroid retention enemas are useful in patients with mucus secretion or tenesmus due to rectal invasion by tumour and anaesthetic jelly applied locally may relieve a painful malignant ulcer.

Drugs

Analgesics (and in particular opioid analgesics) correctly used are the mainstay of treatment of chronic cancer pain. A selection of oral analgesics is given in Table 19.3. Many doctors are, however, afraid to commence patients on opioids because of fears of addiction, tolerance, respiratory depression and excessive sedation. Previous experience of starting a patient on too large a dose of an opioid too late may have compounded a misbelief that introducing opioids is 'active euthanasia'. However, it 'is not necessary to kill the patient to kill pain' (Saunders 1984) and we now know that these other fears are also unfounded in this context (Twycross & Lack 1983). Hospice experience has demonstrated quite clearly the need and effectiveness of giving regular, prophylactic analgesia for the chronic pain of terminal malignancy. Intermittent analgesia, given on an 'as required' (p.r.n.) basis fails to relieve chronic pain. Oral morphine or diamorphine can be given in simple solution with chloroform or tap water on a 4-hourly basis and are equally efficacious if allowance is made for the morphine to diamorphine potency rate of 1:1.5 (Twycross 1977a) (Table 19.4). The so-called 'Brompton Cocktail' has no advantages and definite disadvantages as it contains cocaine and alcohol in addition to the opioid (British National Formulary 1988). If one uses morphine or diamorphine in solution to achieve pain control, the 4-hourly regime allowing a fine degree of titration, one can then subsequently transfer to an equivalent dose of slow release morphine sulphate (MST). The twice daily administration of MST has obvious advantages in terms of convenience and compliance and is especially useful in the home. Because of the linear nature of its dose/response curve (Fig. 19.2), morphine or diamorphine can be introduced in a very small dose when mild analgesics cease to be effective and increased as necessary every 24 to 48 h until pain control is achieved. The following steps are suggested: 5→10→20→30→45→60→80→100→120→160 mg. Most pain will be controlled on a dose of morphine 30 mg or diamorphine 20 mg 4-hourly orally or less (Twycross 1974) although it is occasionally necessary to use very much larger doses. If pain persists despite escalating opioid dosage, the use of adjuvant analgesia or other pain relieving procedures should be considered while asking if the diagnosis of the cause of the pain is correct. Side effects of the

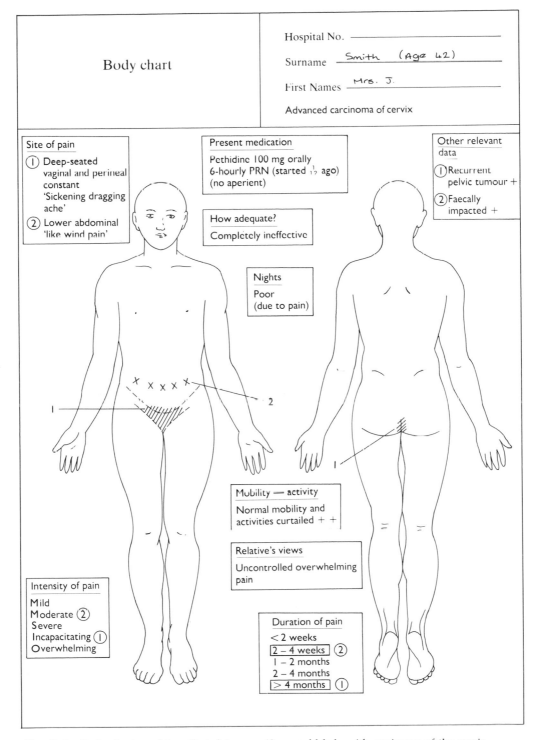

Fig. 19.1. Body chart used to collect data on a 42-year old lady with carcinoma of the cervix

Table 19.3. A selection of oral analgesics

Category	Drug	Dose	Dose interval
Non opioids	Paracetamol	1 g	4-hourly
Weak opioids	Dextropropoxyphene and paracetamol (co-praxamol)	2 tablets	4–6 hourly
	Dihydrocodeine tartrate in controlled release tablets (DHC continus)	60 mg	12-hourly
Strong opioids	Morphine SO$_4$ or HCl exilir	5–30 mg*	4-hourly
	Diamorphine HCl elixir	2.5–20 mg*	4-hourly
	Morphine sulphate in controlled release tablets (MST continus) 10, 30, 60, 100 mg tablets	10–100 mg*	12-hourly

* Recommended 'maximum' doses have no relevance to control of chronic pain. While a majority of patients' pain will be controlled in the dose range listed, a minority of patients will need very much larger doses.

Table 19.4. Morphine and diamorphine equivalents

Oral morphine:oral diamorphine potency ratio 1.5:1
Oral *dia*morphine to injected diamorphine: oral dose mg

$$\frac{}{2} \qquad \text{4-hourly}$$

Oral *mor*phine to injected diamorphine: oral dose mg

$$\frac{}{3} \qquad \text{4-hourly}$$

Morphine in solution to MST: total daily dose mg

$$\frac{}{2} \qquad \text{12-hourly}$$

MST to morphine in solution: total daily dose mg

$$\frac{}{6} \qquad \text{4-hourly}$$

Oral morphine to epidural morphine: total daily dose mg

$$\frac{}{20} \qquad \text{12-hourly}$$

opioids can be minimized by frequent review and fine adjustment of dose against pain. Common side effects that do occur with opioids and need to be anticipated are constipation (requiring a combination of laxatives which both

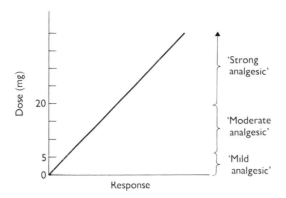

Fig. 19.2. Morphine dose-response curve

induce peristalsis (e.g. senna, bisacodyl) and soften the stool (e.g. lactulose, docusate)) (Drugs and Therapeutic Bulletin 1988) and nausea and vomiting requiring, at least initially, a centrally acting antiemetic.

When oral administration of an analgesic is not appropriate, alternative routes must be considered.

SUBLINGUAL

Buprenorphine 0.2 mg 8-hourly is equivalent to morphine 7 mg 4-hourly and its dose range is 0.2 mg−1.6 mg t.i.d. (Twycross & Lack 1984). However, being an agonist−antagonist, buprenorphine may antagonize the analgesic effect of a pure agonist such as morphine given concurrently (Vere 1978) and has an analgesic 'ceiling' at a daily dose of about 5 mg.

Phenazocine 5 mg is equivalent to 20 mg of oral morphine 4-hourly (Twycross & Lack 1983) and can be given in a dose of 2.5−20 mg 6-hourly. Both these drugs have the advantage of being acceptable to a patient who is unable to swallow analgesics for whatever reason.

RECTAL

Morphine suppositories are available in a range of strengths: 10, 15, 20, 30 and 60 mg. An alternative is oxycodone pectinate by suppository where 30 mg suppositories given 8-hourly are equivalent to 20 mg of oral morphine given 4 hourly (Drugs and Therapeutic Bulletin 1979).

PARENTERAL

Either morphine or diamorphine may be given parenterally when the equivalent dose by injection is half the oral dose of the same opioid the patient has been taking (Table 19.4). As diamorphine hydrochloride is twenty times more soluble than morphine sulphate it has the practical advantage of reducing the volume of the injection (Editorial, *Lancet* 1984).

If diamorphine is being given alone it can be given subcutaneously but if in combination with another drug should be given intramuscularly. It is rarely, if ever, necessary to give diamorphine intravenously and this route is best avoided as it is more likely to induce tolerance. Continuous subcutaneous infusion of diamorphine is useful for the patient who needs parenteral analgesia and has the advantage of avoiding the discomfort of 4-hourly injections and of giving steady plasma drug levels. A syringe pump such as the Graseby Medical Syringe Driver may be used. The 24-h parenteral requirement of opioid is dissolved in 10 ml of sterile water in a 10 ml syringe and the rate on the pump adjusted to deliver this dose via a subcutaneous butterfly needle over a 24-h period (Regnard & Newbury 1983). The mobile patient can carry the pump on a holster worn under the arm or around the neck.

EPIDURAL

Morphine and diamorphine can both be given epidurally on a 12-hourly or continuous basis where the equivalent dose is one-tenth of the oral dose (Hanna 1989) (Table 19.4). The particular indications for giving opioids in this way have not as yet been fully defined but it appears that epidural opioids will have an increasingly important role in the management of intractable pelvic pain.

Drugs to avoid

Dextromoramide and pethidine should be avoided for chronic pain because of their short clinical effect (one-and-a-half to two hours). However, dextromoramide 5–10 mg (p.r.n.) is occasionally useful for the patient with severe breakthrough pain who is already on regular and otherwise effective analgesia. Methadone has a long half-life and tends to accumulate especially in elderly patients and those with impaired renal function (Twycross 1977b). Dipipanone and cyclizine (Diconal) have limited usefulness because of the cyclizine induced side effects which accompany increase in dosage.

Adjuvant analgesia

This is often necessary and will vary according to the underlying pathology.

ANTIBIOTICS

Superimposed infection may contribute to the pain and should be treated appropriately.

NON-STEROIDAL ANTI-INFLAMMATORY DRUGS (NSAID)

These drugs are effective in controlling pain from bone metastases. Useful NSAIDs which should be taken with or immediately after food include ketaprofen slow release 200 mg once daily, naproxen 500 mg—1 g daily in divided doses and indomethacin 75—150 mg daily in divided doses.

ANTISPASMODICS

If pain is due to smooth muscle contraction (e.g. bowel colic) drugs such as loperamide 2—4 mg, diphenoxylade and atropine (Lomotil) 1—2 tablets or hyoscine butylbromide (Buscupan) 10—20 mg are often effective. Pain from skeletal muscle spasm, on the other hand, may be helped by drugs such as diazepam 2—10 mg.

STEROIDS

These are useful coanalgesics where the pain is due to the pressure effects of tumour. They are believed to work by reducing oedema in and around the tumour (Twycross & Lack 1983). A dose of dexamethasone 4—8 mg/day can be introduced for a trial period of one week. Useful side effects of steroid therapy are increased appetite and occasionally an improved sense of well-being.

PSYCHOTROPIC DRUGS

Anxiolytics and antidepressants have a role as coanalgesics in the anxious or depressed patient by helping to elevate the pain threshold. In this group of patients they must not, however, be substituted for reassurance, counselling and diversional therapy (see below). In addition tricyclic antidepressants have been shown to have an intrinsic analgesic activity (Walsh 1986) and are particularly effective in treating deafferentation pain (Glynn 1989).

ANTICONVULSANTS

Drugs such as carbamazepine and sodium valproate used in normal anticonvulsant doses are also of value in treating deafferentation pain.

Nerve blocks

Epidural injection of steroids, epidural infusion of local anaesthetics and procedures to interrupt pain pathways should always be considered for the patient with intractable pelvic pain and a close link with a local pain clinic is essential (Baines & Kirkham 1984). An intrathecal nerve block is useful in this context and in skillful hands side effects can be kept to a minimum (Baxter 1984).

Percutaneous electrical cordotomy (Lipton 1968), cryoanalgesia (Lloyd *et al.*

1976), barbitage of cerebrospinal fluid (Lloyd *et al.* 1972), transcutaneous nerve stimulation (Meyerson 1983) and acupuncture (Chaitow 1976) may each have a place.

Palliative radiotherapy and chemotherapy

In patients who have not had previous radical pelvic radiotherapy, palliative radiotherapy can be considered. While palliative radiotherapy is very effective in the treatment of bone metastases it is less effective in treating pelvic pain caused by advanced or recurrent pelvic gynaecological malignancy. It is necessary to be aware of the risk of precipitating fistulae in patients who have tumour invading neighbouring viscera such as the rectum or bladder where radiotherapy may make symptoms worse (Bates 1984).

Carcinoma of the ovary is the only gynaecological tumour that is particularly sensitive to cytotoxic drugs in current use. At the end of life aggressive chemotherapy is rarely indicated and as a palliative measure it is usually preferable to treat with a single alkylating agent such as oral chlorambucil (Bates & Vanier 1984). Approximately one-third of all carcinomas of the body of the uterus are sensitive to progesterone therapy. If this has not been tried before, oral medroxyprogesterone acetate (Provera) 100 mg t.d.s. may be a helpful adjuvant to treating associated pain and will not be associated with any distressing side effects. (Bleomycin, iphosphamide and cisplatin have shown remarkable pain relief in advanced recurrent cancer of the cervix: Editor's note.)

Nausea and vomiting

Nausea and vomiting occur frequently in this group of patients. Common causes are iatrogenic, metabolic and mechanical. Because treatment depends on the particular cause it is helpful to understand vomiting mechanisms (Fig. 19.3) before choosing the most appropriate antiemetic (Table 19.5). Usually one antiemetic is adequate but if the patient continues to vomit a second antiemetic with a different site of action should be added (Walsh 1982). The oral route is preferable but not always possible. The rectal route is useful but unfortunately the choice of antiemetic suppositories is limited. Parenteral antiemetics may be necessary and a subcutaneous syringe pump can be valuable (Oliver 1985).

Iatrogenic causes

Iatrogenic causes include cytotoxic chemotherapy (via the chemoreceptor trigger zone (CTZ)), abdominal radiotherapy (by local effect), opioids (via CTZ or by causing faecal impaction) and gastric irritants such as steroids or non-steroidal anti-inflammatory drugs. Treatment is discontinuation of the causal agent. If this is not possible an appropriate antiemetic or adjuvant medication may be added,

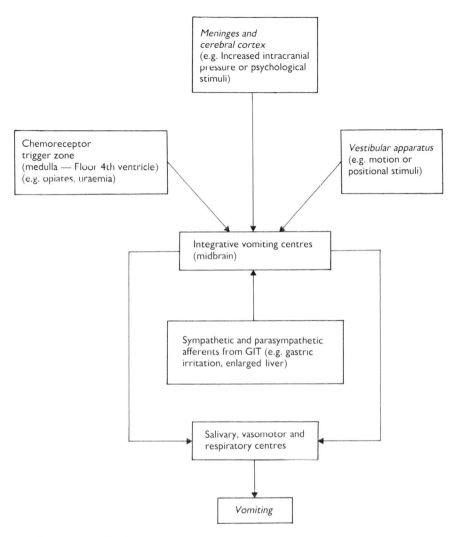

Fig. 19.3. Vomiting mechanisms

e.g. aperient for constipation, antacid or H2 receptor antagonist for gastric irritation.

Metabolic causes

Uraemia is the most frequent metabolic cause of vomiting in terminal gynaecological malignancy and is especially common in the terminal phase of cervical carcinoma (Joslin & Peel 1982). Hypercalcaemia as a cause of vomiting occurs less often and its management is described elsewhere (Wilkinson 1984).

Table 19.5. Useful antiemetic drugs

Category	Drug	Preparations	Dose	Site of action
Pheno-thiazines	Prochlor-perazine	Tablets Syrup Suppositories Injections	15−50 mg daily in divided doses	Chemo-receptor trigger zone
	Chlor-promazine	Tablets Syrup Suppositories Injections	30−200 mg daily in divided doses	
	φ Methotrime-prazine	Tablets Injections	25−100 mg daily in divided doses	
Buty-rophenones	φ Haloperidol	Tablets Elixir Injections	1−10 mg daily	
Antihista-mines	φ Cyclizine	Tablets Injections	50−150 mg daily in divided doses	Vomiting centre
Anti-cholinergics	Atropine sulphate	Tablets Injections	0.6−1.8 mg daily in divided doses	
	Hyoscine hydro-chloride	Tablets Injections	0.3−2.4 daily in divided doses	
Dopamine antagonists	φ Meto-clopramide	Tablets Syrup Injections	10−20 mg before meals	Upper bowel plus chemo-receptor trigger zone
	Domperidone	Tablets Suspension Suppositories	10−30 mg before meals	

Note:
1 An approximate potency ratio for suppository:oral:injections (of antiemetics) is 1:2:4.
2 Suitable antiemetics for subcutaneous administration via a syringe pump are marked φ.

Uraemia

Nausea, vomiting and hiccoughs are often the first symptoms of a rising blood urea which is usually secondary to an obstructive uropathy. Suitable antiemetics are those acting on the chemoreceptor trigger zone or vomiting centre. Ureteric obstruction may be reversed with radiotherapy (possibly in combination with high dose steroids) and should be considered if the patient has not been previously irradiated. Whether or not to surgically bypass the ureteric obstruction can be a difficult decision, particularly in a young otherwise relatively fit patient. Such a procedure, if successful, will relieve the obstruction, possibly reverse the uraemia and prolong life. But in so doing it may substitute a 'uraemic death' where the patient gradually becomes less aware and drifts into unconsciousness for a death dominated by gross local effects from the pelvic tumour such as fungation, fistulae and pain. A temporary nephrotomy will relieve the obstruction and allow time for assessment. There is no 'general rule' for such a complex decision and each case must be carefully and individually determined.

Mechanical causes

Intestinal obstruction

This is a common cause of vomiting in patients with advanced ovarian carcinoma. In one series of 518 patients with ovarian cancer 25% developed intestinal obstruction (Tunca et al. 1981). Although acute mechanical obstruction with its classical features of colicky abdominal pain, distension, vomiting and constipation with increased bowel sounds may occur in these patients, it is less common than subacute or incomplete bowel obstruction where the same symptoms are present but are less marked and often intermittent (Sise & Crichlow 1978). The underlying pathological mechanism of subacute obstruction from extensive intraabdominal malignancy appears to be a combination of 'obstructive' and 'functional' factors (Baines 1987b) (Fig. 19.4). Surgery is the definitive treatment for many obstructed patients. However, the majority of these terminally ill patients are unsuitable for surgery which is associated with a very short postoperative survival. One series showed a medium survival of 2.5 months in a series of 60 patients with ovarian carcinoma undergoing palliative surgery for obstruction (Piver et al. 1982). Traditional conservative measures include intravenous fluids and nasogastric suction, but these may themselves cause the patient discomfort and be of questionable benefit (Glass & Le Duc 1973; Arahna et al. 1981). An alternative which is more appropriate in this context is to manage the symptoms of malignant bowel obstruction on a purely medical basis (Baines 1987b).

DIAGNOSIS

The first step is to establish the diagnosis. This is usually possible on the basis of the history and clinical findings. The absence of abdominal distension in the otherwise clinically obstructed patient with known intraabdominal tumour has been described as a characteristic of widespread intraabdominal disease (Taylor 1985). Erect−supine abdominal X-rays may be helpful in locating the site of the obstruction and in determining if the block is single or multiple. It is important at this stage to rule out a simple reversible cause such as faecal impaction although this may be a difficult differential diagnosis. History (e.g. patient on opioids without a regular aperient), examination and abdominal X-rays will be of help but diagnosis may ultimately depend on what results are achieved by suppositories. Unless one is sure of the diagnosis of faecal impaction, peristalsis inducing aperients and high enemas must be used with great caution.

SYMPTOMATIC MANAGEMENT

Vomiting. 100% of patients with malignant bowel obstruction complain of vomiting of moderate intensity and it is severe in 87% (Baines 1987b). The mechanism of obstructive vomiting is complex but both toxic absorption and reverse peristalsis are thought to play a part (Baines 1987b). It is often accompanied by severe nausea which many patients find worse than the actual vomiting itself. Centrally acting antiemetics are most effective given either by suppository or parenterally. Nausea can almost always be controlled and vomiting reduced to 1−2 episodes a day making a nasogastric tube unnecessary.

Colic. This is reported in 76% of patients with malignant obstruction (Baines 1987b). Peristaltic inducing agents (e.g. senna, bisacodyl, metoclopramide, domperidone) should be discontinued. If the patient can tolerate oral medication the following drugs are effective: loperamide 2−4 mg 6-hourly, diphenoxylate and atropine (Lomotil) 1−2 mg 6-hourly or hyoscine butylbromide (Buscupan) 10−20 mg 6-hourly. If parenteral medication is needed hyoscine butylbromide 40−60 mg by continuous subcutaneous infusion over 24 h is effective. A coeliac plexus block is described as useful in this setting (Baines 1987b) where it causes a reduction in colicky pain, although increased peristalsis continues.

Altered bowel habit. Diarrhoea is common in patients with partial bowel obstruction (34%) (Baines 1987b) and may be treated with one of the antispasmodic drugs mentioned above. Constipation (12%) (Baines 1987b) is best treated with suppositories and stool softening aperients such as docusate sodium (Dioctyl) 200−400 mg/day. Stimulant purgatives may simply increase the patient's colic and should be avoided.

Subcutaneous syringe pump. While it is often possible to manage these patients with oral medications or suppositories or a combination of both along the lines discussed above, parenteral administration is sometimes necessary. The subcutaneous syringe pump is useful and acceptable in these patients and a typical regime might consist of diamorphine (for visceral pain), hyoscine butylbromide (for colic) and haloperidol for vomiting (Oliver 1985).

FEEDING AND HYDRATION

Medical management of the symptoms of malignant obstruction will allow full control of the patient's nausea and reduce her vomiting significantly, perhaps to once or twice a day (Baines 1987b). The patient can then be allowed to take oral fluids and a light diet as she chooses and will not become clinically dehydrated making either intravenous or nasogastric feeding or hydration unnecessary. In the final days of life the patient may be unable to take oral fluids. The most distressing symptom of dehydration at this stage is dry mouth, which is effectively managed by frequent mouth care, crushed ice or small sips of fluid (an activity the patient's family can participate in).

Ascites

Malignant ascites in this context is usually caused by advanced ovarian carcinoma (Souhami & Tobias 1986). Ascites that is asymptomatic need not be treated but if causing vomiting or other symptoms such as abdominal discomfort or breathlessness, consider the following.

Diuretics

Malignant ascites does not usually respond to conventional oral diuretic therapy although a combination of a loop diuretic (e.g. frusemide 40–80 mg/day) with an aldosterone antagonist (e.g. spironolactone 100–200 mg/day) may be helpful. Intravenous infusion of frusemide 100 mg in 500 ml of physiological saline (or less if using a syringe pump) over 24 h has been described as a successful treatment for malignant ascites (Amiel et al. 1984).

Paracentesis

Paracentesis is often necessary symptomatically. It is usually effective if the fluid is not loculated. While there is agreement that too rapid a removal of fluid can be hazardous, too slow a drainage can also cause hypovolaemia. A rate of 1 l over 2 h should not cause problems. To prevent reaccumulation of nonloculated ascites, cytotoxic agents can be instilled into the peritoneum after drainage (e.g. thiotepa or bleomycin). In frail patients removal of large amounts of ascitic fluid can be extremely debilitating and here a 'partial' paracentesis of 1–4 l may be adequate to relieve symptoms.

Cytotoxic chemotherapy

A single cytotoxic agent such as oral chlorambucil may be useful in controlling ascites due to ovarian carcinoma.

Peritoneovenous shunt

A shunt, such as the LeVeen shunt, may be considered if the patient is relatively fit and suffering from repeated episodes of ascites (Osterlee 1980).

Oedema

Dependent oedema is common in these patients who are often hypoalbuminaemic and is managed mechanically (elevation of the end of the bed and feet when sitting and support stockings) occasionally in combination with diuretic therapy. Chronic oedema of the lower limbs is a more difficult management problem. This may be unilateral (unilateral obstruction of veins or lymphatics) or bilateral (possibly due to inferior vena caval obstruction) and is often associated with considerable discomfort and loss of mobility. If possible try to reduce pressure on the veins and lymphatics either by reducing tumour size (radiotherapy) and/or peritumour oedema (dexamethasone 8–16 mg/day initially and subsequently reducing to the smallest possible maintenance dose). Simultaneously one can use a compression stocking device (e.g. Flowtron) on the legs in combination with a diuretic (Gray 1987).

Fistulae

Fistulae are not rare in patients with advanced gynaecological malignancies.

Management

Control pain

Pain is controlled by analgesics and relevant practical measures as described below.

Treat associated infection

Infection exacerbates pain and anaerobic organisms may cause an offensive discharge (see below). The mixed infection of aerobic and anaerobic organisms commonly found is best treated by a combination of appropriate systemic antibiotics, e.g. amoxycillin 250 mg t.d.s. and metronidazole 200 mg t.d.s.

Bulking agent

With any fistula involving bowel, a stool bulking agent (e.g. ispaghula husk (Isogel) 10 ml b.d.) can be tried. By absorbing liquid faeces a bulkier stool is created which will then bypass the fistula tract.

Local measures

The following simple procedures are often helpful: catheterization with a wide bore catheter for vesico—vaginal and vesico—colic fistulae; vaginal packing with tampons (possibly coated with lignocaine gel) or a special prosthesis for recto-vaginal fistulae (Green & Phillips 1986); incontinence pads for vesico—vaginal and rectovaginal fistulae and colostomy bags, if possible, fitted over fistulae connecting with the skin (to absorb offensive odour colostomy bags with charcoal filters are available or alternatively one can use a charcoal or aspirin tablet in an ordinary colostomy bag (Duffield 1989)).

Surgery

Procedures such as closure of the fistula, ureteric diversion or formation of a palliative colostomy should be considered. However, in general, those patients who develop fistulae are iller and have frequently had previous pelvic radiotherapy making them less suitable for surgery.

Offensive vaginal discharge

Many patients with advanced cervical, vaginal and vulval carcinoma have an offensive vaginal discharge causing embarrassment and discomfort.

Management

Treat associated infection

Infection with mixed anaerobic and aerobic organisms is commonly present and is managed along the lines already discussed. In addition metronidazole supposi-tories 500 mg b.d. can be used intravaginally in this instance.

Local cleansing

Antiseptic douches of chlorhexidene gluconate (Hibitane) 1 in 2000 are useful for frequent washdowns of vulval or vaginal lesions.

Local measures

Incontinence pads combined with charcoal pads help by absorbing both discharge and odour. With profuse non-infected discharge steroid enemas inserted into the vagina (e.g. Predsol or Colifoam) may be useful.

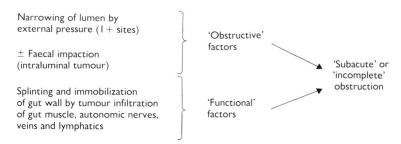

Fig. 19.4. (see text)

Radiotherapy

If the discharge continues despite the above measures a short course of palliative radiotherapy to locally ulcerating or fungating tumour is helpful. The normal precaution of not washing the area of skin being irradiated during treatment need not apply here.

Haemorrhage

Tumour eroding the cervix, body of uterus, bladder, vagina or vulva and metastatic tumour involving inguinal nodes may cause haemorrhage.

Minor bleeding

This is managed by packing locally with gauze soaked in adrenaline 1 in 1000. Oral haemostatic agents such as tranexamic acid or ethamsylate may be of benefit. Palliative radiotherapy is also effective and should be considered (Bates 1984). Embolization using Gelfoam may be necessary for recurrent haemorrhage.

Massive bleeding

An event such as erosion of a femoral artery by inguinal tumour should be anticipated. It is usually more appropriate to manage massive arterial or venous haemorrhage with comforting of that individual, covering locally with a red blanket and parenteral sedation and analgesia (if time allows) than with active resuscitation.

Menopausal symptoms

Radical pelvic surgery or radiotherapy will cause a premature menopause in premenopausal patients. This may be associated with symptoms such as hot flushes, emotional irritability, depression and loss of libido. Oestrogen replacement therapy will help such symptoms in patients with ovarian, cervical or corpus uteri carcinoma.

Psychosocial aspects of care

In this section psychosocial aspects of caring for patients with terminal gynaeco-logical malignancy are discussed under the headings: communication with the patient, caring for the family and specific psychological problems.

Communication with the patient

Good communication is perhaps the single most effective therapeutic tool in treating the previously mentioned non-physical components of 'total pain'. It combats the potentially destructive elements of fear and grief so often present (Parkes 1984) and helps to reconcile the patient and her family to the difficult realities they are facing. Attitudes have changed in the medical profession in regard to communicating with cancer patients so that now a majority of doctors seem to favour a more open approach (Editorial, *Lancet* 1980). However, there is no single best approach, too much or too little information being potentially harmful (Editorial, *Br. Med. J.* 1980). Good communication implies a relationship where trust and openness are found. Consistency is important, so that the patient is not seen by a different doctor on each occasion. Although unhurried time is not always available, a listening attitude is and this must precede any imparting of information (Editorial, *Lancet* 1980). We must first establish what the patient already knows or suspects and listen to what she is asking, consider-ing verbal and non-verbal clues. We often need to clarify what appears to be a very direct question. 'Is it cancer, doctor?' might in fact be an expression of the fear 'Am I going to die in awful pain?'. To discover such 'hidden questions' (as well as to give oneself time to rally an answer!), it is a useful technique to refer the question back to the patient before replying (Parkes 1984). In our listening it may become perfectly clear that the patient is not asking any questions at this point or is actively denying the seriousness of her situation. We must respect this need in the patient (Simpson 1982) while realizing that this same patient may need and be ready for more information at a later date. Coming from this perspective one realizes that the relevant question is not 'whether' to tell the patient but 'how' to tell (West & Kirkham 1981). Indeed it is often the patient who 'tells' the doctor, requiring from us explanation and reassurance. We must never lie to the patient as this will lead to a breakdown in trust at a later stage. What is more, this is unnecessary for even if one has to give bad news more directly, it is possible to impart the 'gentle truth' rather than the 'bitter truth'. To communicate hope by emphasizing some aspects of the present or future situation is always possible and desirable (Brewin 1977). Good communication does not

mean a single 'all or nothing' confrontation, but the giving of appropriate information always combined with reassurance in a continuing relationship.

Caring for the family

In the setting of terminal illness the unit of care is the patient's family with the
patient at its centre. This suggests that the traditional injunction to 'treat the
whole patient' be extended to 'treating the whole family' (Parkes 1984), implying
a sensitivity not just to the terminally ill individual but to those closest to her
whose fate and well-being are inextricably bound up in hers. A multidisciplinary
team approach (doctor, nurse, social worker and counsellor) is helpful. The
family's needs can be examined under the following three headings.

Communication

The same general principles discussed above apply here. If possible, try to
ensure that the patient and those closest to her have the same degree of insight
as otherwise the so-called 'conspiracy of silence' can all too easily develop
adding feelings of isolation to an already stressful situation. Children must be
included also and natural feelings of wanting to protect them countered with the
awareness that even very young children need reassurance, can cope with appropriate explanations and if not included will often subsequently express their
resentment (Stedeford 1981). It may be useful to have a family meeting (including
the patient) where treatment plans, the meanings of different symptoms and
possibly the likely progress of the illness might be discussed. Such a meeting
allows the family to express their fears, anxieties and guilt and to ask questions,
so laying a foundation of trust on which subsequent interviews can build
(Earnshaw-Smith 1981). Fears that the disease is contagious or hereditary or has
been caused by some family 'stress' are common and need to be allayed. In
addition both patients with localized gynaecological malignancy and their families
may find it difficult to accept the gravity of the situation because the patient feels
and looks so well 'from the waist up'. It is helpful to discuss these difficulties
openly with the family. Finally there may be fears of the process of death itself,
most commonly fears of pain, haemorrhage, convulsions or simply not being
able to cope, which may need discussion at some stage, particularly if a home
death is being planned.

Sexual advice

A continuing sexual relationship is important in promoting feelings of acceptance,
warmth and reassurance in the cancer patient (Editorial, *Lancet* 1984). However,
the discussion of sexual matters is generally taboo between cancer patients and
their doctors, if not their gynaecologists, and although a doctor may be at ease in

discussing cancer with his patient this does not necessarily imply an ease in discussing sexual problems. The subject of sex may be particularly problematic in patients with terminal gynaecological malignancy. Dyspareunia and loss of libido are both common. In addition there may be fears of rejection, of the contagiousness of the disease or that intercourse will exacerbate the cancer with additional feelings of self-disgust and embarrassment, particularly if the patient has cervical, vaginal or vulval symptoms. Occasionally the fears are in the healthy partner who may think the patient too ill for intercourse (Golden 1983), or may in fact be repelled by an offensive discharge. As doctors we must be sensitive to this topic, recognizing its importance for the general well-being of the patient. In addition, if the service of a sex counsellor is available, it will be helpful to introduce her to the patient and her partner and to include her as a part of the caring team at as early a stage as possible.

Bereavement counselling

While accepting that good total care and communication from the beginning of the illness are the best possible prophylaxis against a pathological bereavement (Earnshaw-Smith 1981), and that the majority of bereaved individuals will manage without any outside help, a minority will be at risk of psychiatric or social morbidity if unsupported and may need specialist intervention (Parkes 1984). This intervention in the form of bereavement visiting or counselling has been shown to be effective (Parkes 1980a).

Specific psychological problems

The patient with terminal gynaecological disease is subject to psychological stress from many sources. These include the effects of the physical symptoms and their treatment as well as the impact of other forms of palliative treatment. There are also the implications of the illness in terms of increasing dependency, loss of control and separation from loved ones as the patient looks into an uncertain future. Intertwined with these there may be spiritual questioning and doubts. Consequently it is not surprising to encounter feelings of anxiety, fear, helplessness, anger, guilt, sadness, depression and confusion in these patients (Hinton 1963; Parkes 1984). It is important to appreciate the 'normality' of such various emotions and that their presence does not of necessity indicate mental illness (Saunders & Baines 1983). Kubler-Ross (1970) has described the different emotional 'stages' a patient goes through in the process of realization as denial (isolation), anger, bargaining, depression and finally acceptance. This model is helpful only if one appreciates its lack of rigidity; thus the patient may as easily regress as progress and may indeed be at more than one stage at any given point in time (Saunders & Baines 1983). The most important components in caring for patients with psychological symptoms are effective symptom control, good communication, emotional support and counselling. In addition to these measures, psychotropic medication may be indicated, but must not be used as a substitute for the above. A team approach is helpful where one benefits from the observations of those often closest to the patients, the nurses and from the expertise and supervision of a psychiatrist. Actual intervention by the psychiatrist will be necessary in only a small number of patients (Stedeford & Bloch 1979; Parkes 1984).

Anxiety

Anxiety is an understandable response to terminal illness. However, chronic or severe anxiety which does not respond to explanation and reassurance may become incapacitating and exacerbate or cause other symptoms. In this instance the following anxiolytic drugs are useful: diazepam in a single night-time dose of 5–10 mg will not only give night sedation but anxiolysis throughout the following day because of its long effective half-life; haloperidol may also be used in a single night-time dose of 5–10 mg; chlorpromazine 10–50 mg 8-hourly is an alternative if more sedation is required.

Depression

Appropriate sadness including anticipatory grieving must be differentiated from pathological depression and managed appropriately (Parkes 1984). A diagnosis of true depression is made still more difficult because the disease itself may cause overlapping somatic symptoms (e.g. lethargy and anorexia). There is evidence to suggest that depression is more common in patients on narcotic analgesics with a long terminal phase to their illness (Twycross & Wald 1976). This often applies to gynaecological patients with localized pelvic malignancy who may in addition have distressing and intractable symptoms. Medication that may be useful in the depressed patient includes the following.

Corticosteroids

Prednisolone 15–30 mg/24 h or dexamethasone 2–4 mg/24 h are often helpful as they can cause an increase in appetite and an improved sense of well-being.

Antidepressants

If it seems appropriate to use a tricyclic antidepressant, it is important to remember that patients with terminal cancer are particularly sensitive to the side effects of these drugs which may well be potentiated by concurrent medication such as phenothiazines. Amitriptyline 25–100 mg at night is useful in the patient with agitated depression. Imipramine 25–75 mg at night is less sedative. An alternative is mianserin 30—60 mg *nocte* which is a tetracyclic antidepressant that may be sedative initially but has minimal anticholinergic side effects.

Confusion and agitation

Confusion is a common and difficult problem in terminally ill patients and one must attempt to diagnose the underlying cause and treat this appropriately (Stedeford 1984). It may be necessary to initially sedate the agitated confused patient for which the following are useful: diazepam 5—10 mg p.r.; haloperidol 5—20 mg i.m.; chlorpromazine 25—100 mg i.m. or 100 mg p.r. or methotrimeprazine 25—100 mg i.m. The latter is especially useful if more sedation is required. Subsequently the patient may need to be maintained on one of these drugs given orally in a smaller dose on a regular basis. In addition the elderly confused patient may be helped by thioridazine 10—25 mg 8-hourly, trifluoperazine 1—2 mg 8-hourly or if the confusion is mainly nocturnal, chlormethiazole 1—2 capsules at night.

Practical considerations

The 'hospice movement' has focused, in an analytical and positive way, on the needs of the dying and their families. However, 'hospice' does not necessarily imply a distinct specialist unit. It is rather a concept of care applicable in many different settings (Twycross 1980).

From available statistics it is likely that approximately 60% of patients with terminal gynaecological malignancy will die in acute hospitals, 30% at home and a small percentage in hospices (OPCS 1982). In this final section ways of providing the terminal care of such patients are outlined.

Dying in hospital

In hospital terminal care can be provided in one of three ways.

The gynaecological team

The majority of patients with terminal gynaecological malignancy die in hospital under the care of the gynaecological team who have provided their earlier active treatment. In addition, a radiotherapist or oncologist may have been involved and will usually wish to maintain this involvement and offer relevant palliative treatment. It is necessary to work closely with the nursing team and to involve the social worker and other specialists as appropriate (anaesthetist, psychiatrist or specialist counsellor). Given such a team approach and a willingness to learn and apply the principles of symptom control and psychosocial care already discussed, excellent terminal care can be provided in this way. In ensuring continuity of care, such a system is reassuring to both patient and family. The chief disadvantage of such a system is that the gynaecological team will inevitably give priority to those patients who can be cured and often simply does not have enough time to give the sort of care and attention that is required. If this is the case, or if faced with intractable symptoms, one can involve (if available) the hospital's terminal care support team, consider (again if available) referral to the special 'palliative care ward' within the hospital or liaise with a nearby hospice for advice or to arrange patient transfer.

The terminal care support team

There are currently at least 20 such teams in existence in the UK (Hospice Information 1989). The first such team in the UK was established in St Thomas's Hospital, London in 1977 (Bates *et al*. 1981). The aim of such a 'hospice team' working in a general hospital is to 'improve the standard of care of patients dying of cancer and to teach the art of terminal care' (Bates 1982). Such teams consist of between one and four specialist nurses, a medical social worker, a chaplain, a secretary and a part or full time doctor. The teams usually have no beds of their own and their work is advisory so that the patient remains under the gynaecological team and care is shared. Many teams also offer domiciliary support where they work side by side with the patient's own primary care team in the community. The great advantage of such a system is that the teams are relatively inexpensive, have great education potential and provide continuity of patient care (Bates 1982). In addition they assist in liaison and communication between the hospital and the community.

Palliative/continuing care wards

This is where a ward or a certain number of beds are available in the acute hospital for patients needing terminal care. There are currently 14 such wards in the UK (Hospice Information 1989) which are ideally staffed with nurses trained in hospice work with a higher nurse to patient ratio than on the general wards.

   The reintegration of hospice medicine back into acute hospitals in the ways outlined above is seen as important and optimistic (NTCP 1980; Saunders & Baines 1983). In terms of improved standards of symptom control there is evidence that this optimism is justified (Parkes & Parkes 1984).

Dying at home

Although a majority of patients might like to die at home, at present only some 30% do so (OPCS 1982). For those dying at home there is evidence that much terminal distress still exists (Wilkes 1984), pointing to the need for improved symptom control and support for the family. In their report (NTCP 1980), the

Working Group on Terminal Care, under the chairmanship of Professor Eric Wilkes, strongly emphasized the need to increase and improve community based care which may be provided in one of two ways.

Primary care team

The benefits of the patient's own GP providing domiciliary terminal care are obvious. Many such patients will still be well enough to attend gynaecological or radiotherapy outpatient clinics providing opportunity for investigation of intractable symptoms, specialist advice and palliative treatment when appropriate. Such a system of combined care can work well if there is good communication between hospital and home (NTCP 1980). In addition to this contact with the acute hospital, the GP can liaise with a local hospice or hospital based support team on different aspects of management.

Home care teams

Domiciliary terminal care teams are seen as being one of the most important manifestations of the evolving hospice movement (NTCP 1980). There are currently a total of approximately 260 such teams in the UK and they may be free standing community based (170), hospice based (80) or attached to hospital based support teams (approximately 10) (Hospice Information 1989). Such teams are advisory and supplement the care already being provided by the primary care team. In addition to being able to offer expert advice on symptom control, their availability for advice and support 7 days a week and 24 hours a day is much appreciated by the families (Parkes 1980b) and is seen as an important factor in making a home death possible (Wilkes 1984). Hospice and hospital based domiciliary teams usually hold outpatient clinics. In addition there are now 65 terminal care day centres throughout the UK which may be either free standing or attached to a unit or team (Hospice Information 1989) and which provide an otherwise housebound patient with the opportunity of socializing and diversional therapy.

Dying in a hospice

Only a small percentage of terminally ill patients currently die in one of the 92 specialized hospices in the UK (OPCS 1982; Hospice Information 1989). It is important to emphasize that a sizeable percentage (approximately 15%) of patients admitted to such hospices will subsequently be discharged home under the care of their GP and the hospice based domiciliary team (St Christopher's Hospice Statistics 1988). Patients being referred from acute hospital to a hospice must not be told that they are going to a 'convalescent home'. Rather the hospice can be introduced as a smaller hospital specializing in the kind of care they now need. A common fallacy is that if a patient is being transferred to a hospice she must know her diagnosis. There is no such admission stipulation and a patient's right to deny is respected, and possible, in a hospice setting (Saunders & Baines 1983).

Although it is said that the ultimate aim of those working in hospices is to 'do themselves out of a job' there will always be a place for such specialist units to deal with intractable terminal care problems, carry out research and act as specialist training centres for staff to work in home care teams and hospital based support teams (Bates 1985).

Summary

Many patients who currently present with gynaecological cancer will at some stage require terminal care. Terminal care is a continuation of palliative treatment and must be seen as an appropriate, positive treatment option. These patients suffer some of the most intractable symptoms and symptom control is an essential therapeutic aim. Psychosocial factors must be considered, seeing the patient as part of a larger unit, the family. The heightened needs encountered in such patients in the final phase of their illness call for a certain expertise and a team approach. Good terminal care can be provided either in acute hospitals or the community but admission to a specialist hospice will occasionally be necessary.

References

Amiel S.A., Blackburn A.M. & Rubens R.D. (1984) Intravenous infusion of frusemide — a treatment for ascites of malignant disease. *Br. Med. J.*, **288**, 1041.

Aranha G., Folk F. & Greenlee H. (1981) Surgical palliation of small bowel obstruction due to metastatic carcinoma. *Am. Surg.*, **47**, 99.

Baines M. (1981) The principles of symptom control. *In*: Saunders, C., Summers, D.H. & Teller N. (eds), *Hospice: The Living Idea*. Edward Arnold, London. pp. 93—101.

Baines M. (1987a) Terminal illness. *In*: Girdwood R.H. & Petrie J.C. (eds), *Text Book of Medical Treatment*. 1st Edn. Churchill Livingstone, Edinburgh. pp. 325—40.

Baines M. (1987b) Medical management of intestinal obstruction. *In*: Bates T. (ed.), *Contemporary Palliation of Difficult Symptoms*. Balliere Tindall, pp. 357—71.

Baines M. & Kirkham S.R. (1984) Carcinoma involving bone and soft tissue. *In*: Wall P.D. & Melzack R. (eds), *Textbook of Pain*. Churchill Livingstone, Edinburgh. p. 455.

Baker J. & Diggory P. (1982) Vulva, vagina, ovaries and fallopian tube. *In*: Halman K.E. *et al.* (eds), *Treatment of Cancer*. Chapman and Hall, London. p. 537.

Bates T.D. (1982) At home and in the ward: the establishment of a support team in an acute general hospital. *In*: Wilkes E. (ed.), *The Dying Patient*. MTP Press, Lancaster. pp. 263—88.

Bates T.D. (1984) Radiotherapy in terminal care. *In*: Saunders C.M. (ed.), *The Management of Terminal Disease*. Edward Arnold, London. 2nd Edn. pp. 133—38.

Bates T.D. (1985) A clinician's view on palliative care, terminal care and quality of life. *Effective Health Care*, **2** (5), 211—15.

Bates T.D., Hoy A.M., Clarke D.G. & Laird P.P. (1981) The St Thomas's Hospital terminal care support team — a new concept of hospice care *Lancet*, **i**, 1201—03.

Bates T.D. & Vanier T. (1984) Palliation by cytoxic chemotherapy and hormone therapy. *In*: Saunders C.M. (ed.), *The Management of Terminal Disease*. Edward Arnold, London. 2nd Edn. pp. 139—47.

Baxter R.C.H. (1984) Specialised techniques for the relief of pain. *In*: Saunders C.M. (ed.), *The Management of Terminal Malignant Disease*. Edward Arnold, London. 2nd Edn. pp. 91—9.

Brewin T.B. (1977) The cancer patient: communication and morale. *Br. Med. J.*, **283**, 1098—101.

British National Formulary (1988) *Morphine Analgesic Elixirs*. Anonymous No. **15**, p. 172.

Chaitow L. (1976) *The Acupuncture Treatment of Pain*. Thorsons, Wellingborough.

Drugs and Therapeutic Bulletin (1979) *Oxycodone Pectinate (Proladone) and other Opiate Suppositories*. Anonymous. **17** (6), 21—22.

Drugs and Therapeutic Bulletin (1988) **26** (14), 53—56.

Duffield M. (1989) In: Declan Walsh T. (ed.), *Fistulas in Symptom Control*. Blackwell Scientific Publications, Oxford. pp. 203—06.

Earnshaw-Smith E. (1981) Dealing with dying patients and their relatives. *Br. Med. J.*, **282**, 1779.

Editorial (1980) Give sorrow words. *Br. Med. J.*, **280**, 592.

Editorial (1980) In cancer, honesty is here to stay. *Lancet*, **ii**, 245.

Editorial (1984) Sex and the cancer patient. *Lancet*, **i**, 432—33.

Editorial (1984) Heroin for cancer—a great non-issue of our day. *Lancet*, **i**, 1449—50.

Foley K.M. (1979) Pain syndromes in patients with cancer. In: Bonica J.J. & Ventafridda V. (eds), *Advances in Pain Research and Therapy 2*. Raven Press, New York. pp. 59—75.

Glass R.L. & Le Duc R.J. (1973) Small intestinal obstruction from peritoneal carcinomatosis. *Am. J. Surg.*, **125**, 316.

Glynn C. (1989) An approach to the management of the patient with deafferentation pain. *Palliative Medicine*, **3**, 13—21.

Golden J.S. (1983) Sex and the cancer patient. *Dan. Med. Bull.*, **30** (Suppl 2), 4—6.

Gray R.C. (1987) The management of limb oedema in patients with advanced cancer. *Physiotherapy*, **73** (10), 504—6.

Green D.E. & Phillips G.L. (1986) *Gynaecol. Oncol.*, **23**, 119—23.

Hanna M. (1989) Consultant Anaesthetist, Kings College Pain Team, London. Personal communication.

Hinton J. (1963) Mental and physical distress in the dying. *Q. J. Med.*, **32**, 1—21.

Hospice Information (1989) St Christopher's Hospice, London.

Joslin C.A.F. & Peel K.R. (1982) Uterus. In: Halman K.E. *et al.* (eds), *Treatment of Cancer*. Chapman and Hall, London. p. 554.

Kubler-Ross E. (1970) *On Death and Dying*. Tavistock Publications, London.

Lipton S. (1968) Percutaneous electrical cordotomy. In: 'Relief of Intractable Pain'. *Br. Med. J.*, **2**, 210.

Lloyd J.W., Barnard J.D.W. & Glynn C.J. (1976) Cryoanalgesia, a new approach to pain relief. *Lancet*, **ii**, 932—34.

Lloyd J.W., Hughes J.T. & Davies-Jones G.A.B. (1972) Relief of severe intractable pain by barbotage of cerebro-spinal fluid. *Lancet*, **i**, 354—55.

Lunt B. & Jenkins J. (1983) Goal-setting in terminal cancer; a method of recording treatment aims and priorities. *J. Adv. Nursing*, **8**, 495—505.

Meyerson B.A. (1983) Electrostimulation procedures, effects, presumed rationale and possible mechanisms. In: Bonica J.J. *et al.* (eds), *Advances in Pain Research and Therapy*. Raven Press, New York. pp. 405—534.

National Terminal Care Policy — Report of the Working Group on Terminal Care (1980) Chairman Professor E. Wilkes. *J. Roy. Coll. General Practitioners*, **30**, 466—71.

Office of Population Censuses and Surveys (1982) *Mortality Statistics for 1980, England and Wales*. HMSO, London. Series DH 2, No. 7.

Oliver D.J. (1985) The use of the syringe driver in terminal care. *Br. J. Clin. Pharmacol.*, **20**, 515—16.

Osterlee J. (1980) Peritoneovenous shunting for ascites in cancer patients. *Br. J. Surg.*, **67**, 663—66.

Parkes C.M. (1980a) Bereavement counselling: does it work? *Br. Med. J.*, **281**, 3—6.

Parkes C.M. (1980b) Terminal care: evaluation of an advisory domiciliary service at St Christopher's. *Postgrad. Med. J.*, **56** (660), 685—89.

Parkes C.M. (1984) Psychological aspects. In: Saunders C.M. (ed.), *The Management of Terminal Disease*. Edward Arnold, London. 2nd Edn. pp. 43—63.

Parkes C.M. & Parkes J. (1984) Hospice versus hospital care—reevaluation after 10 years as seen by surviving spouses. *Postgrad. Med. J.*, **60**, 120—24.

Piver M.S., Barlow J.J., Lele S.B. & Frank A. (1982) Survival after ovarian cancer induced intestinal obstruction. *Gynaecol. Oncol.*, **13**, 44.

Regnard C. & Newbury A. (1983) Pain and the portable syringe pump. *Nursing Times*, **79** (26), 25—28.

Saunders C.M. (1984) Appropriate treatment, appropriate death. In: Saunders C.M. (ed.), *The Management of Terminal Disease*. Edward Arnold, London. 2nd Edn. pp. 1—2.

Saunders C.M. (1984) The nature and nurture of pain control. *World Medicine*, **19**, 31–32.

Saunders C. & Baines M. (1983) Living with dying. *In*: Saunders C. & Baines M. (eds), *The Management of Terminal Disease*. Oxford University Press, Oxford. pp. Preface, 1, 6–11, 43–66.

Simpson M.A. (1982) Therapeutic uses of truth. *In*: Wilkes E. (ed.), *The Dying Patient*. MTP Press, Lancaster. pp. 260–61.

Sise J. & Crichlow R. (1978) Obstruction due to malignant tumours. *Sem. Oncol.*, **5** (2).

Souhami R.L. & Tobias J.S. (1986) *Cancer and its Management*. Blackwell Scientific Publications, London. pp. 296–300.

St Christopher's Hospice Statistics (1989) Details of Admissions and Discharges. St Christopher's Hospice, London.

Stedeford A. (1981) Couples facing death. ii—Unsatisfactory communication. *Br. Med. J.*, **283**, 1098–101.

Stedeford A. (1984) Confusion. *In*: Stedeford A. (ed.), *Facing Death: Patients, Families and Professionals*. William Heinemann Medical Books, London. pp. 122–36.

Stedeford A. & Bloch S. (1979) The psychiatrist in the terminal care unit. *Br. J. Psychiatry*, **135**, 1–6.

Taylor R.H. (1985) Laparotomy for obstruction with recurrent tumour (letter). *Br. J. Surg.*, **72** (4), 327.

Tobias J.S. & Griffiths C.T. (1976) Management of ovarian carcinoma: current concepts and future prospects. *New Engl. J. Med.*, **294**, 818–23; 877–82.

Tunca J.C., Buchler D.A., Mack E.A., Ruzicka F.F., Crowley J.J. & Carr W.F. (1981) The management of ovarian cancer caused bowel obstruction. *Gynaecol. Oncol.*, **13**, 44.

Twycross R.G. (1974) Clinical experience with Diamorphine in advanced malignant disease. *Int. J. Clin. Pharmacol.*, **9**, 184–98.

Twycross R.G. (1977a) Choice of strong analgesic in terminal cancer: diamorphine or morphine? *Pain*, **3**, 93–104.

Twycross R.G. (1977b) A comparison of diamorphine with cocaine and methadone (letter to the Editor). *Br. J. Clin. Pharmacol.*, **4**, 691–92.

Twycross R.G. (1980) Hospice care—redressing the balance in medicine. *J. Roy. Soc. Med.*, **73**, 475–81.

Twycross R.G. & Lack S.A. (eds) (1983) *Symptom Control in Far Advanced Cancer: Pain Relief*. Pitman Publishing, London. pp. 6, 7–12, 17, 166–88, 223–34, 251, 272.

Twycross R.G. & Lack S. (eds) (1984) *Therapeutics in Terminal Cancer*. Pitman Publishing, London. p. 22.

Twycross R.G. & Wald S.J. (1976) Long term use of diamorphine in advanced cancer. *In*: Bonica J.J. & Alke-Fessand D. (eds), *Advances in Pain Research and Therapy*. Raven Press, New York. p. 653.

Vere D.W. (1978) Pharmacology of morphine drugs used in terminal care. *In*: Vere D.W. (ed.), *Topics in Therapeutics 4*. Pitman Medical, London.

Walsh T.D. (1982) Antiemetic-drug combinations in advanced cancer. *Lancet*, **i**, 1018.

Walsh T.D. (1986) *Controlled study of imipramine and morphine in chronic pain due to advanced cancer*. Paper presented at ASCO annual meeting, Los Angeles, California, May 4–6.

West T.S. & Kirkham S.R. (1981) The family. *In*: Saunders C.M., Summers D.H. & Teller N. (eds), *Hospice—The Living Idea*. Edward Arnold, London. pp. 53–57.

Wilkes E. (1978) A different kind of day hospital—for patients with pre-terminal cancer and chronic disease. *Br. Med. J.*, **2**, 1053–56.

Wilkes E. (1984) Dying now. *Lancet*, **i**, 950–52.

Wilkinson R. (1984) Treatment of hypercalcaemia associated with malignancy (Editorial). *Br. Med. J.*, **288**, 812–13.

Further reading

Baines M. (1987) *Drug Control of Common Symptoms*. St Christopher's Hospice, London.

Bates T.D. (ed) (1987) *Contemporary Palliation of Difficult Symptoms*. Balliere Tindall, London.

Saunders C.M. (1984) *The Management of Terminal Disease*. 2nd Edn. Edward Arnold, London.

Stedeford A. (ed) (1984) *Facing Death: Patients, Families and Professionals*. William Heinemann Medical Books, London.

Twycross R.G. & Lack S. (eds) (1983) *Symptom Control in Far Advanced Cancer: Pain Relief*. Pitman Publishing, London.

Index